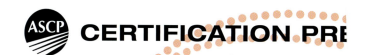

BOC
STUDY GUIDE

Phlebotomy
Certification Examinations

3rd edition

PHLEBOTOMY TECHNICIAN
PBT(ASCP) & PBT(ASCP^i)

QUALIFICATION IN
DONOR PHLEBOTOMY (QDP)

Publishing Team

Erik N Tanck & Annabelle Ulalulae (production)
Joshua Weikersheimer (publishing direction)

Notice

Trade names for equipment and supplies described are included as suggestions only. In no way does their inclusion constitute an endorsement of preference by the ASCP or content contributors. The ASCP and content contributors urge all readers to read and follow all manufacturers' instructions and package insert warnings concerning the proper and safe use of products. The American Society for Clinical Pathology, having exercised appropriate and reasonable effort to research material current as of publication date, does not assume any liability for any loss or damage caused by errors and omissions in this publication. Readers must assume responsibility for complete and thorough research of any hazardous conditions they encounter, as this publication is not intended to be all inclusive, and recommendations and regulations change over time.

NAACLS does not specifically endorse this or any other phlebotomy curriculum.

Copyright © 2022 by the American Society for Clinical Pathology. All rights reserved. No part of this publication may be reproduced, stored in a retrieval system, or transmitted in any form or by any means, electronic, mechanical, photocopying, recording, database, online or otherwise, without the prior written permission of the publisher.

Printed in the Uniited States of America

26 25 24 23 22

Contents

iv Acknowledgments
v The Importance of Certification, CMP, Licensure & Qualification
vii Preparing for & Taking the ASCP BOC Certification Examinations
x Tips for Preparing for the Examinations
xii Index of Phlebotomy Technician (PBT) Questions by Content Outline
xiv Index of Qualification in Donor Phlebotomy (QDP) Questions by Content Outline
xvi Preface

Chapter 1: Circulatory System
1 Questions
18 Answers with Explanations & Citations

Chapter 2: Specimen Collection
29 Questions
128 Answers with Explanations & Citations

Chapter 3: Specimen Handling, Transport & Processing
203 Questions
240 Answers with Explanations & Citations

Chapter 4: Waived & Point-of-Care Testing
271 Questions
282 Answers with Explanations & Citations

Chapter 5: Nonblood Specimens
289 Questions
309 Answers with Explanations & Citations

Chapter 6: Laboratory Operations
321 Questions
372 Answers with Explanations & Citations

Chapter 7: Donor Phlebotomy
409 Questions
457 Answers with Explanations & Citations

Answer Keys
490 Chapter 1: Circulatory System
491 Chapter 2: Specimen Collection
492 Chapter 3: Specimen Handling, Transport & Processing
493 Chapter 4: Waived & Point-of-Care Testing
494 Chapter 5: Nonblood Specimens
495 Chapter 6: Laboratory Operations
496 Chapter 7: Donor Phlebotomy

©ASCP 2022   ISBN 978-089189-6876

Oversight Editor

Susan E Phelan, PhD, MLS(ASCP)[CM]

Adjunct Faculty Lecturer, Hematology
Franciscan Health Hammond School of Medical Laboratory Science

Professor of Phlebotomy and Department Chair of Health Sciences (Retired)
Moraine Valley Community College
Palos Hills, IL

Dedication

To my husband, Robert (Sonny); our sons, Robert and Christopher our daughter and son-in-law, Meghann and Darryl Tyndorf; my parents, the late Selma and William Evers; and my parents-in-law, the late Robert (Sonny) and Phyllis Phelan

Acknowledgements

We thank those whose work contributed to the development of questions, informed the development of explanations, reviewed content, or provided figures/images that enrich this edition:

Rosemarie Brichta, BS, MT(ASCP); Diana Garza, EdD, MT(ASCP)[CM]; Marilyn J Nelson, MT(ASCP); Keith R Nelson, MT(ASCP)PBT; and Tyler Anderson, DPT(ASCP)[CM]

The Importance of Certification, CMP, Licensure & Qualification

Seventy percent of medical decisions are based on results provided by the clinical laboratory. A highly skilled medical team of pathologists, specialists, laboratory scientists, medical laboratory scientists, technicians and phlebotomists works together to determine the presence or absence of disease and provides valuable data needed to determine the course of treatment.

Today's laboratory uses many complex, precision instruments and automated processes. However, the success of the laboratory begins with the laboratorians' dedication to their profession and willingness to help others. Laboratorians must produce accurate and reliable test results, have an interest in science, and be able to recognize their responsibility for affecting human lives.

Role of the ASCP Board of Certification (ASCP BOC)

Founded in 1928 by the American Society of Clinical Pathologists (ASCP—now, the American Society for Clinical Pathology), the ASCP BOC is considered the preeminent certification agency in the US and abroad within the field of laboratory medicine. Composed of representatives of professional organizations and the public, the ASCP BOC mission is to: "Provide excellence in certification of laboratory professionals on behalf of patients worldwide."

The ASCP BOC consists of more than 100 volunteer technologists, technicians, phlebotomists, laboratory scientists, physicians, and professional researchers. These volunteers contribute their time and expertise to the Board of Governors and the Examination Committees. They allow the ASCP BOC to achieve the goal of excellence in credentialing medical laboratory personnel in the US and abroad.

The Board of Governors is the policymaking governing body for the ASCP BOC and is composed of 23 members. These 23 members include technologists, technicians, and pathologists nominated by the ASCP BOC and representatives from the general public as well as from the following societies: the American Association for Clinical Chemistry, the AABB, American Society for Microbiology, American Society for Clinical Laboratory Science, the American Society of Cytopathology, the American Society of Hematology, the American Association of Pathologists' Assistants, Association of Genetic Technologists, the National Society for Histotechnology, and the Clinical Laboratory Management Association .

The Examination Committees are responsible for the planning, development, and review of the examination databases; determining the accuracy and relevancy of the test items; confirming the standards for each examination and performing job or practice analyses.

The Importance of Certification, CMP, Licensure & Qualification

Certification and Credential Maintenance Program (CMP)
www.ascp.org/cmp

Certification is the process by which a nongovernmental agency or association grants recognition of competency to an individual who has met certain predetermined qualifications, as specified by that agency or association. Certification affirms that an individual has demonstrated that he or she possesses the knowledge and skills to perform essential tasks in the medical laboratory. The ASCP BOC certifies those individuals who meet academic and clinical prerequisites and who achieve acceptable performance levels on examinations.

In 2004, the ASCP BOC implemented the Credential Maintenance Program (CMP), which mandates participation every 3 years for newly certified individuals in the US. The goal of this program is to demonstrate to the public that laboratory professionals are performing the appropriate and relevant activities to keep current in their practice. Additional information on ASCP's Credential Maintenance Program may be found on the ASCP website at www.ascp.org/cmp.

United States Certification
www.ascp.org/boc/us-certifications

Specific directions on how to apply for the phlebotomy technician (PBT) or the Qualification in Donor Phlebotomy (QDP) exam are posted on the ASCP web site. The steps are summarized below:

- Identify the examination you are applying for and determine your eligibility.
- Gather your required education and experience documentation.
- Apply for the examination online and pay by credit card. Pay by mail instructions will be available upon the completion of the online application process.
- Submit required documentation.

Upon notification of your eligibility, schedule an appointment to take your examination.

International Certification
www.ascp.org/boc/international-certifications

ASCP offers its gold standard credentials in the form of international certification (ASCPi) to eligible individuals. The ASCPi credential certifies professional competency among new and practicing laboratory personnel in an effort to contribute globally to the highest standards of patient safety. Graduates of medical laboratory science programs outside the United States are challenged with content that mirrors the standards of excellence established by the US ASCP exams. The ASCPi credential carries the weight of over 80 years of expertise in clinical laboratory professional certification. Please visit the ASCP BOC website to view the following:

- Current listing of international certifications.
- Eligibility guidelines.
- Step-by-step instructions to apply for international certification.

The Importance of Certification, CMP, Licensure & Qualification

State Licensure
www.ascp.org/boc/state-licensure

In certain states, phlebotomists must be licensed. Licensure often includes a defined combination of experience and successfully completing a credentialling examination. It is important to identify the state and examination required to determine your eligibility and view the steps for licensure and/or certification. For a list of states that require licensure, please go to the ASCP BOC web site ( ) and click on the specific state licensure of interest.

Qualification
A qualification from the ASCP BOC recognizes the competence of individuals in specific technical areas. Qualifications are available in apheresis, immunohistochemistry, and laboratory safety. To receive this credential, candidates must meet the eligibility requirements and successfully complete an examination (QIA, QBRS, QDP, QIHC, QLS). Candidates who complete the Qualification process will receive a Certificate of Qualification, which is valid for 3 years. The Qualification may be revalidated every 3 years upon completion of the Credential Maintenance Program (CMP) application and fee. (Documentation of acceptable continuing education may be requested). Further information regarding requalification can be found at www.ascp.org/cmp.

Preparing for & Taking the ASCP BOC Certification Examinations
Begin early to prepare for the Certification Examinations. Because of the broad range of knowledge and skills tested by the examination, even applicants with college education and those completing formal laboratory education training programs will find review is necessary, although the exact amount will vary from applicant to applicant. Generally, last minute cramming is the least effective method for preparing for the examination. The earlier you begin, the more time you will have to prepare; and the more you prepare, the better your chance of successfully passing the examination and scoring well.

Study for the Test
Make your preparation for the ASCP BOC Certification Examination part of your daily routine. Set aside a regular time and place to study. It is more beneficial to spend a short time studying every day than to spend several hours in one sitting every week or two. Be sure to allow enough time to cover all of the information specified on the exam Content Outline. Also, be sure to devote some extra time to areas of weakness identified by your initial review.

Examination Content Guidelines and Topic Outlines
www.ascp.org/boc/pbt
www.ascp.org/boc/qdp

The ASCP BOC has developed examination content guidelines and topic outlines to delineate the content included in its tests. **Indices of question numbers by content outline for both PBT and QDP examinations precede the questions in this text, and are located on pages xii-xv.**

Access the PBT content guidelines at this link: www.ascp.org/boc/pbt. Then click on the link for "Content Guideline."

Access the QDP topic outline by going to this link: www.ascp.org/boc/qdp. Then click on the link for "Topic Outline."

Practice Analysis Reports
www.ascp.org/boc/practice-analysis

A practice analysis survey is a formal process for determining or verifying the responsibilities of individuals in the job/profession, the knowledge individuals must possess, and the skills necessary to perform the job at a minimally competent level. The results of the practice analysis inform the specifications and content of the ASCP BOC certification examinations. The practice analysis process ensures that the examinations are reflective of current practices. It also helps guarantee that individuals who become certified are up to date on the state of medical laboratory science practice and are competent to perform as certified laboratory professionals.

Study Guide
The questions in this study guide are in a format and style similar to the questions on the ASCP BOC examinations. The questions are in a multiple choice format with one best answer. Work through each chapter and answer all the questions as presented. Next, review your answers against the answer key. Review the answer explanation for any questions you responded to incorrectly or were uncertain about. Each question is referenced if you require further explanation.

Textbooks
www.ascp.org/content/docs/default-source/boc-pdfs/boc-us-reading-lists/pbt_ipbt_reading_list.pdf
www.ascp.org/content/docs/default-source/boc-pdfs/boc-us-reading-lists/qdp_reading_list.pdf

The references cited in this study guide identify many useful textbooks. The most current reading lists for most of the examinations are available on the ASCP website. Textbooks tend to cover a broad range of knowledge in a given field and may provide expanded explanations, if needed.

Primary Reference Sources Cited in this Study Guide
Garza D & Becan-McBride K [2018] Phlebotomy Handbook: Blood Specimen Collection from Basic to Advanced, 10e. ISBN: 978-0134709321
McCall RE [2020] Phlebotomy Essentials, 7e. ISBN: 978-1496387073

Other Reference Sources
AABB [2020] Standards for Blood Banks and Transfusion Services, 32e. ISBN: 978 156395367-5
ASCLS [2022] American Society for Clinical Laboratory Science Code of Ethics. https://ascls.org/code-of-ethics/
CLSI GP41 [2017] Collection Of Diagnostic Venous Blood Specimens, 7e. ISBN: print 1-562380 812 6, digital 1-56238 813 4
Code of Federal Regulations [2021] Title 21, Food and Drugs, Parts 600, 601,606, 607, 610, 660, 680. Washington DC: US Government Publishing Office. ISBN: 978-1641435741
Cohn CS, et al (eds) [2020] AABB Technical Manual, 20e. ISBN: print 978-1563953705; digital 978-1563953705
Code of Federal Regulations [2021] Title 21, Food and Drugs, Parts 600, 601,606, 607, 610, 660, 680. Washington DC: US Government Publishing Office. ISBN: 978-1641435741
Harmening D [2018] Modern Blood Banking & Transfusion Practices, 7e. ISBN: 978-0803668881

Preparing for & Taking the ASCP BOC Certification Examinations

BOC Interactive Practice Exam

store.ascp.org/productlisting/productdetail?productId=121613463

The BOC Interactive Practice Exam enables the user to build custom quizzes and timed practice test based on topics, difficulty and more, pulling from a library of 1729 study questions. One can compare question-level results to see how your peers are answering. The Practice Exam allows user to set a time limit to simulate a real exam scenario. An PBT-only filter can be applied for those studying for the PBT Qualification Exam. It can be accessed anywhere on desktop or mobile.

Taking the PBT Certification Examination

The ASCP BOC uses computer adaptive testing (CAT), which is criterion referenced. With CAT, provided you answer the question correctly, the next examination question has a slightly higher level of difficulty. The difficulty level of the questions presented to the examinee continues to increase until a question is answered incorrectly. At this point, a slightly easier question is presented. The importance of testing in an adaptive format is that each test is individually tailored to your ability level.

Each question in the examination pool is calibrated for difficulty and categorized into a subtest area, which corresponds to the content guideline for a particular examination. The weight (value) given to each question is determined by the level of difficulty. All certification examinations (with the exception of phlebotomy [PBT] are scheduled for 2 hours and 30 minutes and have 100 questions. The PBT examination is scheduled for 2 hours and has 80 questions. Your preliminary test results (pass/fail) will appear on the computer screen immediately upon completion of your examination. Examination scores will be emailed within 4 business days after the examination administration, provided all required documents have been received. Examination results cannot be released by telephone under any circumstances.

Your official detailed examination score report will indicate a "pass" or "fail" status and the specific scaled score on the total examination. A scaled score is mathematically derived (in part) from the raw score (number of correctly answered questions) and the difficulty level of the questions. Because each examinee has taken an individualized examination, scaled scores are used so that all examinations may be compared on the same scale. The minimum passing score is 400. The highest attainable score is 999.

If you were unsuccessful in passing the examination, your scaled scores on each of the subtests will be indicated on the report as well. These subtest scores cannot be calculated to obtain your total score. These scores are provided as a means of demonstrating your areas of strengths and weaknesses in comparison to the minimum passing score.

Taking the QDP Qualification Examination

www.ascp.org/boc/qualification

The QDP examination is scheduled for 90 minutes and has 50 questions. This examination is self-administered on your own computer. You will receive an email notification to login to view your Admission Notice. Your admission notification will include an authorization number to the online Qualification Examination.

A notification to view your examination score will be emailed to you within 4 business days after completing your exam. If you were unsuccessful in passing the examination, you will be provided with procedures for re-testing.

Tips for Preparing for the Examinations

The ASCP BOC PBT & QDP Study Guide contains over 1700 multiple choice questions and is designed to achieve 2 goals: (1) to assist students in preparing for phlebotomy certification exams and (2) to provide phlebotomy instructors with a resource of examination questions. To achieve the first goal, the ASCP BOC PBT & QDP Study Guide includes a comprehensive set of sample review questions, organized by chapter and further grouped by topic corresponding to the ASCP BOC Examination Content Outlines. Each chapter begins with a set of questions followed by brief explanation for each answer that incorporates references, which may be used to obtain additional information or expanded explanations. Answer keys are grouped at the back of the book for convenience and quick access. Additionally, each question is indexed according to the ASCP BOC Examination Content Outlines for the Phlebotomy Technician and International Phlebotomy Technician, and/or the ASCP BOC Qualification in Donor Phlebotomy Exam.

To determine the set of questions included in the ASCP BOC PBT & QDP Study Guide, 2 criteria were used. First, the ASCP BOC Examination Content Outline for the Phlebotomy Technician and International Phlebotomy Technician and Qualification in Donor Phlebotomy created a framework for content included in the ASCP BOC PBT & QDP Study Guide. The approach outlined below may be transferred to the Qualification in Donor Phlebotomy (QDP) Exam using the QDP Exam Content outline. 6 categories of information are addressed in this guide and correlate to the following chapter headings: Circulatory System; Specimen Collection; Specimen Handling, Transport & Processing; Waived and Point-of-Care Testing; Nonblood Specimens; and Laboratory Operations.

Second, the weighted content of ASCP BOC Examination Content Outline for the Phlebotomy Technician and International Phlebotomy Technician provided direction for content emphasis. Content outline percentages for each examination follow below. The questions in this study guide track this percentage distribution.

ASCP BOC PBT Certification Exam

Content Category	Percentages
Circulatory System	5-10%
Specimen Collection	45-50%
Specimen Handling, Transport & Processing	15-20%
Waived & Point-of-Care Testing (POCT)	5-10%
Nonblood Specimens	5-10%
Laboratory Operations	15-20%

ASCP BOC QDP Qualification Exam

Content Category	Percentages
Basic Science	5-15%
Donor Identification & Selection	25-35%
Donor Blood Collection & Handling	30-40%
Donor Considerations	10-20%
Donor Center Operations	10-15%

Tips for Preparing for the Examinations

In summary, the ASCP BOC PBT & QDP Study Guide is a comprehensive tool designed to assist phlebotomy students with preparing for phlebotomy certification or qualification exams, and secondly, to assist phlebotomy instructors in developing written competency assessments (tests). Questions with images will appear as they would on the certification examination. Laboratory results will be presented in both conventional and SI units. The practice questions are presented in a format and style similar to the questions included on the ASCP BOC examinations. The ASCP BOC Examination Content Outline for the Phlebotomy Technician and International Phlebotomy Technician and Qualification in Donor Phlebotomy served as the framework for the ASCP BOC PBT & QDP Study Guide. Responses providing explanations to the answer key were based in a number of resources, including Clinical and Laboratory Standards Institute GP41 Collection of Diagnostic Specimens by Venipuncture, 7th edition.

Please note: None of these exact questions will appear on any ASCP BOC examination. This book is not a product of the ASCP BOC; rather, it is a product of the ASCP Press, the independent publishing arm of the American Society for Clinical Pathology. Use of this book does not ensure passing an examination. The ASCP BOC's evaluation and credentialing processes are entirely independent of this study guide; however, this book should significantly help students prepare to challenge the ASCP BOC examination.

PBT Index of Questions by Content Outline

Numbers shown are question numbers, not page numbers

Chapter 1: Circulatory System
A. structure/function of the circulatory system 1-27, 29-34, 37
 1. heart 1-18, 33-34 and arteries 15-24
 2. capillaries 19-20, 25-28
 3. veins 29-34, 37
B. composition/function of blood 35-36, 38-64
 1. plasma/serum 35-45
 2. cellular elements 46-50
C. terminology 65-90

Chapter 2: specimen collection
A. review & clarification of orders 1-19, 69-70
B. patient communication 20-34, 108-109, 112, 114
C. patient identification 48-68
D. patient assessment/preparation 34-43, 71-81, 86-96, 99-100, 102-107, 110-111, 113, 115-117, 119, 124-131, 286-290
E. site selection 101, 132-154, 156-157, 159-165, 170, 172-189, 191-197, 286-290, 404-408, 410-411, 424, 454-456
F. techniques 45-47, 155, 166-169, 171, 198-217, 219, 221-256, 263-270, 272-285, 291-296, 297, 304, 306-322, 323-329, 339, 341-349, 352, 414-416, 435-437, 442-443, 453, 506
G. common tests 82, 102, 277-278, 301-303, 322, 339, 346-349, 448-450, 510, 534
H. order of draw 353-384, 396-398, 412
I. complications & considerations 83-85, 90, 97-98, 121, 158, 190, 218, 220, 257-258, 260-262, 271, 298-300, 305, 330-337, 351, 385-395, 399-403, 409, 417-423, 425-434, 438-441, 444-447, 451-452, 461
J. equipment 118, 120, 122-123, 338, 340, 457-460, 462-505, 507-509, 511-524
K. terminology 350, 525-633, 535-561
skin puncture 18-197, 286, 336, 338, 345-349, 351, 382, 384, 444-447, 451-453, 484, 518-524
venipuncture 101, 121, 132-185, 198-263, 260-285, 340-344, 352-381, 385-444, 454-483, 485-517

Chapter 3: Specimen Handling, Transport & Processing
A. specimen types 9-10, 53 60, 62-73, 75-76, 85 /suitability 12-52, 61
 1. routine specimens 9-62, 124 125
 2. unusual specimen types 63-73, 75-76
 3. newborn screening 77-78, 81-84
 4. chain-of-custody specimens 86-90
B. accessioning, 91-94
C. labeling 102-107
D. assess specimen quality 11, 74, 98-100, 108 123, 160, 161, 169, 171, 173, 175 186
E. transport & storage 95

  transport 126 135, 144-159, 162-168, 190-192

  storage 79-80, 137-143, 174, 199
 1. temperature 79, 144-159
 2. light 162-168
 3. time 79-80, 96-97, 101, 137, 170, 187 189
 4. shipping 193-195

PBT Index of Questions by Content Outline

Chapter 3: specimen handling, transport & processing (continued)
F. equipment 136, 196-198, 200-202
G. terminology 1-8, 203-230

Chapter 4: waived & point-of-care testing
A. urinalysis 1-7
B. hemoglobin & hematocrit 8-11
C. coagulation (introduced in Chapter 1 35-38, 42-45; eg, bleeding time 12-21, PT 22)
D. glucose 23-27, 30, 39
E. kit tests (eg, strep screen, rapid flu test, pregnancy test) 61-70
F. performance/operations 28-29, 31-38, 40-50
G. terminology 51-60

Chapter 5: nonblood specimens
A. physiology 1-8, 12-15, 92, 97-98, 102-103, 108-109, 113, 116, 118-120, 122, 124, 126
B. patient preparation 19-20, 33, 36, 38-41, 47-53, 63-67, 93-94, 104
C. patient collection 16-18, 21-24, 26-29, 31 32, 34-35, 37, 43-45, 54-60, 62, 68-70, 84-86, 96, 99-100, 105, 110-111, 114-115, 121, 123
D. processing & handling 30, 42, 46, 61, 71-72, 95, 101, 106-107, 112, 125
E. terminology 9-11, 25, 77-83, 87-91, 117

Chapter 6: laboratory operations
A. quality control
  1. techniques 2, 6-7
  2. equipment 8-17
B. quality improvement 3-5, 18-26, 88, 98-101
C. interpersonal relations 27-44, 46-48, 51-61
D. professional ethics 62-73
E. regulatory applications (eg. OSHA, CLSI, CDC, CLIA) 74-87, 89-94, 103-282
  1. safety 1, 119
    a. patient 1, 45, 49-50, 95-96
    b. personal 103, 110-111, 282
    c. equipment 112, 115-118, 120-125, 157-160, 236-237
    d. laboratory/hospital 113-114, 126-156, 161
  2. infection control 89-94, 106, 163-164, 167, 169, 172, 119-183, 185-188, 213, 232-235
    a. protective equipment 108, 189-195, 197-205, 207-212, 214, 216-234, 238, 249
    b. disposal of contaminated equipment 109, 119, 196, 239-248, 251
    c. hand hygiene 185, 215, 256-265
  3. coding/billing 266-270
  4. patient confidentiality 97, 271-280
F. terminology 102, 104-105, 107, 162, 165-166, 168, 170-171, 173-178, 206, 250, 252-255, 282-299

QDP Index of Questions by Content Outline

Numbers shown are question numbers, not page numbers

The Qualification in Donor Phlebotomy examination questions encompass different topics or content areas within the area of Donor Phlebotomy: Basic Science, Donor Identification and Selection, Donor Blood Collection and Handling, Donor Considerations, and Donor Center Operations. Each of these content areas comprises a specific percentage of the overall 50-question qualification exam.

Exam questions may be both theoretical and/or procedural. Theoretical questions measure skills necessary to apply knowledge. Procedural questions measure skills necessary to evaluate donor eligibility, prepare donor and equipment, perform collection, and follow quality assurance protocols. Additionally, regulatory questions are based on US sources (eg, AABB, FDA, CLIA). The content areas and percentages are described in detail below.

IMPORTANT NOTE ABOUT COVID-19: FDA guidance for changes in donor eligibility during the COVID-19 pandemic are to ensure an adequate blood supply and only apply for the duration of the pandemic. Donor eligibility questions are based on pre-pandemic requirements and will not reflect temporary changes.

Chapter 7: Donor Phlebotomy

I. BASIC SCIENCE
A. structure/function of the circulatory system
   1. heart 17-22, 32-33
   2. arteries 23
   3. veins 28-32
B. composition/function of blood
   1. types of blood (eg, venous, capillary, arterial) 13, 23, 25, 28, 30-31, 35-44
   2. plasma/serum 14, 34-47
   3. serum
   4. cellular elements (RBC, WBC, platelets) 11-12, 15, 38-44
C. blood compatibility
   1. ABO 1-8, 10, 13, 16
   2. Rh 10, 13
   3. HLA antibodies 9
D. terminology 23-29, 36-40, 55-57, 79

Other related questions that might be useful for further studies can be found in Chapter 1: 2-23, 38, 42-45, 49-52, 56-62

II. DONOR IDENTIFICATION & SELECTION
A. donor identification/verification 45, 49-50, 52-53, 98, 120-123
B. donor selection 58-97, 105-112, 145
   1. interview
      a. whole blood 12, 58-61, 66-67, 72-75, 85, 210
      b. platelets 11, 65, 68, 70-71, 107, 210
   2. physical assessment 54, 58, 112, 132, 198
      a. Hgb/Hct evaluation 101-102, 196-197
      b. pulse 104
      c. blood pressure 103
      d. temperature 99-100, 200
C. terminology 46-48, 51, 55-57, 113

QDP Index of Questions by Content Outline

Chapter 7: donor phlebotomy (continued)

III. DONOR BLOOD COLLECTION & HANDLING (30-40%)
A. phlebotomy process
  1. site selection 125, 152-167
  2. site preparation 124, 126-128
  3. labeling 120-123, 138
  4. venipuncture 139, 172-186
  5. post-donation instructions 140-143, 183-184
B. supplies/equipment (eg, additives, collection kits, scales) 115, 129-133, 146, 185-187
C. handling 118, 145
  1. transport 144
  2. storage 114-118
D. terminology 149-151, 159, 188-191

Other related questions that might be useful for further studies can be found in Chapter 2: 135-136, 143-144, 146-151, 166, 168-169, 259

IV. DONOR CONSIDERATIONS (10%-20%)
A. special donor categories
  1. directed 48, 201-202
  2. autologous 47, 192-200
  3. therapeutic 203-204
  4. concerns 58-97, 105-106, 202
B. concerns (eg, petechiae, occluded veins, scarring, edema) 58-97, 105-106, 202
C. adverse effects
  1. low volume/incomplete collection 135-136, 199
  2. arterial puncture 206
  3. donor reactions (eg, hematoma, fainting) 140, 147, 207, 211
D. terminology 209

Other related questions that might be useful for further studies can be found in Chapter 2: 414

V. DONOR CENTER OPERATIONS
A. safety (eg, OSHA guidelines)
  1. personal (PPE, Standard precautions) 221, 237-240, 242, 246, 270
  2. equipment 222-223
  3. donor center (eg, fire, chemical) 247-256
  4. infection control 242-246, 258-265, 268-292
B. quality assurance and control
  1. techniques 119-121, 129-131, 134, 225-226,
  2. equipment and materials 129-131, 135-136, 219
  3. variance/incident/error reports 133, 220, 227-228
C. donor related regulatory compliance (eg, HIPAA, CDC, FDA) 51-52, 119-122, 137-138, 215-218, 229-236
D. terminology 51, 224, 227-228, 241, 245, 257, 265, 266-267

Other related questions that might be useful for further studies can be found in Chapter 6: 14-17, 23, 26, 66-70, 76, 81, 84-86, 110-112, 120, 128-133, 135-154, 158, 171, 198

Preface

The ASCP *Board of Certification Study Guide for Phlebotomy Certification Examinations*, third edition (BOC PBT & QDP Study Guide 3e) is designed to assist phlebotomy students and practitioners in their preparation for taking a phlebotomy certification exam. Obtaining certification, and its corollary, maintaining certification, are the foundations of a professional's career. The goal of this edition is to support candidates for phlebotomy certification in their preparation endeavors.

The ASCP BOC PBT & QDP Study Guide is expanded and reflects the most recent changes to the Clinical Laboratory and Standards Institute-GP41 Collection of Diagnostic Venous Blood Specimens, seventh edition, published in April 2017.

Changes include increased detail in patient identification strategies, specimen handling, approaches to difficult draws and guidelines for acceptable sites for venipuncture. Additionally, the ASCP BOC PBT & QDP Study Guide was expanded to include a chapter of questions addressing the Content Outline for the Qualification in Donor Phlebotomy Examination.

Each chapter is arranged to include a series of questions corresponding to each exam's content outline followed by an answer key. Following the answer key is a brief explanation for the correct answer. Resources with additional information are included at the end of each explanation. Questions with images appear as they would on the certification examination. Laboratory results are presented within the context of both conventional and SI units. The practice questions are presented in a format and style similar to the questions included on the ASC BOC examinations. Questions are cross-referenced to exam content outlines following the introductory material (see pxii-xv).

Please note: None of these exact questions will appear on any ASCP BOC examination. This book is not a product of the ASCP BOC; rather, it is a product of the ASCP Press, the independent publishing arm of the American Society for Clinical Pathology. Use of this book does not ensure passing of an examination. The ASCP BOC's evaluation and credentialing processes are entirely independent of this study guide; however, this book should significantly support your preparation strategies for the ASCP BOC examination.

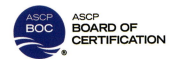

To the examinee,

Certification is an important first step in your professional career. It is my hope that you find your career in laboratory medicine a rewarding one.

Good luck on your certification exam and on your future endeavors.

—Patricia A Tanabe, MPA, MLS(ASCP)^{CM}
Executive Director, Board of Certification (retired)

Circulatory System

The following items have been identified as appropriate for those preparing for both PBT & QDP examinations.

1. In the figure below, the structure indicated by the arrow is the:

   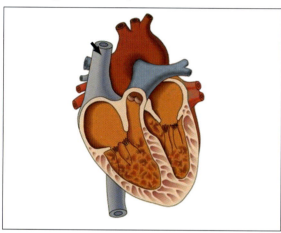

   a   pulmonary artery
   b   pulmonary vein
   c   inferior vena cava
   d   superior vena cava

2. In the figure below, the structure indicated by the arrow is the:

   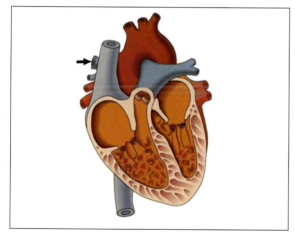

   a   pulmonary artery
   b   pulmonary vein
   c   inferior vena cava
   d   superior vena cava

Circulatory System — Questions

3. In the figure below, the structure indicated by the arrow is a:

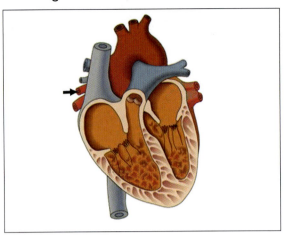

    a   pulmonary artery
    b   pulmonary vein
    c   inferior vena cava
    d   superior vena cava

4. In the figure below, the structure indicated by the arrow is the:

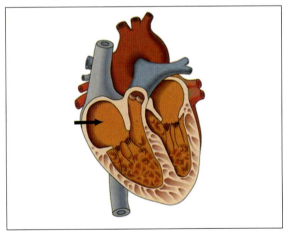

    a   right atrium
    b   left atrium
    c   right ventricle
    d   left ventricle

Questions

Circulatory System

5. In the figure below, the structure indicated by the arrow is the:

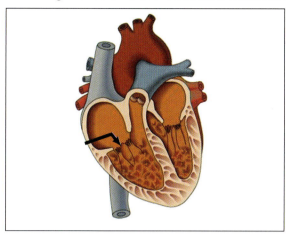

   a   aortic valve
   b   bicuspid valve
   c   superior vena cava
   d   tricuspid valve

6. In the figure below, the structure indicated by the arrow is the:

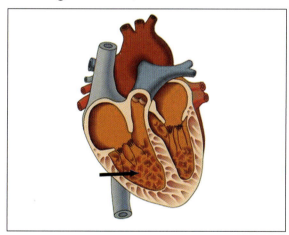

   a   right atrium
   b   left atrium
   c   right ventricle
   d   left ventricle

Circulatory System

Questions

7. In the figure below, the structure indicated by the arrow is the:

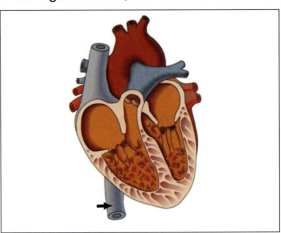

    a   pulmonary artery
    b   pulmonary vein
    c   inferior vena cava
    d   superior vena cava

8. In the figure below, the structure indicated by the arrow is the:

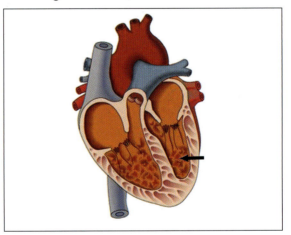

    a   right atrium
    b   left atrium
    c   right ventricle
    d   left ventricle

Questions

Circulatory System

9. In the figure below, the structure indicated by the arrow is the:

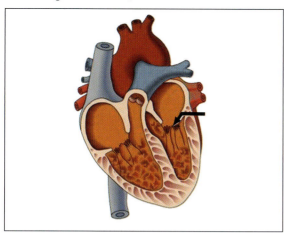

   a   aortic valve
   b   bicuspid valve
   c   superior vena cava
   d   tricuspid valve

10. In the figure below, the structure indicated by the arrow is the:

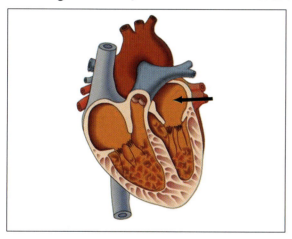

   a   right atrium
   b   left atrium
   c   right ventricle
   d   left ventricle

Circulatory System

11. In the figure below, the structure indicated by the arrow is the:

    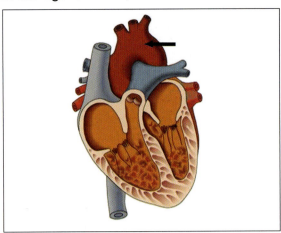

    a   aorta
    b   coronary artery
    c   pulmonary artery
    d   pulmonary vein

12. Blood exits the right atrium through the following valve:
    a   aortic
    b   mitral
    c   pulmonic
    d   tricuspid

13. Blood exits the left ventricle through the following valve:
    a   aortic
    b   mitral
    c   pulmonic
    d   tricuspid

14. Which of the following structures contains deoxygenated blood?
    a   aorta
    b   left atrium
    c   left ventricle
    d   right atrium

15. Which of the following structures contains oxygenated blood?
    a   aorta
    b   right atrium
    c   right ventricle
    d   superior vena cava

16. Which of the following structures is included in the pulmonary circuit?
    a   aorta
    b   coronary artery
    c   pulmonary artery
    d   right atrium

Questions Circulatory System

17. Which of the following structures is included in the systemic circuit?
    a   aorta
    b   pulmonary artery
    c   right atrium
    d   right ventricle

18. Which of the following structures contains oxygenated blood?
    a   inferior vena cava
    b   superior vena cava
    c   pulmonary artery
    d   aorta

19. What is the blood flow sequence from the aorta?
    a   arteries, arterioles, capillaries, venules, veins
    b   arterioles, arteries, capillaries, veins, venules
    c   venules, veins, capillaries, arterioles, arteries
    d   veins, venules, capillaries, arterioles, arteries

20. The interior of a blood vessel is called the:
    a   lumen
    b   lunar caustic
    c   tunica adventitia
    d   tunica intima

21. The blood vessel with the thickest tunica media is the:
    a   arteriole
    b   artery
    c   capillary
    d   vein

22. Blood vessels that carry blood away from the heart are the:
    a   arteries
    b   capillaries
    c   veins
    d   venules

23. Which of the following blood vessels contains oxygenated blood?
    a   arteries
    b   pulmonary arteries
    c   veins
    d   venules

Circulatory System — Questions

24. After performing a routine venipuncture, the phlebotomist noticed the blood in the evacuated tube was bright, cherry red. What vessel did the phlebotomist likely puncture?
    a artery
    b capillary
    c pulmonary artery
    d vein

25. The blood vessel whose wall is 1 cell layer thick is the:
    a arteriole
    b artery
    c capillary
    d vein

26. Which of the following blood vessels contains a mixture of oxygenated and deoxygenated blood?
    a arteries
    b capillaries
    c pulmonary arteries
    d veins

27. Which of the following structures connect arterioles and venules?
    a arteries
    b pulmonary arteries
    c capillaries
    d veins

28. Which of the following blood vessels allows gas and solute exchange between blood and tissues?
    a capillaries
    b pulmonary arteries
    c pulmonary veins
    d veins

29. Which of the following specimens has the lowest concentration of oxygen?
    a arterial
    b arterialized capillary
    c capillary
    d venous

30. The blood vessels with 1-way valves in the lumen are called:
    a arterioles
    b arteries
    c capillaries
    d veins

Questions

Circulatory System

31. Which of the following blood vessels contains deoxygenated blood?
    a   arteries
    b   arterioles
    c   veins
    d   pulmonary veins

32. After performing a routine venipuncture, the phlebotomist noticed that the blood in the evacuated tube was dark red. What vessel did the phlebotomist likely puncture?
    a   artery
    b   capillary
    c   pulmonary artery
    d   vein

33. Blood enters the right side of the heart through the:
    a   aorta
    b   pulmonary artery
    c   pulmonary vein
    d   superior vena cava

34. Blood enters the left side of the heart through the:
    a   aorta
    b   pulmonary arteries
    c   pulmonary veins
    d   inferior & superior vena cava

35. The substance that causes fibrinogen to convert to fibrin is:
    a   prothrombin
    b   thrombin
    c   antihemophilic factor
    d   tissue thromboplastin

36. An element critical to coagulation function *in vivo* and *in vitro* is:
    a   calcium
    b   nitrogen
    c   phosphorous
    d   potassium

37. The 3 components of hemostasis are:
    a   blood vessels, platelets, coagulation factors
    b   tissue thromboplastin, platelets, antihemophiliac factor
    c   fibrin split products, blood vessels, platelets
    d   blood vessels, fibrin degradation products, platelets

Circulatory System — Questions

38. Which of the following proteins is found in plasma, but not serum?
    a albumin
    b fibrinogen
    c fibrin
    d globulins

39. Normal plasma is composed of primarily:
    a antibodies
    b fibrinogen
    c solutes
    d water

40. A blood specimen was collected into an evacuated tube containing an anticoagulant. What is the fluid portion of this blood specimen called?
    a fibrin
    b fibrinogen
    c plasma
    d serum

41. A blood specimen was collected into an evacuated tube without anticoagulant and allowed to clot. What is the fluid portion of this blood specimen called?
    a fibrin
    b fibrinogen
    c plasma
    d serum

42. Which of the following coagulation pathways is initiated through the activation of Factor XII?
    a extrinsic pathway
    b intrinsic pathway
    c common pathway
    d fibrinolytic pathway

43. Which of the following coagulation pathways is initiated through the release of tissue thromboplastin?
    a extrinsic pathway
    b intrinsic pathway
    c common pathway
    d fibrinolytic pathway

44. The coagulation pathway initiated by a combination of the intrinsic and extrinsic pathways is the:
    a extrinsic pathway
    b intrinsic pathway
    c common pathway
    d fibrinolytic pathway

Questions

Circulatory System

45. Fibrin degradation products are the end result of the:
    a extrinsic pathway
    b intrinsic pathway
    c common pathway
    d fibrinolytic pathway

46. The cellular element of the blood responsible for the transport of oxygen to the tissues is:
    a erythrocyte
    b leukocyte
    c megakaryocyte
    d thrombocyte

47. The cellular element of the blood responsible for the transport of carbon dioxide from the tissues is:
    a erythrocyte
    b leukocyte
    c megakaryocyte
    d thrombocyte

48. The substance that transports oxygen in the blood is called:
    a hemoglobin
    b hematocrit
    c plasma
    d serum

49. The reference range for hematocrit levels in adult females is:
    a 30-40%
    b 35-47%
    c 40-52%
    d 50-60%

50. The reference range for hematocrit levels in adult males is:
    a 30-40%
    b 35-47%
    c 40-52%
    d 50-60%

51. The reference range for hemoglobin levels in adult females is:
    a 8-10 g/100 mL
    b 10-12 g/100 mL
    c 12-16 g/100 mL
    d 14-16 g/100 mL

Circulatory System — Questions

52. The reference range for hemoglobin levels in adult males is:
    a 8-10 g/100 mL
    b 10-12 g/100 mL
    c 12-14 g/100 mL
    d 14-18 g/100 mL

53. Blood group antigens are located:
    a on the surface of erythrocytes
    b on the surface of lymphocytes
    c in plasma
    d in serum

54. The reference range for white blood cells is:
    a 1,000-3,000/µL
    b 2,500-5,000/µL
    c 4,400-11,000/µL
    d 15,000-17,500/µL

55. The cellular element of the blood that functions in fighting infection is:
    a erythrocyte
    b leukocyte
    c megakaryocyte
    d thrombocyte

56. Leukocytes may be classified as:
    a agranulocytes & granulocytes
    b agranulocytes & erythrocytes
    c granulocytes & erythrocytes
    d granulocytes & thrombocytes

57. Leukocytes that destroy pathogens by phagocytosis are:
    a basophilic segmented cells
    b eosinophilic segmented cells
    c neutrophilic segmented cells
    d plasma cells

58. The largest leukocyte in the peripheral circulation is the:
    a basophilic segmented cells
    b lymphocytes
    c monocytes
    d neutrophilic segmented cells

59. Lymphocytes exist in 2 forms. They are:
    a A & B lymphocytes
    b A & O lymphocytes
    c A, B, AB & O lymphocytes
    d B & T lymphocytes

Questions
Circulatory System

60. The leukocyte that functions in antibody production is the:
    a   A lymphocyte
    b   B lymphocyte
    c   AB lymphocyte
    d   T lymphocyte

61. Leukocytes that defend against parasites are:
    a   basophilic segmented cells
    b   eosinophilic segmented cells
    c   neutrophilic segmented cells
    d   plasma cells

62. The granules of this leukocyte release heparin and histamine:
    a   basophilic segmented cells
    b   eosinophilic segmented cells
    c   neutrophilic segmented cells
    d   plasma cells

63. The cellular element of the peripheral blood that functions in coagulation is the:
    a   erythrocyte
    b   leukocyte
    c   megakaryocyte
    d   thrombocyte

64. The layer of cells that forms between red cells and plasma during centrifugation is called:
    a   agglutination
    b   buffy coat
    c   γ globulin
    d   erythropoietin

65. The term for an abnormally enlarged heart is:
    a   bradycardia
    b   cardiomegaly
    c   pericarditis
    d   tachycardia

66. The condition in which a healthy body through constant changes and functioning remains the same is:
    a   hematoma
    b   hemoconcentration
    c   hemostasis
    d   homeostasis

Circulatory System — Questions

67. The term for all of the chemical reactions necessary to sustain life is:
    a anabolism
    b catabolism
    c embolism
    d metabolism

68. The process by which complex substances in food are broken down into simple substances while releasing energy is:
    a anabolism
    b catabolism
    c embolism
    d metabolism

69. The process by which body cells use energy to make complex substances from simpler ones is called:
    a anabolism
    b catabolism
    c embolism
    d metabolism

70. A blood clot occurring in a blood vessel is called a(n):
    a aneurysm
    b embolus
    c thrombus
    d turgent

71. A foreign body such as a blood clot, bacteria, or fibrin clot, causing an obstruction in a blood vessel is called a(n):
    a embolus
    b thrombocyte
    c thrombus
    d turgent

72. The body plane that runs lengthwise from front to back, dividing the body into right and left halves, is called:
    a frontal plane
    b lateral plane
    c sagittal plane
    d transverse plane

73. Which term describes a patient lying on his back?
    a anatomic position
    b distal position
    c proximal position
    d supine position

Questions

Circulatory System

74. Which term describes a patient standing erect, with palms facing forward?
    a anatomic position
    b distal position
    c proximal position
    d supine position

75. The directional term that refers to the front of the body is:
    a anterior
    b lateral
    c medial
    d posterior

76. The directional term that refers to the back of the body is:
    a anterior
    b dorsal
    c lateral
    d medial

77. The directional term that refers to the front of the body is:
    a dorsal
    b medial
    c posterior
    d ventral

78. The directional term that refers to the back of the body is:
    a anterior
    b medial
    c posterior
    d ventral

79. The directional term that refers to the midline of the body is:
    a dorsal
    b medial
    c posterior
    d ventral

80. The directional term that refers to the side of the body is:
    a lateral
    b medial
    c posterior
    d proximal

81. The directional term that means nearest to the center of the body, point of attachment, or origin is:
    a distal
    b lateral
    c medial
    d proximal

Circulatory System

82. The directional term that means farthest from the center of the body, point of attachment, or origin is:
    a   distal
    b   lateral
    c   medial
    d   proximal

83. The directional term that means above, higher, or toward the head is:
    a   dorsal
    b   inferior
    c   superior
    d   ventral

84. The directional term that means lower, beneath, or away from the head is:
    a   dorsal
    b   inferior
    c   superior
    d   ventral

85. A 200 pound adult male will have a blood volume of:
    a   4 liters
    b   5 liters
    c   637 mL
    d   6,363 mL

86. A 10-year-old female patient who weighs 55 pounds will have a blood volume of:
    a   875 mL
    b   1,000 mL
    c   1,875 mL
    d   6,363 mL

87. Which of the following structures is located on the midsagittal plane?
    a   intestines
    b   left kidney
    c   right lung
    d   sternum

88. Which of the following structures is located on the posterior side of the frontal plane?
    a   bladder
    b   diaphragm
    c   epididymis
    d   spinal cord

Questions

Circulatory System

89. Which of the following structures is located superior to the transverse plane?
    - a appendix
    - b bladder
    - c epididymis
    - d heart

90. The process by which the body stops the leakage of blood from the vascular system is called:
    - a hematoma
    - b hemoconcentration
    - c hemostasis
    - d homeostasis

Circulatory System — Explanations

Please consult the diagram below for questions 1-11 regarding identification of anatomical structures of the heart.

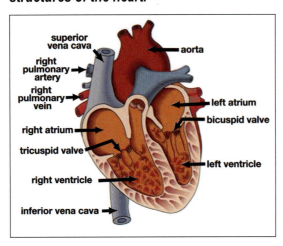

1. **d** The superior vena cava brings deoxygenated blood from the arms, chest, head and neck to the right atrium.
   [Garza 10e, p219]

2. **a** The pulmonary artery, specifically the right pulmonary artery on this diagram, carries deoxygenated blood to the lungs. The pulmonary arteries begin the pulmonary circuit. Unlike arteries in the systemic circuit, pulmonary arteries carry deoxygenated blood.
   [Garza 10e, p219-221]

3. **b** The pulmonary vein, specifically branches of the right pulmonary vein on this diagram, carries oxygenated blood to the heart and enters the heart via the left atrium. Unlike veins in the systemic circuit, pulmonary veins carry oxygenated blood.
   [Garza 10e, p219-221]

4. **a** The inferior and superior vena cava deliver deoxygenated blood from the tissues into the right atrium.
   [Garza 10e, p219-221]

5. **d** Deoxygenated blood flows from the right atrium into the right ventricle through the tricuspid valve.
   [Garza 10e, p219]

6. **c** The right ventricle contracts, forcing blood through the pulmonary semilunar valve and closing the tricuspid valve. The pulmonary circuit begins when blood exits the right ventricle.
   [Garza 10e, p219-221]

7. **c** The inferior vena cava brings deoxygenated blood from the lower trunk and legs to the right atrium.
   [Garza 10e, p219]

Explanations

Circulatory System

8. **d**   The left ventricle fills with oxygenated blood from the left atrium though the mitral valve. Contraction of the left ventricle forces blood through the aortic valve into the aorta.
[Garza 10e, p219]

9. **b**   The left ventricle fills with oxygenated blood from the left atrium though the bicuspid (mitral) valve. Contraction of the left ventricle forces the bicuspid valve to close and blood through the aortic valve into the aorta.
[Garza 10e, p219]

10. **b**   Pulmonary veins deposit oxygenated blood from the lungs into the left atrium.
[Garza 10e, p219]

11. **a**   The left ventricle empties oxygenated blood into the aorta, the largest artery in the body.
[Garza 10e, p219, 222]

12. **d**   Deoxygenated blood flows from the right atrium into the right ventricle through the tricuspid valve.
[Garza 10e, p219]

13. **a**   Oxygenated blood exits the left ventricle through the aortic valve.
[Garza 10e, p219]

14. **d**   The inferior and superior vena cava bring deoxygenated blood from the body to the right atrium.
[Garza 10e, p219]

15. **a**   Contraction of the left ventricle forces oxygenated blood through the aortic valve into the aorta.
[Garza 10e, p219]

16. **c**   The inferior and superior vena cava deliver deoxygenated blood from the tissues to the right atrium. Deoxygenated blood moves through the right atrium and ventricle and exits the heart to begin the pulmonary circuit through the right and left pulmonary arteries. The pulmonary circuit begins when blood exits the right ventricle and travels into the left or right pulmonary arteries.
[Garza 10e, p219, 221]

17. **a**   The systemic circuit begins when blood exits the left ventricle and travels into the ascending aorta.
[Garza 10e, p221]

18. **d**   The inferior and superior vena cava deliver deoxygenated blood from the tissues to the right atrium. Deoxygenated blood moves through the right atrium and ventricle and exits the heart to begin the pulmonary circuit through the right and left pulmonary arteries. Oxygenated blood is returned to the heart by pulmonary veins, which empty into the left atrium and then the left ventricle. Oxygenated blood exits the heart via the aorta.
[Garza 10e, p219-221]

Circulatory System — Explanations

19. **a** The systemic circuit begins when oxygenated blood enters the ascending aorta. The aorta branches into smaller structures called arteries, which branch into smaller structures called arterioles, which branch into capillaries. In the capillaries, oxygen passes from the hemoglobin molecule in the red blood cells to the tissues and carbon dioxide from the tissues attaches to the hemoglobin molecule in the red blood cells. Deoxygenated blood exits the capillary beds and moves to venules, which contribute to larger structures called veins. Ultimately, deoxygenated blood returns to the heart via the inferior or superior vena cava.
    [Garza 10e, p220-221]

20. **a** The center of a blood vessel (either artery or vein) is called a lumen.
    [Garza 10e, p225]

21. **b** The middle layer of tissue constituting the wall of veins and arteries is called the tunica media and is composed of smooth muscle. The tunica media is much thicker in arterioles and arteries than in veins.
    [Garza 10e, p225]

22. **a** Arteries in the systemic circuit carry oxygenated blood away from the heart. The pulmonary arteries uniquely carry deoxygenated blood away from the heart to the lungs as part of the pulmonary circuit.
    [Garza 10e, p225]

23. **a** Arteries in the systemic circuit carry oxygenated blood away from the heart. The pulmonary arteries uniquely carry deoxygenated blood away from the heart to the lungs as part of the pulmonary circuit.
    [Garza 10e, p225]

24. **a** When arterial blood is oxygenated to normal levels, it is bright cherry red in color. If a phlebotomist inadvertently punctures an artery, the blood in the collection tube will be bright cherry red. If the phlebotomist believes an artery has been accidentally punctured, he should immediately remove the needle, apply continuous pressure to the site for at least 5 minutes. Once the bleeding has stopped, a supervisor should be notified per the policies at the facility.
    [Garza 10e, p224, 335]

25. **c** Capillary vessel walls are 1 cell layer thick to allow diffusion of oxygen and nutrients from the blood to the tissues and carbon dioxide and waste products from the tissues into the bloodstream. In contrast, vessel walls of veins and arteries have 3 distinct layers (tunica adventitia, tunica media, and tunica intima).
    [Garza 10e, p225]

26. **b** Gas and solute exchange occurs in the capillaries across the 1 cell layer thick vessel wall. As a result, blood in the capillaries is a mixture of deoxygenated and oxygenated blood.
    [Garza 10e, p229]

Explanations

Circulatory System

27. c Capillaries are the blood vessels that connect the circuit of blood vessels by linking arterial and venous circulation.
[Garza 10e, p229]

28. a Capillary vessel walls are 1 cell layer thick to allow diffusion of oxygen and nutrients from the blood to the tissues and carbon dioxide and waste products from the tissues into the bloodstream. Capillaries are the only blood vessels that allow this exchange with the tissues.
[Garza 10e, p229]

29. d Veins in the systemic circuit return deoxygenated blood to the heart. Consequently, venous specimens obtained by venipuncture contain the lowest concentration of oxygen.
[Garza 10e, p226]

30. d Blood moves through most of the venous network against the force of gravity. Many veins include valves composed of epithelial tissue. The valves prevent backflow of blood and ensure blood continues to move toward the heart.
[Garza 10e, p226]

31. c Veins in the systemic circuit carry deoxygenated blood to the heart. The pulmonary veins uniquely carry oxygenated blood from the lungs to the heart as part of the pulmonary circuit.
[Garza 10e, p220]

32. d Deoxygenated blood is dark red in color verifying that the phlebotomist punctured a vein.
[Garza 10e, p220]

33. d The superior vena cava brings deoxygenated blood from the arms, chest, head, and neck to the right atrium.
[Garza 10e, p220]

34. c Pulmonary veins deposit oxygenated blood from the lungs into the left atrium.
[Garza 10e, p220]

35. b Activation of intrinsic, extrinsic, and common coagulation pathways culminate in the activation of thrombin. Thrombin functions in numerous ways to achieve coagulation, including converting fibrinogen to fibrin.
[Garza 10e, p244-245]

36. a Calcium is a crucial element in the coagulation cascade. Calcium assists in promoting adhesion of coagulation factors to platelet and other membranes, ultimately culminating in a stable fibrin clot.
[Garza 10e, p244]

37. a There are 3 elements contributing to hemostasis *in vivo,* including blood vessels, platelets, and coagulation factors.
[Garza 10e, p243-244]

Circulatory System — Explanations

38. **b** If a blood specimen is collected into an evacuated tube and allowed to clot, the fibrinogen is converted to fibrin to form the clot. Therefore, fibrinogen is not found in serum. If a blood specimen is collected into an anticoagulant and clotting is prevented, fibrinogen remains in the plasma.
[Garza 10e, p234-235]

39. **d** Approximately 90% of plasma is water (H_2O).
[Garza 10e, p234]

40. **c** If coagulation is prevented, the fluid portion of the blood specimen is called plasma. A variety of substances function as anticoagulants in evacuated tubes and prevent coagulation of the specimen, yielding plasma.
[Garza 10e, p233-234]

41. **d** If a blood specimen is collected into an evacuated tube and allowed to clot, the fluid portion of the specimen is called serum. Fibrinogen cannot be found in serum because it was converted to fibrin in the clotting process.
[Garza 10e, p233-234]

42. **b** There are 3 pathways used to describe the coagulation phase of hemostasis, namely the intrinsic, extrinsic, and common pathways. The factors included in the intrinsic pathway are found inside, ie, intrinsic to the blood vessels. Factor XII circulates in the plasma and is activated by changes to the endothelial lining of the blood vessel. The activation of Factor XII initiates the intrinsic pathway.
[Garza 10e, p244-245]

43. **a** There are 3 pathways used to describe the coagulation phase of hemostasis, namely the intrinsic, extrinsic, and common pathways. The factors included in the extrinsic pathway are found outside, ie, extrinsic to the blood vessels. Tissue damage releases tissue thromboplastin which activates the extrinsic pathway.
[Garza 10e, p244-245]

44. **c** There are 3 pathways used to describe the coagulation phase of hemostasis, namely the intrinsic, extrinsic, and common pathways. The intrinsic and extrinsic pathways combine to initiate the common pathway, which ultimately generates fibrin, the foundation of a stable fibrin clot.
[Garza 10e, p244]

45. **d** Fibrinolysis, the final stage in hemostasis, is the dissolution of the fibrin clot as healing to the injury occurs. The activation of certain coagulation factors convert plasminogen to plasmin. Plasmin is an enzyme that enzymatically converts fibrin into fibrin split products, the end result of fibrinolysis.
[Garza 10e, p244]

46. **a** Erythrocytes (red blood cells or RBCs) contain hemoglobin, which transports oxygen to the tissues and carbon dioxide away from tissues.
[Garza 10e, p236-237]

Explanations   Circulatory System

47. **a** Erythrocytes (red blood cells or RBCs) contain hemoglobin, which transports oxygen to the tissues and carbon dioxide away from tissues.
[Garza 10e, p236-237]

48. **a** Red blood cells (RBCs) transport hemoglobin molecules, which transport oxygen to the tissues and carbon dioxide away from tissues.
[Garza 10e, p236-237]

49. **b** Reference ranges specify results expected for laboratory tests in healthy patient populations and some variation between laboratories is likely. Based on combined data, the reference range for HCT level in adult females is 35-47%. Please note: Hemoglobin (HGB or Hb) and hematocrit (Hct or HCT) reference ranges may be specified by gender.
[Garza 10e, p236-237]

50. **c** Reference ranges specify results expected for laboratory tests in healthy patient populations and some variation between laboratories is likely. Based on combined data, the reference range for Hct level in adult males is 40-52%. Please note: hemoglobin (HGB or Hb) and hematocrit (Hct or HCT) reference ranges may be specified by gender.
[Garza 10e, p240]

51. **c** Reference ranges specify results expected for laboratory tests in healthy patient populations and some variation between laboratories is likely. Based on combined data, the reference range for hemoglobin level in adult females is 12-16 g/dL. Please note: hemoglobin (HGB or Hb) and hematocrit (Hct or HCT) reference ranges may be specified by gender.
[Garza 10e, p240]

52. **d** Reference ranges specify results expected for laboratory tests in healthy patient populations and some variation between laboratories is likely. Based on combined data, the reference range for hemoglobin level in adult males is 14-18 g/dL. Please note: hemoglobin (HGB or Hb) and hematocrit (Hct or HCT) reference ranges may be specified by gender.
[Garza 10e, p240]

53. **a** Blood group antigens are proteins found on the red cell membrane. The presence of blood group antigens on red cell membranes is determined genetically.
[Garza 10e, p236-237-238]

54. **c** Reference ranges specify results expected for laboratory tests in healthy patient populations and some variation between laboratories is likely. Based on combined data, the reference range for white blood cell counts in adults is $4.4-11 \times 10^3/\mu L$. Please note: unlike hemoglobin (HGB or Hb) and hematocrit (Hct or HCT) values, reference ranges for white cell counts do not vary by gender.
[Garza 10e, p240]

Circulatory System — Explanations

55. **b** Leukocytes or white blood cells (WBCs) function in fighting infection.
[Garza 10e, p236-239]

56. **a** There are 5 different types of leukocytes or white blood cells (WBCs) normally found in the peripheral blood and each type is categorized as either an agranulocyte or a granulocyte. If a peripheral blood smear is stained with Wright stain, agranulocytes are WBCs without discernible granules in the cytoplasm and granulocytes are WBCs with granules in the cytoplasm easily identified following Wright stain.
[Garza 10e, p235]

57. **c** Neutrophilic segmented cells are granulocytes with fine, purple granules in the cytoplasm. Neutrophilic segmented cells ("segs") destroy pathogens by phagocytosis.
[Garza 10e, p235]

58. **c** The largest WBC in peripheral circulation is the monocyte, which is an agranulocyte. Monocytes are approximately 2-2.5× larger than a red blood cell.
[Garza 10e, p234-235]

59. **d** Lymphocytes are agranulocytes that exist as B & T lymphocytes. B & T lymphocytes look very similar on a peripheral blood smear, but have very different functions. B lymphocytes function in antibody production. T lymphocytes function in cellular immunity.
[Garza 10e, p249]

60. **b** Lymphocytes are agranulocytes that exist as B & T lymphocytes. B & T lymphocytes look very similar on a peripheral blood smear, but have very different functions. B lymphocytes function in antibody production. T lymphocytes function in cellular immunity.
[Garza 10e, p249]

61. **b** Eosinophilic segmented cells (eosinophils or "eos") are granulocytes with bright, red-orange granules in the cytoplasm. Eosinophilic segmented cells function in allergic reactions and parasitic infections.
[Garza 10e, p235]

62. **a** Basophilic segmented cells (basophils or "basos") are granulocytes with very dark blue granules in the cytoplasm. The granules in basophilic segmented cells contain histamine and heparin.
[Garza 10e, p235]

Explanations
Circulatory System

63. **d** Thrombocytes (platelets) are the smallest cellular element in the peripheral blood. Following an injury to a blood vessel and during the second phase of hemostasis, thrombocytes aggregate and adhere to form a plug over the site of injury, reducing blood flow.
[Garza 10e, p242]

64. **b** Blood separates into 3 distinct layers following centrifugation of a blood specimen collected in anticoagulant. The heaviest cellular elements, erythrocytes, are at the bottom of the evacuated tube and the lightest element, plasma, at the top. White cells and platelets form a thin layer called a buffy coat between the erythrocytes and the plasma.
[Garza 10e, p233]

65. **b** By identifying the meaning of the root word and suffix, the meaning of the word can be surmised. The root word *cardi-* means "heart." The suffix *-megaly* means "enlargement." The vowel "o" serves as the combining vowel joining the 2 word components. Therefore, *cardiomegaly* means "enlargement of the heart."
[Garza 10e, p167-168, 248]

66. **d** The prefix *homeo-* means "the same" and the suffix *-stasis* means "standing." Therefore, *homeostasis* means "standing the same." Homeostasis is the process by which the body, through constant change, consistently maintains internal balance.
[Garza 10e, p169]

67. **d** Metabolism is the term that refers to all of the processes associated with using or releasing energy, a critical component in maintaining homeostasis.
[Garza 10e, p171]

68. **b** Catabolism is the process the body uses to convert complex substances to simpler substances while releasing energy.
[Garza 10e, p171]

69. **a** Anabolism is the process by which the body uses energy to create complex substances from simpler ones.
[Garza 10e, p171]

70. **c** A thrombus (thrombi is the plural form) is a blood clot lodged in a blood vessel. Thrombi may partially or completely obstruct a blood vessel.
[Garza 10e, p246]

71. **a** An embolus (emboli is the plural form) is any foreign material, such as a blood clot, bacteria, or fibrin clot which obstructs a blood vessel. Emboli may partially or completely obstruct a blood vessel.
[Garza 10e, p248]

Circulatory System — Explanations

72. **c** Body planes are invisible flat surfaces that divide the body sections. The use of body planes provides health care workers with reference points used to describe a patient's condition in a standardized manner. The sagittal plane divides the body into right and left sides. The midsagittal plane intersects the body at midline and divides the body into equal right and left halves.
[Garza 10e, p174-177]

73. **d** Vocabulary used to describe patient body positioning assists health care workers by standardizing the descriptive language. When a patient is in a supine position, she is horizontal, resting on her back, face up. Most patients in hospital beds are in a supine position during venipuncture.
[Garza 10e, p174-175]

74. **a** Vocabulary used to describe patient body positioning assists health care workers by standardizing the descriptive language. Anatomic position describes a patient who is standing erect, facing forward, arms relaxed at the patient's side, and palms facing forward.
[Garza 10e, p172-175]

75. **a** Directional terms describe the location of a body part relative to other parts of the body or the body as a whole and often have antonyms and synonyms. One directional term referring to the front of the body is anterior. An antonym for anterior is posterior and a synonym is ventral.
[Garza 10e, p172-175]

76. **b** Directional terms describe the location of a body part relative to other parts of the body or the body as a whole and often have antonyms and synonyms. One directional term referring to the back of the body is dorsal. An antonym for dorsal is ventral and a synonym is posterior.
[Garza 10e, p175]

77. **d** Directional terms describe the location of a body part relative to other parts of the body or the body as a whole and often have antonyms and synonyms. One directional term referring to the front of the body is ventral. An antonym for ventral is dorsal and a synonym is anterior.
[Garza 10e, p175]

78. **c** Directional terms describe the location of a body part relative to other parts of the body or the body as a whole and often have antonyms and synonyms. One directional term referring to the back of the body is posterior. An antonym for posterior is anterior and a synonym is dorsal.
[Garza 10e, p175-177]

79. **b** Directional terms describe the location of a body part relative to other parts of the body or the body as a whole. The directional term referring to the midline of the body is medial.
[Garza 10e, p173-175]

Explanations

Circulatory System

80. **a**   Directional terms describe the location of a body part relative to other parts of the body or the body as a whole. The directional term referring to the side of the body is lateral.
[Garza 10e, p173-175]

81. **d**   Directional terms describe the location of a body part relative to other parts of the body or the body as a whole. The directional term meaning nearest to the center of the body, point of attachment or origin is proximal.
[Garza 10e, p173-175]

82. **a**   Directional terms describe the location of a body part relative to other parts of the body or the body as a whole. The directional term meaning farthest to the center of the body, point of attachment, or origin is distal.
[Garza 10e, p173-175]

83. **c**   Directional terms describe the location of a body part relative to other parts of the body or the body as a whole and often have antonyms and synonyms. One directional term referring to above, higher or toward the head is superior. An antonym for superior is inferior and a synonym is cranial.
[Garza 10e, p175]

84. **b**   Directional terms describe the location of a body part relative to other parts of the body or the body as a whole and often have antonyms and synonyms. One directional term referring to lower, beneath, or away from the head is inferior. An antonym for inferior is superior and a synonym is caudal.
[Garza 10e, p175]

85. **d**   If a 200-lb man's weight is converted to kg, he weighs 90.9 kg. (2.2 lb = 1 kg, so 200 lb ÷ 2.2 = 90.9 kg). To calculate adult blood volume, 70 mL/kg × 90.9 kg = 6,363 mL total blood volume, which is approximately 3× the volume of a 2 L bottle of soda.
[Garza 10e, p600]

86. **c**   If a 55-lb female patient is converted to kg, she weighs 25 kg. (2.2 lb = 1 kg, so 55 lb ÷ 2.2 = 25 kg). To calculate pediatric blood volume, 75 mL/kg × 25 kg = 1,875 mL total blood volume, which is approximately the volume of a 2 L bottle of soda.
[Garza 10e, p600]

87. **d**   The midsagittal plane intersects the body at midline and divides the body into equal right and left halves. The sternum is located on the midsagittal plane.
[Garza 10e, p175]

88. **d**   The frontal plane divides the body into front and back parts. The spinal cord is encased in vertebrae located in the dorsal cavity.
[Garza 10e, p176]

Circulatory System — Explanations

89. **d** The transverse plane divides the body into upper and lower parts. The heart is located above the transverse plane.
[Garza 10e, p174]

90. **c** The root *hem-* means "blood" and the suffix *-stasis* means "stopping." Therefore, *hemostasis* literally means "stopping blood." Hemostasis is the process by which blood remains in the fluid state within the blood vessels and also the complex response to control bleeding following an injury.
[Garza 10e, p243-244]

Specimen Collection

The following items have been identified as appropriate for those preparing for both PBT & QDP examinations.

1. The process ensuring that a patient specimen and corresponding documentation definitely refer to the same patient is called:
   a   accession
   b   adulteration
   c   aliquot
   d   ambulatory care

2. What form is used to notify the laboratory that a test has been ordered?
   a   chain of custody
   b   references
   c   requisition
   d   *res ipsa loquitor*

3. A laboratory information system (LIS) is offline. What method may be used to order laboratory tests and report results?
   a   bar codes
   b   computerized requisitions
   c   multipart manual requisition forms
   d   radio frequency identification (RFID)

4. In the figure below, what information is provided by the item indicated by the arrow?

   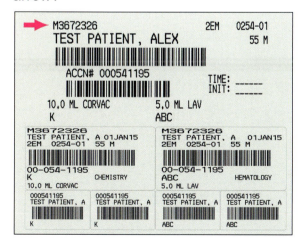

   a   accession number
   b   medical record number
   c   patient age & sex
   d   specimen label

5. In the figure below, what information is provided by the item indicated by the arrow?

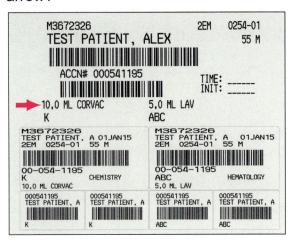

   a   analysis required
   b   medical record number
   c   specimen label
   d   specimen volume required

6. In the figure below, what information is provided by the item indicated by the arrow?

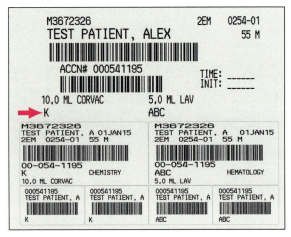

   a   analysis requested
   b   patient age & sex
   c   specimen label
   d   specimen volume required

Questions

Specimen Collection

7. In the figure below, what information is provided by the item indicated by the arrow?

   a accession number
   b medical record number
   c patient age & sex
   d patient location

8. In the figure below, what information is provided by the item indicated by the arrow?

   a analysis requested
   b patient age & sex
   c patient location
   d specimen volume required

9. In the figure below, what information is provided by the item indicated by the arrow?

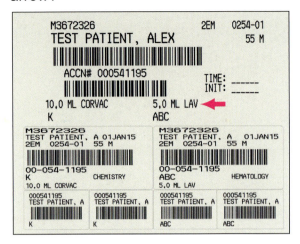

   a analysis required
   b patient location
   c plasma specimen required
   d evacuated tube required by stopper color

10. In the figure below, what is the function of the box highlighted in pink?

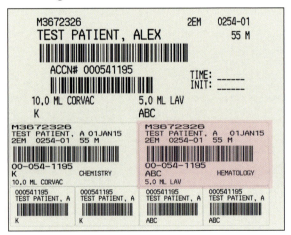

   a quality assurance
   b quality control
   c requisition from the patient's physician
   d specimen label

11. Which of the following requisition types is most accurate and error-free?

   a requisitions created manually
   b verbal requisitions
   c computer-generated requisitions
   d barcode requisitions

Questions
Specimen Collection

12. Once a blood specimen has been collected and analyzed, the requisitions are:
    a   archived as evidence
    b   discarded in the trash
    c   included with the patient's medical record
    d   shredded

13. Requisitions typically originate with the patient's:
    a   certified nurse assistant
    b   Medical Records Department
    c   nurse
    d   physician

14. What information is characteristically included on an outpatient requisition form but not usually included on an inpatient requisition?
    a   patient's first name
    b   patient's last name
    c   physician's name
    d   billing and/or coding information

15. How are requisitions for laboratory tests generated?
    a   by the health care facility's computer system or via smart phone text
    b   delivered by the US postal service or via smart phone text
    c   manually or by the health care facility's computer system
    d   manually or verbally

16. Which of the following requisitions is employed when computer systems are offline?
    a   bar codes
    b   computerized requisitions
    c   multipart manual requisition forms
    d   radio frequency identification (RFID)

17. Which of the following requisitions typically do not include information on the specimen required?
    a   bar codes
    b   computerized requisitions
    c   multipart manual requisition forms
    d   radio frequency identification (RFID)

18. Bar codes represent:
    a   patient name & identification numbers
    b   physician name & identification numbers
    c   patient's room number & availability
    d   billing & coding data

Specimen Collection   **Questions**

19. A computer generates a bar code label. The phlebotomist affixes the label to the tube. What additional information may be required and handwritten on the label?
    a date of collection
    b phlebotomist signature
    c time of collection, room number
    d date and time of collection, phlebotomist initials

20. Which of the following information should never be provided to the patient by the phlebotomist?
    a an explanation of the clinical purpose of the test
    b if the phlebotomist is a student
    c the department the phlebotomist works in
    d the phlebotomist's name

21. A phlebotomist enters a patient's room at 5:30 AM, but the patient is asleep. The phlebotomist should:
    a ask the nurse to wake the patient
    b gently wake the patient and proceed
    c mark the slip "Can't get," and return to the lab
    d turn on the lights and noisily set up equipment

22. A phlebotomist is about to collect a blood specimen from a patient in ICU, but the patient is unconscious. The phlebotomist should:
    a call a code
    b call a nurse or family member to verbally verify the patient's identity
    c proceed as though the patient were conscious
    d return when the patient awakens

23. If a patient is not in his room, how should the phlebotomist locate the patient?
    a ask the patient's nurse
    b page the patient
    c refer to the patient's chart
    d search the laboratory's computer

24. When approaching the patient, the first thing the phlebotomist should do is:
    a assemble his/her equipment and tie the tourniquet
    b identify himself as a phlebotomist sent to collect the patient's blood
    c identify himself as a "vampire" sent to collect the patient's blood
    d loudly knock on the patient's door and announce the name of the test

25. Which of the following laboratory professionals has the greatest public relations responsibility for the laboratory?
    a pathologist
    b phlebotomist
    c medical laboratory technician
    d medical technologist

Questions
Specimen Collection

26. What will determine the quality of a patient encounter?
    a   the first 3 seconds
    b   the last 6 seconds
    c   the amount of pain associated with the venipuncture
    d   the success of the venipuncture

27. A patient has hearing impairment. To approach the patient, the phlebotomist should:
    a   get as close as possible and speak loudly directly into the patient's ear
    b   look directly at the patient and speak slowly and slightly louder than normal
    c   look directly at the patient and speak quickly and very loudly
    d   not attempt to speak to the patient because it will cause patient frustration

28. The rate and urgency of a phlebotomist's speech is:
    a   pace
    b   placebo
    c   tenor
    d   tone

29. The pitch of a phlebotomist's speech is:
    a   pace
    b   placebo
    c   tenor
    d   tone

30. A patient is blind. To approach the patient, the phlebotomist should:
    a   get as close as possible and speak loudly directly into the patient's ear
    b   look directly at the patient and speak slowly using a normal tone of voice
    c   look directly at the patient and speak quickly and very loudly
    d   not attempt to speak to the patient because it will startle him/her

31. A phlebotomist releases a blind patient after collecting his blood specimen and says, "It was nice to see you." The supervisor should:
    a   do nothing because this is totally acceptable
    b   refer the employee for sensitivity training
    c   reprimand the employee for discrimination
    d   reprimand the employee for insensitivity

32. A phlebotomist ushers a blind patient into a draw station, which is very small. The phlebotomist should:
    a   provide the patient with a white cane
    b   firmly hold the patient's arm just above the elbow to steer him/her about a half-step ahead
    c   refrain from identifying any hazards in the patient's path
    d   offer the patient his/her arm and allow the patient to follow about a half-step behind

33. What percentage of communication is nonverbal?
    a 10-20%
    b 20-40%
    c 40-60%
    d 80-90%

34. A phlebotomist enters the room of a 16-year-old female patient to collect a blood specimen for human gonadotropin (HCG) analysis. The patient asks what the test is for. The phlebotomist should respond:
    a I have no idea
    b This test is commonly ordered but please ask your physician how it applies to your case
    c This test is ordered on every patient admitted to the hospital
    d This is a pregnancy test

35. A phlebotomist enters the room of a 10-year-old male patient to collect a complete blood count (CBC) by venipuncture. The patient asks, "Will this hurt?" The phlebotomist should reply:
    a No, not at all
    b No, because I am the best phlebotomist in the hospital!
    c Yes, a little bit but will be over in a jiffy
    d Yes, very much but please hold very still

36. Patient permission allowing a phlebotomist to collect a blood specimen is called:
    a battery
    b implied consent
    c informed consent
    d refusal

37. An unconscious trauma patient is admitted to the emergency department and the physician orders a type and crossmatch "STAT"! The phlebotomist draws the patient's blood. This is legally acceptable because it is:
    a implied consent
    b informed consent
    c *respondeat superior*
    d statute of limitations

38. A 6-year-old child, accompanied by his mother, is extremely unwilling to have his blood drawn. The mother understood the procedure and agreed the blood should be drawn. The phlebotomists use a papoose to restrain him. The phlebotomists may be charged with:
    a assault
    b battery
    c nothing—informed consent was given
    d nothing—implied consent was given

Questions

Specimen Collection

39. A phlebotomist has a requisition to collect a hemoglobin electrophoresis from a 45-year-old female, paralyzed from the neck down. The phlebotomist approaches the patient, introduces herself, and asks for permission to obtain a blood sample. The patient responds, "No, I would like to speak with my physician first." The phlebotomist ignores the request and collects the specimen. The phlebotomist may be charged with:
   a assault & battery
   b malpractice
   c nothing—informed consent was given
   d nothing—implied consent was given

40. A phlebotomist receives a STAT order for a type and crossmatch on a patient admitted through the emergency department and scheduled for immediate surgery. When the phlebotomist arrives in the patient's room, the patient refuses to give consent for the blood test. The phlebotomist should:
   a call the nurse to restrain the patient and draw the blood
   b call the nurse and inform her of the patient's refusal; make a note on the requisition
   c discard the requisitions
   d discuss approaches to obtain the patient's consent with the physician

41. An outpatient arrives at the laboratory for a prenatal screen. As the phlebotomist is assembling equipment needed for the venipuncture, the patient expresses her tremendous fear of needles and indicates she has a history of fainting during blood draw. The phlebotomist should:
   a ignore the information—it is irrelevant
   b place the patient in a reclining position, using a bed or reclining chair
   c refuse to draw the patient's blood
   d roll her eyes and jokingly tell the patient, "Don't be such a baby!"

42. A patient arrives at the outpatient draw station chewing bubble gum and creating bubbles. The phlebotomist should:
   a encourage the patient to create larger bubbles to take her mind off the procedure
   b encourage the patient to create small, frequent bubbles to take her mind off the procedure
   c politely ask the patient to stop creating bubbles
   d politely ask the patient to discard her gum before starting the procedure

43. Once the venipuncture is completed, the specimen labeled and waste discarded, the phlebotomist should:
   a leave the specimen at the patient's bedside for the nurse to deliver to the lab
   b leave without saying anything—the patients are unwell and will not want to talk
   c notify the nurse that the specimen was collected
   d thank the patient politely

Specimen Collection — **Questions**

44. Once a routine venipuncture is completed, the specimen labeled, and waste discarded, the phlebotomist should remove his/her:
    a   gloves
    b   gown
    c   N95 fit-tested mask
    d   safety goggles

45. When a phlebotomist removes his/her gloves following a procedure, the gloves should be removed:
    a   aerobically
    b   anaerobically
    c   anaphylactically
    d   aseptically

46. If gloves are removed properly, the end result is:
    a   1 glove inside the other with contaminated surfaces on the inside
    b   1 glove inside the other with contaminated surfaces on the outside
    c   2 gloves discarded separately
    d   2 gloves discarded separately inside out

47. The last task a phlebotomist must complete before moving to the next patient is to:
    a   confirm that the specimen arrived in the laboratory
    b   discard his/her gloves
    c   sanitize his/her hands
    d   sanitize his/her tourniquet

48. According to The Joint Commission (TJC), what is the minimal number of steps in proper patient identification?
    a   1
    b   2
    c   3
    d   4

49. What is the first step in proper patient identification?
    a   the patient is asked to state and spell his/her first and last name
    b   the phlebotomist asks, "Are you Mrs. Smith?"
    c   the phlebotomist reads the card above the bed
    d   the nurse identifies the patient from the nurse's station by room number

50. After an outpatient states his or her name, the phlebotomist should ask the patient to:
    a   confirm his/her address
    b   extend his/her arm
    c   spell his/her email address
    d   spell his/her first and last names

Questions
Specimen Collection

51. In a three-way identification reprocess, the phlebotomist must match the:
    a. physician listed on the requisition to the physician posted on the patient's whiteboard
    b. requisition information to the patient's whiteboard
    c. specimen label to the patient's message board
    d. specimen label to the patient's wristband

52. A phlebotomist enters the room of an 18-month-old pediatric patient. The baby's mother is also in the room. The baby's mother stated and spelled the baby's first and last names. The identification bracelet is affixed to the baby's ankle and the information matched with the requisition. The phlebotomist should:
    a. ask a nurse to affix the identification band on the baby's wrist
    b. discard the requisition
    c. discard the wristband
    d. draw the patient's blood

53. Where is the risk of patient identification errors the greatest?
    a. emergency department
    b. intensive care unit
    c. nursery
    d. pediatric department

54. Which of the following information is unique to each patient?
    a. date of birth
    b. first names
    c. last names
    d. medical record number

55. A patient's wristband matches the requisition entirely except for the medical record number. The phlebotomist should:
    a. change the number on the requisition
    b. change the number on the wristband
    c. contact the nurse's station
    d. draw the patient's blood

56. A patient's identification bracelet is on her nightstand and it matches the requisition exactly. The phlebotomist should:
    a. ask a nurse to affix the correct wristband on the patient
    b. discard the requisition and ask the lab to generate a correct requisition
    c. discard the wristband and complete an incident report
    d. draw the patient's blood

57. Which of the following tests may require an extra step in patient identification?
    a. blood cultures
    b. cold agglutinin titers
    c. glucose tolerance testing
    d. type and crossmatch

Specimen Collection   **Questions**

58. The most important step in a specimen collection procedure is:
    a. adequate specimen
    b. patient identification
    c. site preparation
    d. site selection

59. How many patient identifiers are required for proper patient identification?
    a. 1
    b. 2
    c. 3
    d. 4

60. A phlebotomist enters the room of a pediatric patient to collect a blood specimen. The toddler is in a crib and her patient identification band is secured around the crib handles. The phlebotomist should:
    a. collect the specimen and complete an incident report upon return to the lab
    b. notify the baby's nurse and refuse to collect the specimen
    c. report the incident to the quality assurance committee
    d. use the identification bracelet as part of standard patient identification protocols

61. A phlebotomist enters the room of a comatose patient to collect a blood specimen. The patient is unable to provide identification information. The phlebotomist should:
    a. ask the nurse to identify the patient and document the nurse's name
    b. collect the specimen and complete an incident report upon return to the lab
    c. report the incident to the patient's physician
    d. use the information posted to the patient's message board as patient identification

62. A phlebotomist enters the room of a comatose patient to collect a blood specimen. The requisition lists the patient's name as John J Smith. The patient's wristband lists the patient's name as John W Smith. The phlebotomist should:
    a. collect the blood specimen and report the discrepancy to the patient's nurse
    b. collect the specimen and label using the labels generated with the requisition
    c. notify the nurse of the discrepancy and wait to collect the blood specimen until the discrepancy is resolved
    d. use the information posted to the patient's white board as confirmation of patient identification

Questions   Specimen Collection

63. A jogger is brought to the emergency room via ambulance. The jogger is unconscious and no personal identification is available. The physician orders a troponin and cardiac enzymes. How should the phlebotomist proceed?
    a   use the patient information posted to the white board as patient identification
    b   ask the nurse to identify the patient and document the nurse's name on the specimen label
    c   request that a temporary identification bracelet be affixed to the patient
    d   collect the specimen and complete an incident report upon return to the lab

64. A phlebotomist enters the room of a patient in the emergency department to collect a CBC. The patient has an identification bracelet attached to the railing of his cart issued by the emergency department documenting his name, age, and medical record number. The phlebotomist should:
    a   draw the patient's blood using the available documents
    b   draw the specimen and notify the nurse that the specimen has been collected
    c   notify the nurse and refuse to draw the specimen until the identification band is affixed to the patient
    d   refuse to draw the specimen and notify the hospital's quality assurance department

65. A phlebotomist enters the room of a patient named Robert Smith, age 60. The patient has an identification bracelet attached to his wrist issued by the emergency department identifying him as Robert Smith. The age is not listed on the temporary identification band, but the patient looks much older than 60. The phlebotomist should:
    a   draw the patient's blood using the available documents
    b   draw the specimen and notify the nurse of the potential clerical error
    c   notify the nurse of the discrepancy and refuse to draw the specimen until the discrepancy is resolved
    d   refuse to draw the specimen and notify the hospital's quality assurance department

66. Patient admission to which of the following areas may exempt the patient from having an identification wristband affixed to their person?
    a   emergency department
    b   medical intensive care unit
    c   neonatal unit
    d   psychiatric unit

67. A phlebotomist may appropriately identify an outpatient using the patient's:
    a   identification bracelet and a computer-generated label
    b   identification bracelet and a handwritten requisition and label
    c   state and spell first and last name and provide a photo ID
    d   verbal confirmation of first and last name and date of birth

Specimen Collection — **Questions**

68. Which of the following methods for patient identification and specimen labeling is most accurate?
    a   bar code requisitions & labels
    b   color-coded requisitions & labels
    c   computer-generated requisitions & labels
    d   manually generated requisitions & labels

69. Which of the following automated methods of generating requisitions and specimen labels employs light or laser technology to enter information into the laboratory information system?
    a   bar code
    b   radio frequency identification
    c   manual
    d   verbal

70. Which of the following automated methods of generating requisitions and specimen labels employs silicon chips and wireless receivers to enter information into the laboratory information system?
    a   bar code
    b   radio frequency identification
    c   manual
    d   verbal

71. A patient is scheduled for a blood test which requires fasting. The patient is usually required to fast for a period of:
    a   4-8 hours
    b   8-12 hours
    c   12-14 hours
    d   14-18 hours

72. A patient is scheduled to have his blood drawn for triglyceride analysis. How long is the patient expected to fast?
    a   4-8 hours
    b   8-12 hours
    c   12-14 hours
    d   14-18 hours

73. If a patient is fasting, he or she must refrain from ingesting:
    a   all beverages
    b   all food
    c   all beverages and food except water unless contraindicated
    d   all beverages, including water, and all food

Questions

Specimen Collection

74. Which of the following tests will be falsely elevated if the patient fasted for longer than 14 hours?
    a glucose
    b HDL cholesterol
    c lactic dehydrogenase
    d triglycerides

75. Which of the following tests will be falsely elevated if the patient fasted for longer than 14 hours?
    a bilirubin
    b HDL cholesterol
    c lactic dehydrogenase
    d T3

76. Which of the following tests will be falsely elevated if the patient fasted for longer than 14 hours?
    a glucagon
    b HDL cholesterol
    c lactic dehydrogenase
    d T3

77. Which of the following tests will be falsely decreased if the patient fasted for longer than 14 hours?
    a bilirubin
    b glucagon
    c glucose
    d triglycerides

78. Which of the following tests will be falsely decreased if the patient fasted for longer than 14 hours?
    a bilirubin
    b glucagon
    c HDL cholesterol
    d triglycerides

79. Which of the following tests will be falsely decreased if the patient fasted for longer than 14 hours?
    a amino acids
    b bilirubin
    c glucagon
    d lactic dehydrogenase

Specimen Collection — Questions

80. An outpatient arrives at the laboratory to have her blood drawn for a complete blood count. She is carrying a designer coffee containing cream and topped with whipped cream. The coffee is 3/4 empty and the patient confirms she drank the coffee. What specimen characteristic is likely to result?
    a hemoconcentration
    b hemolysis
    c lipemia
    d QNS

81. A patient on chemotherapy arrives in the laboratory. When asked if he was fasting, he replied yes except for one nutrition supplement drink. What specimen characteristic is likely to result?
    a hemoconcentration
    b hemolysis
    c lipemia
    d QNS

82. A morbidly obese patient was admitted to the hospital. The phlebotomist attempted to draw blood specimens for electrolytes and a complete blood count (CBC), but was unsuccessful. She experienced great difficulty finding a vein suitable for venipuncture. Who should the phlebotomist enlist next to assist her with finding a vein?
    a another phlebotomist
    b the nurse
    c the physician
    d the patient

83. Sclerosed veins may be caused by:
    a energy drinks
    b excessive vitamins
    c multiple venipunctures
    d prolonged tourniquet application

84. A phlebotomist notes a patient's antecubital area (antecubital fossa) was recently burned. What is true of the affected area?
    a the area is very sensitive and prone to infection
    b the area may be treated like normal skin
    c the veins are sclerosed
    d the veins are occluded

85. A phlebotomist notes burn scars on a patient's antecubital area (antecubital fossa). What is true of the affected area?
    a scarring will result in hemolysis of the specimen
    b the area may be treated like normal skin
    c palpating is more difficult through burn scars
    d palpating is much easier through burn scars

Questions Specimen Collection

86. A phlebotomist notes tattoo "sleeves" covering a patient's antecubital area (antecubital fossa). What is true of the affected area?
    a   the area is resistant to infection
    b   palpating is more difficult through tattoos
    c   palpating is much easier through tattoos
    d   the tattoo dye may be introduced into the specimen and interfere with laboratory results

87. The Chicago Marathon is usually held on a Sunday in October. A marathoner presents at the outpatient department Monday following the race to have his blood drawn as part of his wellness physical. What impact will this have on his results?
    a   none
    b   potassium, sodium and osmolality will be decreased
    c   blood urea nitrogen (BUN), creatinine, and bilirubin will be increased
    d   hematocrit, mean corpuscular hemoglobin (MCH) and mean corpuscular hemoglobin concentration (MCHC) will be increased

88. A phlebotomist approaches a patient prior to venipuncture. The phlebotomist determines that the patient is very anxious about the procedure. What effect will the patient's high anxiety have on her results?
    a   all analytes will be adversely affected
    b   decreased white cell count
    c   increased white cell count
    d   none

89. A phlebotomist approaches a patient prior to venipuncture. The phlebotomist determines that the patient is very anxious about the procedure. What effect will the patient's high anxiety have on her results?
    a   all analytes will be adversely affected
    b   decreased serum iron
    c   increased serum iron
    d   none

90. A phlebotomist performs a skin puncture on an infant, who proceeds to cry violently. What effect will this have on the baby's white cell count?
    a   increase the white cell count by 113%
    b   increase the white cell count by 125%
    c   increase the white cell count by 140%
    d   no effect

91. Which of the following analyte categories is most likely to fluctuate during the day due to diurnal rhythms?
    a   antibodies
    b   hormones
    c   electrolytes
    d   enzymes

Specimen Collection

92. Which of the following analyses will yield higher results if the specimen is collected in the afternoon?
    a adrenocorticotropic hormone
    b cortisol
    c eosinophil counts
    d insulin

93. What effect will occur if a patient's position changes from supine to standing?
    a lipid molecules will shift from the bloodstream to the tissues
    b lipid molecules will shift from the tissues to the bloodstream
    c water molecules will shift from the bloodstream to the tissues
    d water molecules will shift from the tissues to the bloodstream

94. A patient returned from an extensive vacation spanning over 10 time zones. The day after she arrives home she arrives at the laboratory for her wellness screen. Which of the following may be impacted by the time zone changes?
    a diurnal rhythms
    b dissociation
    c dizygotic
    d dolichocolon

95. Which of the following analytes will be higher in a 20-year-old female than in an 85-year-old female?
    a bilirubin
    b blood cholesterol
    c estrogen
    d triglycerides

96. Which of the following analytes will be higher in an 85-year-old female than in a 20-year-old female?
    a bilirubin
    b estrogen
    c growth hormone
    d triglycerides

97. A phlebotomist receives a requisition to collect electrolytes from a patient in renal failure. The patient's arms are markedly swollen due to edema. The phlebotomist should:
    a collect the specimen following standard protocol
    b collect the specimen from the dorsal vein of the patient's wrist
    c consult with the patient's physician to determine the most appropriate course of action
    d immediately notify the institution's epidemiologist

Questions Specimen Collection

98. A phlebotomist receives a requisition to collect electrolytes from a patient in renal failure. The patient's arms are markedly swollen due to edema. The patient has an IV in his right arm so the phlebotomist collects the specimen from the patient's left arm. What effect will this have on the specimen?
    a   none because the phlebotomist drew the specimen from the arm without the IV
    b   concentrated because the arm used was edematous
    c   diluted because the arm used was edematous
    d   hemolyzed because the arm used was edematous

99. A phlebotomist would most likely choose a winged infusion needle to perform a venipuncture procedure on a(n):
    a   18-year-old college freshman
    b   46-year-old high school teacher
    c   53-year-old construction worker
    d   85-year-old grandmother

100. A syringe would most likely be used on which of the following patients?
    a   female patient following a mastectomy
    b   female patient following a miscarriage
    c   male patient following an angioplasty
    d   male patient using a heparin lock

101. What criterion does a phlebotomist use when selecting needle gauge prior to a venipuncture procedure?
    a   direction of the patient's vein
    b   if the specimen is arterial or venous
    c   the lumen size of the patient's vein
    d   the physician's order

102. Which of the following levels will remain elevated for at least 24 hours following exercise?
    a   arterial blood gas (ABG)
    b   blood urea nitrogen (BUN)
    c   complete blood count (CBC)
    d   creatine kinase (CK)

103. A patient is being treated with a thiazide diuretic. Which health care professional is responsible for recognizing potential drug interferences with test results?
    a   medical technologist
    b   nurse
    c   phlebotomist
    d   physician

Specimen Collection — Questions

104. What test requires a patient to eat balanced meals that include approximately 150 g of carbohydrates for 3 days prior to the test?
    a   2-hour postprandial
    b   3-hour glucose tolerance
    c   lactose tolerance
    d   sweat chloride test

105. Which of the following procedures requires a patient to refrain from strenuous exercise for 12 hours prior to the test?
    a   blood culture
    b   cold agglutinin titer
    c   3-hour glucose tolerance test
    d   type and screen

106. Which of the following tests requires that a patient fast prior to collection of the blood specimen?
    a   blood culture
    b   cold agglutinin titer
    c   glucose tolerance testing
    d   type and crossmatch

107. The sign above the patient's bed indicates that the patient is NPO. Before drawing the patient's blood, the phlebotomist should confirm that the patient is:
    a   being discharged
    b   fasting
    c   going to surgery
    d   resting, fasting, and in a supine position

108. A phlebotomist enters a patient's room to collect a STAT specimen. The curtain is drawn around the patient's bed. The phlebotomist should:
    a   announce himself and wait a moment before approaching the bedside
    b   call the nurse and ask for instructions
    c   leave the requisition at the nurse's station for the nurse to draw
    d   loudly announce himself and immediately open the curtain

109. A phlebotomist is about to enter the room of a patient to draw a STAT test. The phlebotomist notices that the patient's priest is in with the patient. The phlebotomist should:
    a   come back to draw the patient's blood after the priest has left
    b   leave the slips for the nurse to draw blood
    c   politely knock on the door, excuse herself, and explain that she must collect a STAT specimen
    d   throw out the requisition

Questions

Specimen Collection

110. Which of the following patients may be a candidate for a syringe draw?
    a comatose patient
    b combative patient
    c patient with exceptionally large veins
    d patient with exceptionally small veins

111. Which of the following blood collection procedures must be completed by specifically trained health care workers, such as nurses, in collaboration with phlebotomists?
    a blood collection from a central venous access device (CVAD)
    b venipuncture performed on the palmar surface of the patient's wrist
    c venipuncture performed on a patient's hand vein
    d venipuncture performed on a patient's vein in the antecubital area (antecubital fossa)

112. A phlebotomist is about to enter the room of a patient to draw a STAT test. The phlebotomist notices that the patient's physician is in conference with the patient. The phlebotomist should:
    a come back to draw the patient's blood after the physician has left
    b leave the slips for the doctor to draw blood
    c politely knock on the door, excuse herself, and ask if the physician would like the blood collected now or after her conference with the patient
    d throw out the requisition

113. Changing a patient's position from supine to standing will cause which physiologic change?
    a no change will occur
    b plasma glucose will increase
    c water will filter from the plasma to the tissues
    d water will filter from the tissues to the plasma

114. A phlebotomist is about to enter the room of a patient to draw a STAT specimen. The phlebotomist notices that the patient's extended family is in the room with the patient. The phlebotomist should:
    a come back to draw the patient's blood after the family has left
    b leave the slips for the doctor to draw blood
    c notify security immediately
    d politely knock on the door, introduce himself, indicate that he is there to collect a blood specimen, and politely ask the family to wait outside the room

115. A phlebotomist has a requisition to collect a specimen for triglyceride analysis from a patient. When the phlebotomist enters the patient's room, the patient is eating breakfast, including oatmeal and a banana. The phlebotomist should:
    a   draw the patient's blood following standard procedure
    b   draw the specimen and notify the nurse of the patient's breakfast
    c   notify the nurse of the potential error and ask that the test be rescheduled
    d   refuse to draw the specimen and notify the hospital's quality assurance department

116. A phlebotomist is to collect a blood specimen from a patient for a glucose analysis. When the phlebotomist enters the patient's room, the patient's family is visiting and the patient is eating breakfast, including eggs, bacon, and toast with butter. The phlebotomist should:
    a   draw the patient's blood following standard procedure
    b   draw the specimen and notify the nurse of the patient's breakfast
    c   notify the nurse the patient is not fasting
    d   politely knock on the door, introduce himself, indicate that he is there to collect a blood specimen, and politely ask the family to wait outside the room

117. A phlebotomist enters a patient's room and notices that the sign above the patient's bed indicates that the patient has an "adhesive allergy." The phlebotomist should use the following supplies to administer postpuncture care:
    a   70% isopropyl alcohol
    b   90% isopropyl alcohol
    c   bandage
    d   self-adhesive gauze

118. Wearing gloves during phlebotomy procedures is mandated by:
    a   College of American Pathologists
    b   National Accrediting Agency for Clinical Laboratory Sciences
    c   Occupational Safety & Health Administration
    d   The Joint Commission (TJC)

119. A phlebotomist enters a patient's room and notices petechiae on both arms. After the venipuncture, the phlebotomist can expect that the:
    a   patient will bleed less than usual
    b   patient will bleed longer than usual
    c   specimen will be contaminated
    d   specimen will be hemolyzed

Questions

Specimen Collection

120. A phlebotomist must enter the room of a patient diagnosed with active tuberculosis, per the isolation sign posted outside the patient's door. The phlebotomist should wear the following mask into the patient's room:
    a   National Institute of Health approved N75 mask
    b   National Institute of Health approved N95 mask
    c   National Institute for Occupational Safety & Health approved N75 fit-tested mask
    d   National Institute for Occupational Safety & Health approved N95 fit-tested mask

121. A patient had a mastectomy of the left breast. The phlebotomist notices her left arm is markedly swollen. What is the name of this condition?
    a   lymphadenia
    b   lymphadenitis
    c   lymphatology
    d   lymphedema

122. A patient requires droplet precaution isolation. In addition to gloves, what personal protective equipment should the phlebotomist wear into the patient's room?
    a   gown
    b   mask
    c   gown and mask
    d   National Institute of Health approved N95 mask

123. A patient is in contact precaution isolation. In addition to gloves, what personal protective equipment should the phlebotomist wear into the patient's room?
    a   gown
    b   mask
    c   gown and mask
    d   National Institute of Health approved N95 mask

124. Which of the following values is higher in the morning?
    a   cortisol levels
    b   eosinophil counts
    c   iron levels
    d   WBC counts

125. Eating which of the following foods can cause lipemic serum in a patient's blood specimen?
    a   apple
    b   butter
    c   carrot
    d   hard candy

Specimen Collection — Questions

126. Which of the following can affect cortisol levels?
    a   caffeine
    b   glucose
    c   lipids
    d   saccharin

127. A phlebotomist entered a patient's room to collect a specimen for glucose. The nurse was in the patient's room adjusting an IV and the patient was eating breakfast when the phlebotomist entered the room. The phlebotomist informed the nurse that she was there to collect a glucose level. The nurse instructed the phlebotomist to draw the specimen. The phlebotomist should:
    a   collect the specimen as instructed and write "Nonfasting" on the requisition
    b   report the nurse to The Joint Commission (TJC)
    c   report the nurse to the patient's doctor
    d   submit an incident report to the laboratory supervisor

128. A phlebotomist is called to the emergency department to collect electrolytes and a complete blood count (CBC) from a patient suffering from hyperemesis. The patient's condition may cause which of the following specimen characteristics?
    a   hemoconcentration
    b   hemolysis
    c   lipemia
    d   reflux

129. What method of blood collection is preferred for infants?
    a   accessing indwelling lines
    b   arterial puncture
    c   skin puncture
    d   venipuncture

130. Which of the following patients is a candidate for skin puncture instead of venipuncture for blood specimen collection?
    a   6-month-old baby for a blood culture
    b   25-year-old female for type and crossmatch
    c   new admit, for a chemistry profile
    d   oncology patient, for a WBC count and platelet count

131. Why is skin puncture preferred over venipuncture for infants for the collection of blood specimens?
    a   continuous quality indicator
    b   increased accuracy of test results
    c   prevent anemia
    d   prevent infection

Questions

Specimen Collection

132. "Antecubital" means:
    a behind the elbow
    b below the skin
    c in front of the elbow
    d on the surface of the skin

133. "Fossa" means:
    a deep depression
    b deep exterior
    c shallow depression
    d thin superficial

134. The antecubital fossa is the:
    a deep depression located behind the elbow
    b deep exterior located in front of the elbow
    c superficial surface located behind the elbow
    d shallow depression located in front of the elbow

135. Antecubital veins characteristically present in the shape of which letters?
    a H & E
    b H & M
    c M & N
    d M & W

136. Which of the following venous distribution patterns is most prevalent?
    a E
    b H
    c M
    d W

137. Approximately 70% of the population displays a venous pattern resembling which of the following letters?
    a E
    b H
    c M
    d N

138. In the figure below, what is the structure indicated by the arrow?

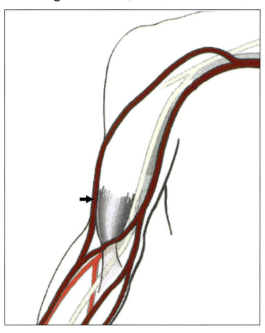

a basilic vein
b brachial artery
c cephalic vein
d median nerve

139. In the figure below, what is the structure indicated by the arrow?

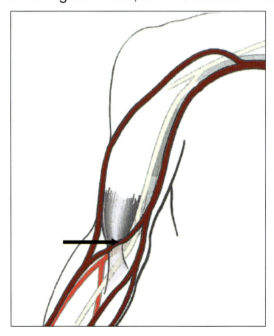

a basilic vein
b brachial artery
c median nerve
d median cubital vein

Questions
Specimen Collection

140. In the figure below, what is the structure indicated by the arrow?

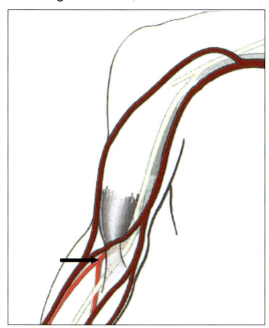

- a basilic vein
- b brachial artery
- c cephalic vein
- d median cubital vein

141. In the figure below, what is the structure indicated by the arrow?

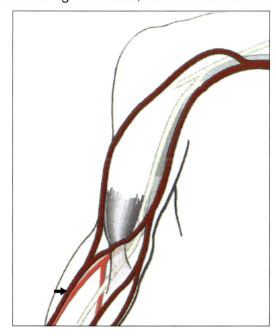

- a basilic vein
- b brachial artery
- c cephalic vein
- d median nerve

142. In the figure below, what is the structure indicated by the arrow?

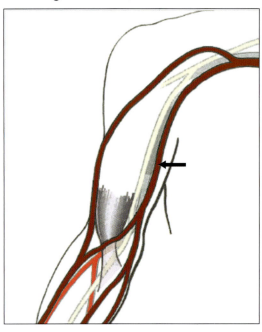

- a basilic vein
- b bicipital aponeurosis
- c brachial artery
- d median nerve

143. In the figure below, what is the structure indicated by the arrow?

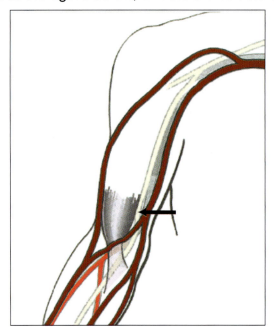

- a basilic vein
- b bicipital aponeurosis
- c brachial artery
- d median nerve

Questions
Specimen Collection

144. In the figure below, what is the structure indicated by the arrow?

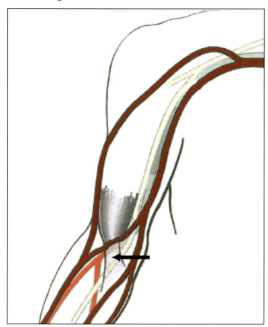

- a   basilic vein
- b   bicipital aponeurosis
- c   brachial artery
- d   median nerve

145. In the figure below, what is the structure indicated by the arrow?

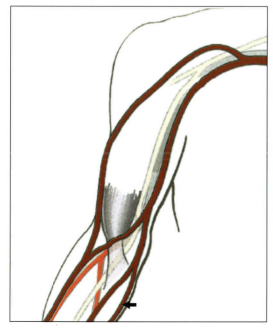

- a   basilic vein
- b   bicipital aponeurosis
- c   brachial artery
- d   median nerve

146. In the figure below, what is the structure indicated by the arrow?

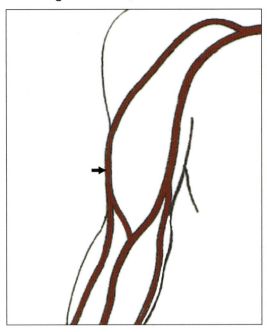

    a   basilic vein
    b   brachial artery
    c   cephalic vein
    d   median nerve

147. In the figure below, what is the structure indicated by the arrow?

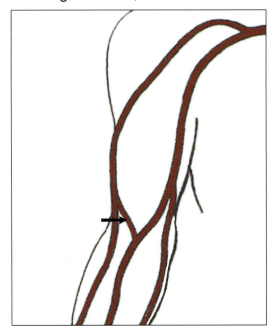

    a   basilic vein
    b   cephalic vein
    c   median basilic vein
    d   median cephalic vein

Questions

Specimen Collection

148. In the figure below, what is the structure indicated by the arrow?

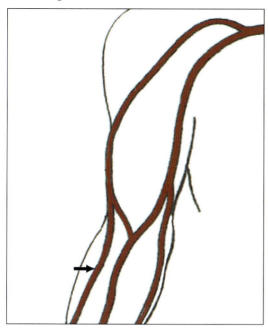

- a basilic vein
- b cephalic vein
- c median basilic vein
- d median cephalic vein

149. In the figure below, what is the structure indicated by the arrow?

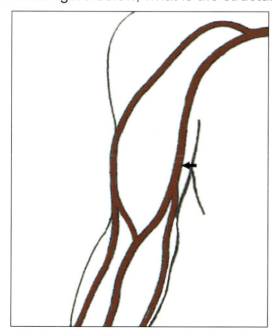

- a basilic vein
- b cephalic vein
- c median basilic vein
- d median cephalic vein

150. In the figure below, what is the structure indicated by the arrow?

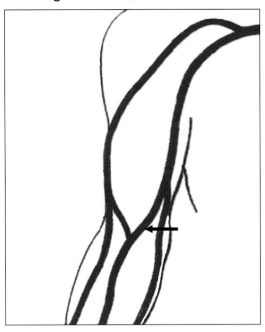

- a basilic vein
- b cephalic vein
- c median basilic vein
- d median cephalic vein

151. In the figure below, what is the structure indicated by the arrow?

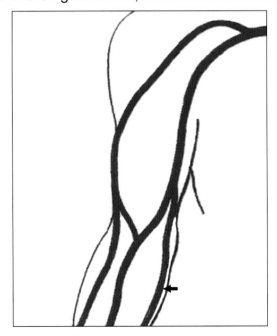

- a basilic vein
- b cephalic vein
- c median basilic vein
- d median cephalic vein

Questions

Specimen Collection

152. In the figure below showing the back of the right hand, what is the structure indicated by the arrow?

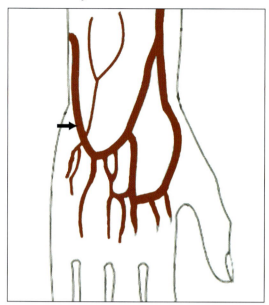

   a   basilic vein
   b   dorsal metacarpal veins
   c   cephalic vein
   d   palmar venous arch

153. In the figure below showing the back of the right hand, what is each of the structures indicated by the arrows?

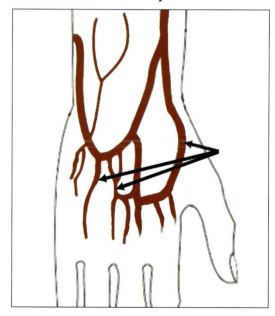

   a   basilic vein
   b   dorsal metacarpal veins
   c   cephalic vein
   d   palmar venous arch

154. In the figure below showing the back of the right hand, what is the structure indicated by the arrow?

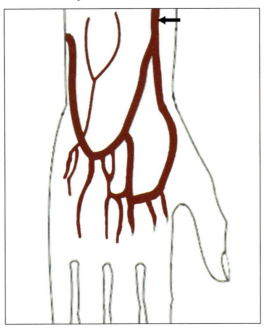

- a basilic vein
- b dorsal metacarpal veins
- c cephalic vein
- d palmar venous arch

155. The most effective method for applying alcohol to cleanse a venipuncture site is:
- a by cleansing the site with back-and-forth friction motion
- b in concentric circles, beginning away from the puncture site
- c parallel to the antecubital crease
- d perpendicular to the antecubital crease

156. To examine by touch or feel is to:
- a palate
- b palpate
- c palpitate
- d patency

157. Which of the following veins is often the most accessible in obese patients?
- a basilic vein
- b brachial vein
- c cephalic vein
- d median vein of the forearm

Questions

Specimen Collection

158. If a phlebotomist must collect a blood specimen from a patient's arm that has an intravenous line (IV), the phlebotomist should draw from:
    a proximal to (above) the IV
    b distal to (below) the IV
    c directly from the IV
    d the patient's CVC

159. A phlebotomist ties a tourniquet on a patient's arm. The phlebotomist palpates the vessels listed below. All of the vessels are the same size. Which is the MOST suitable for venipuncture?
    a basilic vein
    b cephalic vein
    c median vein of the forearm
    d median cubital vein

160. A phlebotomist ties a tourniquet on a patient's arm. The phlebotomist palpates the vessels listed below. All of the vessels are the same size. Which is the LEAST suitable for venipuncture?
    a basilic vein
    b cephalic vein
    c median vein of the forearm
    d median cubital vein

161. A phlebotomist ties a tourniquet on a patient's left arm. The phlebotomist cannot palpate any veins suitable for venipuncture in the antecubital area (antecubital fossa). What site should the phlebotomist examine next for a suitable vein?
    a left antecubital area
    b right antecubital area
    c left wrist
    d right wrist

162. A phlebotomist ties a tourniquet on a patient's right arm. The phlebotomist cannot palpate any veins suitable for venipuncture in the antecubital area (antecubital fossa). What site should the phlebotomist examine next for a suitable vein?
    a left antecubital area
    b palmar surface right forearm
    c left wrist
    d right wrist

Specimen Collection — Questions

163. After tying a tourniquet, the phlebotomist examines the antecubital area (antecubital fossa) in a patient's right and left arms for a suitable site for venipuncture. The phlebotomist cannot palpate any veins suitable for venipuncture either antecubital area. What area should the phlebotomist examine next for a suitable vein?
    a left antecubital area
    b right antecubital area
    c left foot
    d right hand

164. A patient has a fistula in his right forearm. What area should the phlebotomist examine first for a suitable vein for venipuncture?
    a left antecubital area (antecubital fossa)
    b right antecubital area
    c left foot
    d right hand

165. A phlebotomist palpates a vein the patient's antecubital area (antecubital fossa) and notes the vein feels hard and cordlike. The vein is likely:
    a collapsed
    b hemolyzed
    c sclerosed
    d superficial

166. During a venipuncture procedure, a tourniquet should be applied:
    a away from skin lesions
    b for at least 2 minutes before releasing
    c tight enough to stop all blood flow
    d 12 inches above the intended puncture

167. During a venipuncture procedure, a tourniquet should be tied:
    a 3-4 inches above the intended puncture site
    b for at least 2 minutes before releasing
    c like a shoelace
    d tight enough to stop all blood flow

168. During a venipuncture procedure, a tourniquet is applied to increase veins by:
    a diminishing venous blood flow
    b diminishing arterial blood flow
    c increasing venous blood flow
    d increasing arterial blood flow

169. When is it appropriate to tie a tourniquet over an open sore?
    a always
    b if the open sore is covered with the patient's gown
    c if the open sore is covered with a towel
    d never

Questions

Specimen Collection

170. Which of the following senses will the phlebotomist rely on most when selecting a site for venipuncture?
    a   hearing
    b   seeing
    c   smell
    d   touch

171. When palpating for a vein, the phlebotomist should use her:
    a   index finger
    b   middle finger
    c   ring finger
    d   thumb

172. When examining a venipuncture sight, what vein characteristics does the phlebotomist palpate for?
    a   depth, direction, ease of visual recognition
    b   depth, direction, shape
    c   depth, direction, size
    d   depth, ease of visual recognition, size

173. According to CLSI Standards, which vessel must a phlebotomist attempt to locate in both arms before considering alternative venipuncture sites?
    a   brachial artery
    b   basilic vein
    c   median vein of the forearm
    d   median cubital vein

174. Which of the following veins of the antecubital area (antecubital fossa) is characteristically most stationary?
    a   basilic vein
    b   cephalic vein
    c   dorsal metacarpal vein
    d   median cubital vein

175. According to CLSI Standard GP41, the phlebotomist must examine both arms in an attempt to locate which of the following before considering alternative venipuncture sites?
    a   basilic vein
    b   bicipital aponeurosis
    c   cephalic vein
    d   median cephalic vein

176. Which of the following veins of the antecubital area (antecubital fossa) is typically less painful during needle insertion?
    a   basilic vein
    b   bicipital aponeurosis
    c   cephalic vein
    d   median cephalic vein

Specimen Collection — Questions

177. What structure provides support to the median cubital vein in the antecubital area (antecubital fossa)?
    a   bicipital aponeurosis
    b   brachial artery
    c   median cutaneous nerve
    d   radial artery

178. Which of the following veins is located on the lateral aspect of antecubital area (antecubital fossa) and may also be palpated on the lateral side of the wrist leading to the dorsal side of the hand?
    a   basilic vein
    b   cephalic vein
    c   dorsal metacarpal vein
    d   median cubital vein

179. Which of the following veins is located on the medial aspect of antecubital area (antecubital fossa) and may also be palpated on the medial side of the wrist leading to the dorsal side of the hand?
    a   basilic vein
    b   cephalic vein
    c   dorsal metacarpal vein
    d   median cubital vein

180. Which of the following veins is located on the medial aspect of antecubital area (antecubital fossa) and is located in proximity to the median cutaneous nerve?
    a   basilic vein
    b   cephalic vein
    c   dorsal metacarpal vein
    d   median cubital vein

181. Which of the following veins is located on the medial aspect of antecubital area (antecubital fossa) and is located in proximity to the brachial artery?
    a   basilic vein
    b   cephalic vein
    c   dorsal metacarpal vein
    d   median cubital vein

182. Which of the following veins would be the safest choice for venipuncture?
    a   basilic vein
    b   cephalic vein
    c   dorsal metacarpal vein
    d   median cubital vein

Questions
Specimen Collection

183. Which of the following veins located in the antecubital area (antecubital fossa) is associated with the highest risk for nerve injury if selected for venipuncture?
   a   basilic vein
   b   cephalic vein
   c   dorsal metacarpal vein
   d   median cubital vein

184. Which of the following veins may move (roll) most frequently during venipuncture?
   a   basilic vein
   b   cephalic vein
   c   dorsal metacarpal vein
   d   median cubital vein

185. Which of the following sites should never be used for venipuncture?
   a   dorsal metacarpal vein
   b   dorsal wrist veins
   c   dorsal cephalic vein
   d   palmar wrist veins

186. Which of the following describes the best site to select for skin puncture on an infant's foot?
   a   arch area of the foot
   b   lateral portion of the palmar surface of the heel
   c   lateral portion of the plantar surface of the heel
   d   posterior curvature of the heel

187. Which of the following sites is acceptable to use for skin puncture on an infant's foot?
   a   arch of the foot
   b   lateral portion of the palmar surface of the heel
   c   medial portion of the palmar surface of the heel
   d   medial portion of the plantar surface of the heel

188. A heelstick procedure for blood collection must be employed until the child is at least how old?
   a   6 months
   b   12 months
   c   18 months
   d   24 months

189. Which of the following sites should never be used for heelstick on an infant?
   a   central area of the infant's heel or the great toe
   b   lateral portion of the plantar surface of the heel
   c   medial portion of the plantar surface of the heel
   d   medial or lateral portion of the plantar surface of the heel

Specimen Collection — **Questions**

190. Which of the following complications may result from multiple heelsticks in an infant?
     a cellulitis and osteomyelitis
     b hemoconcentration and hemolysis
     c hemolysis and lipemia
     d icterus and lipemia

191. Capillary beds at the dermal-subcutaneous junction are typically located how far below the skin surface of an infant's heel?
     a 0.00-0.35 mm
     b 0.35-1.6 mm
     c 1.6-2.0 mm
     d 2.0-2.5 mm

192. The best site to select for skin puncture in adults is the palmar surface and distal segment of the:
     a index finger
     b little finger
     c middle finger
     d thumb

193. The best site to select for skin puncture is the palmar surface and distal segment of the:
     a index finger
     b little finger
     c ring finger
     d thumb

194. The best site to select for skin puncture is the palmar surface and distal segment of the:
     a thumb, dorsal surface
     b index finger, dorsal surface
     c little finger, palmar surface
     d middle finger, palmar surface

195. Skin punctures performed on patients' fingers should be made:
     a at the crease between the first and second phalanx
     b on the very tip of the finger
     c parallel to the fingerprints
     d perpendicular to the fingerprints

196. Why is the fifth finger of a patient's hand routinely eliminated as a potential site for skin puncture?
     a it has a pulse
     b it has an increased number of nerve endings
     c the tissue is thinner than other fingers
     d it is usually calloused

Questions
Specimen Collection

197. Why is the index finger of a patient's hand routinely eliminated as a potential site for skin puncture?
    a it has a pulse
    b it has an increased number of nerve endings
    c the tissue is thinner than other fingers
    d it is usually calloused

198. What is the correct sequence of the following steps in the venipuncture procedure?
    a apply the tourniquet, palpate for a median cubital vein in the patient's right arm; if a suitable vein is not located, palpate for a median cubital vein in the patient's right wrist
    b locate a suitable vein in the patient's right antecubital area (antecubital fossa), release the tourniquet, use ethyl alcohol to prepare the site
    c locate a suitable vein in the patient's right antecubital area, release the tourniquet, use isopropyl alcohol to prepare the site
    d palpate for a median cubital vein in the patient's right arm; apply the tourniquet; if a suitable vein is not located, palpate for a suitable dorsal metacarpal vein in the patient's right hand

199. What is the correct sequence of the following steps in the venipuncture procedure?
    a apply the tourniquet, locate a suitable vein; prepare the site; release the tourniquet;
    b apply the tourniquet, locate a suitable vein; release the tourniquet; prepare the site
    c locate a suitable vein in the patient's right antecubital area (antecubital fossa), apply the tourniquet, prep the site; release the tourniquet
    d locate a suitable vein in the patient's right antecubital area, release the tourniquet, use ethyl alcohol to prepare the site

200. What is the correct sequence of the following steps in the venipuncture procedure?
    a apply the tourniquet; prepare the site; release the tourniquet, put on gloves
    b ask the patient to make a fist; put on gloves; prepare the site; repalpate the vein; reapply the tourniquet;
    c repalpate the vein; reapply the tourniquet; prepare the site; put on gloves
    d release the tourniquet; put on gloves; prepare the site; reapply the tourniquet

201. What is the correct sequence of the following steps in the venipuncture procedure?
    a put on gloves; prepare the site; reapply the tourniquet; uncap the needle
    b put on gloves; release the tourniquet; anchor the vein; uncap the needle
    c uncap the needle; put on gloves; reapply the tourniquet; anchor the vein
    d release the tourniquet; put on gloves; uncap the needle; anchor the vein

Specimen Collection — Questions

202. What is the correct sequence of the following steps in a routine venipuncture procedure?
   a   apply alcohol, palpate site, apply tourniquet
   b   apply tourniquet, palpate site, release tourniquet
   c   palpate site, apply alcohol, apply tourniquet
   d   palpate site, apply tourniquet, apply alcohol

203. What is the correct sequence of the following steps in a routine venipuncture procedure?
   a   anchor the vein, insert the needle, uncap the needle
   b   anchor the vein, uncap the needle, insert the needle
   c   uncap the needle, anchor the vein, insert the needle
   d   uncap the needle, insert the needle, anchor the vein

204. What is the correct sequence of the following steps in a routine venipuncture procedure?
   a   release tourniquet, engage tube, release vein
   b   release tourniquet, release the vein, engage the tube
   c   release vein, engage tube, release tourniquet
   d   release vein, release tourniquet, engage tube

205. What is the correct sequence of the following steps in a routine venipuncture procedure?
   a   confirm blood flow is established, engage the first evacuated tube, release the tourniquet, fill subsequent evacuated tubes
   b   confirm blood flow is established, release the tourniquet, engage the first evacuated tube, fill subsequent evacuated tubes
   c   engage the first evacuated tube, confirm blood flow is established, release the tourniquet, fill subsequent evacuated tubes
   d   release the tourniquet, engage the first evacuated tube, confirm blood flow is established, fill subsequent evacuated tubes

206. What sequence should be followed after withdrawing the needle following venipuncture?
   a   activate the safety mechanism, label the tubes
   b   apply a bandage to the venipuncture site, activate the safety feature
   c   complete mixing the evacuated tubes, activate the safety feature
   d   label the tubes, activate the safety feature

207. A phlebotomist attempts a venipuncture on a patient's basilic vein. If the blood that appears in the evacuated tube is dark purple-red, the phlebotomist should:
   a   allow the tube to fill, following standard procedures
   b   immediately release the tourniquet and withdraw the needle
   c   insert the needle deeper
   d   withdraw the needle, and apply pressure for 5 minutes

Questions
Specimen Collection

208. A phlebotomist selects a 4.5 mL sodium citrate tube to collect a patient's specimen. The patient's specimen was difficult to draw, but the phlebotomist successfully collected approximately 3.0 mL of specimen into the sodium citrate tube. The phlebotomist should next:
   a   gently invert the specimen 5-10×
   b   label the specimen
   c   recollect the specimen
   d   shield the specimen from light

209. Which of the following would generate the best quality specimen?
   a   hand vein using a 25 gauge butterfly needle and a 10 mL evacuated tube
   b   hand vein using a 25 gauge syringe and a 10 mL evacuated tube
   c   using routine venipuncture equipment above an IV and drawing from the cephalic vein
   d   using a blood pressure cuff as a tourniquet and the cephalic vein

210. What should the phlebotomist check for before using an evacuated tube? The:
   a   expiration date
   b   label is firmly affixed to the tube
   c   label is positioned on the tube horizontally
   d   label is affixed to the tube vertically

211. Positioning a patient's arm downward prior to venipuncture will help prevent:
   a   hemoconcentration
   b   hemolysis
   c   reflux
   d   syncope

212. How should a patient's arm be positioned during venipuncture using a vein in the antecubital area (antecubital fossa)? The bicep to forearm should create a:
   a   30° angle
   b   45° angle
   c   90° angle
   d   straight line from shoulder to wrist

213. Positioning the patient's arm correctly and supporting the elbow with a pillow or rolled towel will help to:
   a   allow the veins to roll
   b   anchor the veins
   c   prevent hemolysis
   d   prevent syncope

Specimen Collection — **Questions**

214. When should the patient be instructed to relax his/her fist by opening his/her hand?
    a   after blood flow is established and when the last tube is half-filled
    b   after the needle is inserted, but before engaging the first evacuated tube
    c   after the needles is inserted and blood flow is established in the first evacuated tube
    d   after the vein is anchored, but before inserting the needle

215. What is the maximum length of time that a tourniquet may be left on a patient's arm without adversely affecting test results?
    a   1 minute
    b   3 minutes
    c   5 minutes
    d   7 minutes

216. When performing venipuncture on a hand vein, the tourniquet should be applied on the:
    a   ankle
    b   forearm
    c   upper arm
    d   wrist

217. Once the tourniquet is in place, the patient should be instructed to:
    a   close his/her fist
    b   clench his/her fist very tightly
    c   hold his/her breath
    d   pump his/her fist vigorously throughout the procedure

218. Hemoconcentration of the specimen may be caused by:
    a   drawing from a hematoma
    b   prolonged tourniquet application
    c   residual alcohol on the site
    d   shaking additive tubes

219. When should the tourniquet be released during venipuncture? After the:
    a   blood flow is established and when the last tube is half-filled
    b   needle is inserted, but before engaging the first evacuated tube
    c   needle is inserted and blood flow is established in the first evacuated tube
    d   vein is anchored, but before inserting the needle

220. What change in cholesterol levels can occur if tourniquet application exceeds 2 minutes?
    a   5% decrease
    b   7% decrease
    c   5% increase
    d   7% increase

Questions

Specimen Collection

221. What compound is commonly used to prepare a site prior to venipuncture?
    a   30% isopropyl alcohol
    b   50% isopropyl alcohol
    c   70% isopropyl alcohol
    d   quaternary ammonia compound

222. Why must a venipuncture site be cleansed prior to venipuncture? To prevent:
    a   glycolysis
    b   hemolysis
    c   contamination of the needle with microorganisms on the skin
    d   contamination of the needle with microorganisms on the tube

223. Following decontamination of a venipuncture site with alcohol, the phlebotomist should:
    a   allow the site to air dry
    b   blow on the site to facilitate drying
    c   dry the site with a gauze pad
    d   dry the site with a tissue

224. How long will it take for a venipuncture site to air dry following alcohol application?
    a   10-15 seconds
    b   15-30 seconds
    c   30-60 seconds
    d   the site should never be allowed to air dry

225. When anchoring a vein in the antecubital area (antecubital fossa) prior to venipuncture, the phlebotomist should place the thumb approximately 2 inches:
    a   above the puncture site
    b   below the puncture site
    c   below the puncture site and the index finger above the puncture site
    d   below the puncture site and the middle finger above the puncture site

226. When anchoring a vein in the antecubital area (antecubital fossa) prior to venipuncture, the phlebotomist should pull the skin toward the:
    a   lateral side of the arm
    b   medial side of the arm
    c   patient's shoulder
    d   patient's wrist

227. To anchor a hand vein prior to venipuncture, the phlebotomist may place the thumb:
    a   2 inches above the wrist
    b   4 inches below the wrist
    c   above the vein selected
    d   across the patient's knuckles

Specimen Collection — Questions

228. During routine venipuncture, the needle should be inserted with the bevel turned:
    a   down
    b   up
    c   toward the left
    d   toward the right

229. During routine venipuncture, what angle should the needle be inserted, relative to the patient's arm?
    a   0-10 degrees
    b   5-10 degrees
    c   15-30 degrees
    d   30-45 degrees

230. During routine venipuncture, how should the needle be positioned immediately before the puncture, relative to the vein selected?
    a   parallel, 1 inch above
    b   parallel, 1 inch below
    c   perpendicular
    d   same direction

231. During routine venipuncture, how deep should the needle be inserted?
    a   1 inch
    b   1½ inches
    c   until the phlebotomist feels a slight decrease in resistance
    d   until the phlebotomist feels a slight increase in resistance

232. Which of the following presents the greatest safety risk to phlebotomists?
    a   evacuated tubes
    b   multisample needles greater than 20 gauge
    c   multisample needles less than 25 gauge
    d   winged infusion needles

233. After the needle is uncapped, the phlebotomist should inspect the needle:
    a   by retracting the sheath to be sure it will spring back after the needle is disengaged
    b   by touching the shaft to be sure there are no burrs or gouges
    c   by touching the tip to be sure there are no burrs or filaments
    d   visually

234. A phlebotomist uncaps a needle and determines that a burr is present. She should:
    a   determine the size of the burr; if it is small, use that needle
    b   determine the size of the burr, if it is large, discard it
    c   discard the needle and take another to use
    d   discard the needle and notify the hospital's safety officer

Questions

Specimen Collection

235. When holding an evacuated tube system, the phlebotomist's thumb should be positioned on the holder at the:
    a   bottom
    b   left
    c   right
    d   top

236. A phlebotomist wanted to be sure the blood she collected in an EDTA tube was well mixed so she inverted the tube gently 8 times. What adverse effect will this have on the patient's specimen?
    a   clotting of the patient's specimen
    b   hemolysis
    c   hemoconcentration
    d   no adverse effect

237. Evacuated tubes containing additives should be mixed with the patient's blood:
    a   after labeling the tube
    b   before placing in the pneumatic tube system
    c   immediately upon removal from the evacuated tube holder
    d   in the lab before centrifugation

238. How should evacuated tubes containing additives be mixed with the patient's blood?
    a   forcefully shaking the evacuated tube
    b   gentle inversion
    c   never
    d   using a vortex

239. Most evacuated tubes containing anticoagulants should be mixed with the patient's blood by inverting the tube at least:
    a   0×
    b   2×
    c   4×
    d   8×

240. A phlebotomist collects a specimen by venipuncture into an evacuated tube containing an additive. She vigorously shakes the evacuated tube to ensure adequate mixing of the blood with the tube additive. What specimen characteristic may result?
    a   hemoconcentration
    b   hemolysis
    c   lipemia
    d   nothing—this is the appropriate method of specimen inversion

241. A phlebotomist performs a venipuncture on a patient and engages the evacuated tube. No blood appears in the evacuated tube. The phlebotomist should:
    a abort the procedure immediately and start over
    b call the patient's nurse
    c establish vein location, advance the needle slightly farther if needle placement is too deep
    d establish vein location, advance the needle slightly farther if needle placement is too shallow

242. A phlebotomist performs a venipuncture on a patient and engages the evacuated tube. No blood appears in the tube. The phlebotomist should first:
    a abort the procedure immediately and start over
    b call the patient's nurse
    c establish vein location relative to the needle
    d immediately reposition the needle

243. A phlebotomist performs a venipuncture on a patient and engages the evacuated tube. No blood appears in the evacuated tube. The phlebotomist should:
    a abort the procedure immediately and start over
    b call the patient's nurse
    c probe aggressively for the vein
    d replace the evacuated tube

244. What is the maximum number of venipuncture attempts a phlebotomist should make to secure a specimen?
    a 1
    b 2
    c 3
    d as often as necessary to secure the specimen

245. A phlebotomist was unable to obtain a blood specimen by venipuncture after 2 attempts. Her colleague offers to attempt. How many attempts may the second phlebotomist make?
    a 0
    b 2
    c 3
    d as many attempts as needed to obtain the blood specimen

246. After the last evacuated tube to be collected is filled, the phlebotomist should disengage the tube from the back of the needle by:
    a disengaging the tube is not necessary because it is the last tube
    b pulling straight back forcibly
    c unscrewing the tube off of the back of the needle
    d using the flange of the holder as a brace

Questions

Specimen Collection

247. Before withdrawing the needle from the patient's arm, the phlebotomist should cover the site with:
    a 70% isopropyl alcohol
    b 90% isopropyl alcohol
    c clean, dry gauze
    d self-adherence wrap (Coban)

248. Which of the following is most suitable to apply to a venipuncture site after needle withdrawal?
    a 70% isopropyl alcohol pad
    b 90% isopropyl alcohol pad
    c clean, dry gauze pad
    d cotton ball

249. When inspecting a venipuncture site before leaving the patient's bedside, the phlebotomist noted a scratch on the patient's arm below the venipuncture site. What likely caused the scratch?
    a failure to apply pressure following phlebotomy
    b pushing down on the gauze while withdrawing the needle
    c withdrawing the needle too quickly
    d withdrawing the needle too slowly

250. After needle withdrawal, patients should be instructed to apply pressure to the puncture site using the gauze and:
    a a bandage
    b by bending the arm at the elbow, securing the gauze
    c keeping the arm straight
    d while holding the arm below the heart

251. Specimen labels should be affixed to evacuated tubes:
    a at the nurse's station
    b immediately before drawing the specimen
    c immediately after drawing the specimen
    d in the lab when preparing equipment

252. What information is optional on a specimen label?
    a date of collection
    b patient's first name
    c patient's last name
    d physician's name

253. What information is never included on a specimen label?
    a date of collection
    b patient diagnosis
    c patient's first name
    d time of collection

Specimen Collection

254. Specimen labels must be affixed in a specific manner. Why?
    a to ensure the labels are not torn off in transit
    b the laboratory supervisor likes things neat
    c so the analyzer can detect patient information
    d so the tube will fit in the centrifuge

255. Before leaving the patient's bedside, the specimen label should be confirmed with which of the following?
    a message board above the patient's bed
    b nurse
    c patient's wristband
    d requisition

256. Following needle withdrawal, the patient should be instructed to keep his arm:
    a bent with an alcohol prep pad positioned over the puncture site
    b bent with a dry gauze pad positioned over the puncture site
    c straight and apply pressure using an alcohol prep pad
    d straight and apply pressure using a dry gauze pad

257. Residual alcohol on the patient's skin following site preparation may result in specimen:
    a glycogenesis
    b glycolysis
    c hemoconcentration
    d hemolysis

258. Residual alcohol on the patient's skin following site preparation may result in the patient experiencing:
    a a burning sensation
    b a tingling sensation
    c no change
    d shooting pain

259. Which of the following veins has the greatest tendency to roll or move upon needle insertion during venipuncture?
    a basilic vein
    b cephalic vein
    c dorsal metacarpal vein
    d median cubital vein

260. Patients are at increased risk for thrombosis when venipuncture is performed on the following:
    a basilic vein
    b cephalic vein
    c dorsal metacarpal vein
    d great saphenous vein

Questions
Specimen Collection

261. During venipuncture, the evacuated tube should be positioned so the non-stoppered end of the tube is:
    a   above the puncture site
    b   at a 90 degree angle to the puncture site
    c   below the puncture site
    d   the position of the tube has no impact on patient results

262. Which of the following has been implicated most frequently in adverse patient reactions to reflux?
    a   acid citrate dextrose
    b   EDTA
    c   sodium citrate
    d   sodium heparin

263. Which step in the venipuncture procedure must the phlebotomist exercise extra care in performing when collecting blood by venipuncture from a hand vein?
    a   anchoring the vein
    b   labeling the specimen
    c   needle insertion
    d   patient identification

264. Specimens transported to the laboratory using a pneumatic tube system should be:
    a   discarded once they arrive in the laboratory
    b   labeled with a 'contact isolation' sticker
    c   placed in a test tube rack
    d   wrapped in shock-absorbent material and placed in a primary transport container

265. Which of the following blood collection techniques requires sterile technique to prepare a venipuncture site?
    a   blood culture
    b   cold agglutinin titers
    c   glucose tolerance testing
    d   type and crossmatch

266. A phlebotomist must collect a specimen for a blood culture analysis. The phlebotomist should prepare the venipuncture site using:
    a   alcohol only
    b   iodine only
    c   alcohol and iodine
    d   tincture of green soap

267. Which of the following actions may result in a false-positive blood culture result?
    a   collecting blood in an SPS evacuated tube
    b   introducing iodine into the collection container
    c   leaving the tourniquet on too long
    d   repalpating the site

268. Prior to blood specimen collection, a disinfectant solution must be applied using a friction scrub technique for a minimum of:
    a   10 seconds
    b   20 seconds
    c   30 seconds
    d   40 seconds

269. According to the American Society for Microbiology (ASM), what is the recommended volume of blood required from an adult patient for quality blood culture results?
    a   5-10 mL
    b   10-20 mL
    c   20-30 mL
    d   30-40 mL

270. A facility recommends the use of a 1-step site preparation procedure prior to blood culture specimen collection. What are the active ingredients in the 1-step preparation solution?
    a   chlorhexidine gluconate and ethyl alcohol
    b   chlorhexidine gluconate and isopropyl alcohol
    c   chloramphenicol and ethyl alcohol
    d   chloramphenicol and isopropyl alcohol

271. When using a winged infusion needle for venipuncture, the volume of blood collected in the first evacuated tube engaged will be decreased by:
    a   0.005 mL
    b   0.05 mL
    c   0.5 mL
    d   5.0 mL

272. When using a winged infusion needle to perform venipuncture, small-volume evacuated tubes should be used to prevent specimen:
    a   contamination
    b   glycolysis
    c   hemolysis
    d   platelet clumping

Questions

Specimen Collection

273. To reduce the risk associated with using a winged infusion needle, phlebotomists should carefully adhere to manufacturer's guidelines regarding:
    a   activation of the safety device
    b   needle gauge
    c   needle length
    d   wing color

274. A phlebotomist selected a patient's dorsal metacarpal vein as a venipuncture site. At what angle should a needle be inserted during venipuncture with a winged infusion needle?
    a   0-10°
    b   10-15°
    c   15-30°
    d   30-45°

275. When using a winged infusion needle for blood collection, what is often the first indication that the needle is successfully inserted in the vein?
    a   blood in the evacuated tube
    b   lack of blood in the evacuated tube
    c   small amount of blood in the tubing
    d   the patient says "ouch"!

276. When using a winged infusion needle for blood collection, what is critically important to obtain a quality specimen for analysis?
    a   anchoring the vein
    b   drawing a discard tube
    c   holding the needle securely
    d   securing the tourniquet

277. A phlebotomist must collect a sodium citrate tube from a patient for a prothrombin time (PT). The phlebotomist assesses the patient and determines that a winged infusion needle is required. What evacuated tube should the phlebotomist use first?
    a   lavender top (EDTA)
    b   light blue top (sodium citrate)
    c   green top (sodium heparin)
    d   red discard tube

278. A phlebotomist uses a winged infusion needle to collect an activated partial thromboplastin time (APTT) from a patient. A discard tube is not used. As a result, the specimen will be:
    a   discarded because the blood:anticoagulant ratio will be inaccurate
    b   discarded due to hemoconcentration
    c   discarded due to hemolysis
    d   used for testing

Specimen Collection — Questions

279. A phlebotomist uses a winged infusion needle to collect a blood specimen. What specimen requires a discard tube collected?
    a   PT/APTT
    b   erythrocyte sedimentation rate (ESR)
    c   fasting blood glucose
    d   type and screen

280. A phlebotomist collects a blood specimen using a winged infusion needle and several tubes containing anticoagulants. While filling, the evacuated tubes should be held so the tube:
    a   fills from the bottom up
    b   fills from the top down
    c   is held vertically
    d   is rocked gently back and forth in the holder

281. When using a syringe for blood draw, what must a phlebotomist have ready for blood transfer into evacuated tubes?
    a   graduated cylinder
    b   graduated pipette
    c   safety transfer device
    d   test tube rack

282. The device used to aliquot blood from syringe into evacuated tubes eliminates the need for:
    a   gloves
    b   gown
    c   using the syringe needle to aliquot specimen into evacuated tubes
    d   using the syringe plunger to aliquot specimen into evacuated tubes

283. To comply with OSHA standards, syringes used for blood collection must:
    a   be at least a 21 gauge
    b   be at least a 22 gauge
    c   be equipped with a resheathing device
    d   never be used

284. When using a syringe for blood collection, what is often the first indication that the needle is successfully inserted in the vein?
    a   blood appears in the barrel of the syringe
    b   blood appears in the hub of the syringe
    c   blood appears in the needle
    d   the patient says "ouch"!

285. When using a syringe for blood collection, what mechanism results in blood collection?
    a   inserting the needle and allowing the barrel to fill
    b   inserting the needle and untying the tourniquet
    c   pulling back gently on the plunger
    d   untying the tourniquet and pulling back on the plunger

Questions
Specimen Collection

286. Which of the following patient circumstances would indicate blood specimen collection via skin puncture instead of venipuncture?
    a   erythrocyte sedimentation rate (ESR) from a 60-year-old female outpatient
    b   blood culture specimen from a 25-year-old male
    c   blood culture specimen from a 2-day-old infant
    d   platelet and white cell (WBC) counts from a 75-year-old oncology patient

287. A physician orders a basic metabolic panel (BMP) and complete blood count (CBC) for the patients listed below. Which of the following patient circumstances would indicate blood specimen collection via skin puncture instead of venipuncture?
    a   8-month-old toddler
    b   32-year-old obstetrics patient pre-delivery
    c   32-year-old obstetrics patient post-delivery
    d   65-year-old male on the cardiac floor

288. Assuming the tests ordered may be collected by skin puncture, which of the following patient circumstances would indicate blood specimen collection via skin puncture instead of venipuncture?
    a   16-year-old female in the psychiatric floor suffering from anorexia
    b   50-year-old female suffering from lupus erythematosus
    c   car crash victim with IVs in both the right and left hands and casts on both legs
    d   postoperative patient with IVs in the right hand and left antecubital area (antecubital fossa)

289. Which of the following patient circumstances would indicate blood specimen collection via skin puncture instead of venipuncture?
    a   16-year-old female scheduled for a series of blood culture collections
    b   35-year-old male scheduled for a series of point-of-care blood glucose levels
    c   50-year-old female for erythrocyte sedimentation rate
    d   85-year-old male for activated partial thromboplastin time (PTT) requiring plasma

290. Which of the following patient circumstances would indicate blood specimen collection via skin puncture instead of venipuncture?
    a   neonate for phenylketonuria (PKU) screen
    b   60-year old male for a lipid profile
    c   70-year-old female for prothrombin time using a specimen collected in sodium citrate
    d   90-year-old female for blood culture

291. The correct sequence in the skin puncture procedure for an infant is to:
    a   apply a heel warmer, sanitize hands, identify the patient, select appropriate lancet
    b   identify the patient, select appropriate lancet, apply a heel warmer, sanitize hands
    c   identify the patient, sanitize hands, apply a heel warmer, select appropriate lancet
    d   sanitize hands, identify the patient, apply a heel warmer, select appropriate lancet

292. The correct sequence in the skin puncture procedure for an infant is to:
    a   apply a heel warmer, sanitize hands, cleanse the skin puncture site with alcohol, use a dry, sterile gauze pad to wipe away the first drop of blood
    b   apply a heel warmer, cleanse the skin puncture site with alcohol, sanitize hands, use a dry sterile gauze pad to dry the site
    c   cleanse the skin puncture site with alcohol, apply a heel warmer, sanitize hands, use a dry gauze pad to dry the site
    d   sanitize hands, apply a heel warmer, cleanse the skin puncture site with alcohol, allow the site to air dry

293. The correct sequence in the skin puncture procedure for an infant is to:
    a   cleanse the site with 70% isopropyl alcohol, allow the site to air dry, verify sterility of the lancet, wipe away the first drop of blood using the alcohol pad
    b   cleanse the site with 70% isopropyl alcohol, allow the site to air dry, verify sterility of the lancet, wipe away the first drop of blood using a dry sterile gauze pad
    c   cleanse the site with 90% isopropyl alcohol, allow the site to air dry, verify sterility of the lancet, wipe away the first drop of blood using the alcohol pad
    d   cleanse the site with 90% isopropyl alcohol, allow the site to air dry, verify sterility of the lancet, wipe away the first drop of blood using a dry gauze pad

294. The correct way to hold an infant's foot during heelstick is to:
    a   place the thumb around the bottom of the foot, the index finger across the arch of the foot, and the remaining fingers across the top of the foot
    b   place the index finger around the bottom of the foot, the thumb across the arch of the foot, and the remaining fingers across the top of the foot
    c   place the fingers around the bottom of the foot, the thumb across the arch of the foot, and the index finger across the top of the foot
    d   place the thumb around the bottom of the foot, the fingers across the arch of the foot and the index finger across the top of the foot

Questions

Specimen Collection

295. The correct sequence in the skin puncture procedure for an infant is to deploy the safety lancet, gently squeeze the baby's foot and:
    a wipe away the first drop of blood using a sterile gauze pad and gently squeeze the baby's foot to generate the specimen for collection
    b wipe away the first drop of blood using an alcohol pad and gently squeeze the baby's foot to generate the specimen for collection
    c wipe away the first drop of blood using a sterile gauze pad and "milk" the baby's foot to generate the specimen for collection
    d gently squeeze the baby's foot to immediately generate the specimen for collection

296. Which of the following collection procedures will yield a specimen composed of arterial, capillary, and venous blood?
    a arterial puncture
    b drawing from an indwelling line
    c skin puncture
    d venipuncture

297. Which of the following skin puncture specimens is most likely to be adversely affected by excessive squeezing of the site?
    a bedside glucose test from a 75-year-old female
    b electrolyte panel from a 12-hour-old neonate
    c microhematocrit determination from a 30-year-old donor
    d WBC and platelet count from a 65-year-old oncology patient

298. A phlebotomist experiences great difficulty when securing a specimen from a neonate following a heelstick. She aggressively squeezes the site, employing a technique commonly referred to as "milking" to secure the specimen. What effect will this most likely have on specimen quality?
    a hemoconcentration
    b hemolysis
    c none
    d QNS

299. A phlebotomist experiences great difficulty when securing a specimen from a neonate following a heelstick. She aggressively squeezes the site, employing a technique commonly referred to as "milking" to secure the specimen. What effect will this most likely have on specimen quality?
    a hemoconcentration
    b hemodilution
    c QNS
    d tissue fluid contamination

300. A phlebotomist submits a skin puncture specimen collected from a neonate to the laboratory for bilirubin analysis. Following centrifugation, it was determined that the specimen was hemolyzed. The appropriate course of action is to:
    a   analyze the specimen
    b   dilute the specimen prior to analysis
    c   recollect the specimen by skin puncture
    d   recollect the specimen by venipuncture

301. Which of the following reference ranges will be higher for capillary blood specimens than for venipuncture specimens?
    a   calcium
    b   glucose
    c   rubella antibodies
    d   total protein

302. Which of the following reference ranges will be lower for capillary blood specimens than for venipuncture specimens?
    a   calcium
    b   glucose
    c   rubella antibodies
    d   rubeola antibodies

303. A phlebotomist experiences great difficulty when securing a specimen for electrolyte analysis from a neonate following a heelstick. She employs a technique commonly referred to as "milking" the site to secure the specimen. What effect will this technique most likely have on potassium levels?
    a   falsely decreased
    b   falsely increased
    c   none
    d   QNS

304. A phlebotomist receives a requisition to collect a bilirubin on an 18-hour-old neonate. What collection container should she use?
    a   amber microcollection container with a lavender red stopper
    b   amber microcollection container with a red stopper
    c   clear microcollection container with a gold stopper
    d   clear microcollection container with a lavender stopper

Questions
Specimen Collection

305. A phlebotomist has a requisition to collect a prothrombin time from a 75-year-old patient. The methodology used by the laboratory conducting the analysis uses the plasma portion of the specimen. The phlebotomist attempted venipuncture twice and was unsuccessful. She asked a second phlebotomist for assistance, who completed a skin puncture on the patient and collected a microcollection tube with a blue stopper. The specimen will likely be:
- a accepted for testing
- b rejected for testing
- c clotted
- d QNS

306. Prior to performing a heelstick, the infant's foot should be positioned:
- a above his torso
- b lower than his torso
- c parallel to his torso
- d perpendicular to his torso

307. Prior to performing a fingerstick on an adult patient, the patient's:
- a arm should be bent at the elbow with the palm facing forward
- b arm should be bent at the elbow with the palm facing backward
- c arm should be extended with the palm facing up
- d arm should be extended with the palm facing down

308. A commercial heel warmer is applied to a skin puncture site. This will:
- a decrease blood flow to the site
- b increase blood flow to the site
- c prevent hemoconcentration of the specimen
- d prevent hemolysis of the specimen

309. By how much can blood flow to a skin puncture site be increased if a commercial heel warmer is applied prior to skin puncture?
- a 4×
- b 5×
- c 6×
- d 7×

310. What portion of the capillary circulation is increased when a commercial heel warmer is applied to a skin puncture site?
- a arterial
- b capillary
- c interstitial fluid
- d venous

Specimen Collection — Questions

311. At least how long should a commercial heel warmer be applied to a skin puncture site prior to making a skin puncture?
    a 0-2 minutes
    b 2-4 minutes
    c 3-5 minutes
    d 4-6 minutes

312. Which of the following tests requires warming the site prior to skin puncture?
    a bilirubin
    b calcium
    c capillary blood gases
    d reticulocyte count

313. The temperature of commercial heel warmers should not exceed:
    a 22°C
    b 37°C
    c 42°C
    d 47°C

314. What compound should be used to cleanse a skin puncture site?
    a 70% isopropyl alcohol
    b 90% isopropyl alcohol
    c povidone-iodine
    d tincture of iodine

315. A phlebotomist cleanses a skin puncture site with povidone iodine. Which of the following tests will most likely be adversely affected?
    a bilirubin
    b rubella titer
    c red cell count
    d white cell count

316. A phlebotomist cleanses a skin puncture site with povidone iodine. Which of the following tests will most likely be adversely affected?
    a blood culture
    b capillary blood gases
    c red cell count
    d uric acid

317. A phlebotomist cleanses a skin puncture site with povidone iodine. Which of the following tests will most likely be adversely affected?
    a blood culture
    b capillary blood gases
    c potassium
    d white cell count

Questions
Specimen Collection

318. A phlebotomist cleanses a skin puncture site with povidone iodine. Which of the following tests will most likely be adversely affected?
    a capillary blood gases
    b phosphorous
    c platelet count
    d reticulocyte count

319. Following skin puncture, the blood specimen should be collected by:
    a applying gentle pressure proximal to the site while holding the puncture site in a downward position
    b applying gentle pressure with your thumb away from the puncture site to the patient's fingernail
    c holding the collection container under the puncture site and allowing the blood to flow into the microcollection container
    d holding the collection container under the puncture site and scooping the blood into the collection container

320. A phlebotomist performs a skin puncture on a 59-year-old female patient. She activates the safety lancet and blood appears at the puncture site. The phlebotomist should first:
    a place the collection container below the puncture site and immediately begin specimen collection
    b scoop the specimen into the specimen collection container
    c wipe away the first drop of blood using the alcohol prep pad
    d wipe away the first drop of blood using a dry gauze pad

321. A phlebotomist is performing a heelstick using an automated heel incision device. Most manufacturers recommend positioning the device at an angle of:
    a 45° to the length of the infant's foot
    b 45° to the width of the infant's foot
    c 90° to the length of the infant's foot
    d 90° to the width of the infant's foot

322. A phlebotomist collects a specimen for platelet count from a neonate using a heelstick procedure. She employs a scooping method to collect the specimen from the infant, repeatedly scraping the scoop along the infant's skin. What effect will this have on the specimen?
    a dilute the platelets, requiring a redraw of the specimen
    b stimulate platelet clumping, requiring a redraw of the specimen
    c QNS
    d this is the appropriate method to use to generate a quality specimen

323. A phlebotomist collects a microcollection tube with a lavender stopper following skin puncture. Following collection, the phlebotomist should gently invert the tube minimally:
   a   1-3×
   b   3-6×
   c   4-8×
   d   8-10×

324. What is the maximum number of times an infant's heel may be punctured to collect a blood specimen?
   a   1
   b   2
   c   3
   d   4

325. When should specimen labels be affixed to skin puncture specimen tubes?
   a   before collecting the specimen, while preparing supplies
   b   before collecting the specimen, at the patient's bedside
   c   after collecting the patient's specimen and after arriving in the laboratory
   d   after collecting the patient's specimen and before leaving the patient

326. Which of the following pieces of information must always be included on skin puncture specimen labels?
   a   patient address
   b   patient blood type
   c   phlebotomist initials
   d   physician name

327. A phlebotomist collects 6 capillary tubes following heelstick. How should the specimen be labeled?
   a   label each tube individually, following standard labeling procedures
   b   remove the stopper from a red evacuated tube, place the capillary tubes in the evacuated tube, and label the evacuated tube, following standard labeling procedures
   c   remove the stopper from a red SST evacuated tube, place the capillary tubes in the evacuated tube, and label the evacuated tube, following standard labeling procedures
   d   transport the capillary tubes in the sealant tray and label the tray, following standard labeling procedures

328. What should the phlebotomist apply to a skin puncture site on an adult to stop bleeding following specimen collection?
   a   heel warmer
   b   ice
   c   pressure using an alcohol prep pad
   d   pressure site using a dry, clean gauze pad

Questions — Specimen Collection

329. What should the phlebotomist apply to the puncture site after blood collection following heelstick?
    a   bandage
    b   heel warmer
    c   ice
    d   pressure using a dry, sterile gauze pad

330. A phlebotomist completes a heelstick on a neonate. The site continues to bleed 7 minutes following the procedure. The phlebotomist should:
    a   apply a bandage
    b   call a code
    c   complete an incident report
    d   inform the baby's nurse or physician

331. Which of the following is one of the most common reasons for neonatal blood transfusion?
    a   iatrogenic blood loss
    b   idiopathic thrombocytopenia
    c   hemolytic disease of the newborn
    d   hemophilia

332. What percentage of blood volume loss over a short period of time can be life threatening?
    a   2%
    b   4%
    c   5%
    d   10%

333. A neonate weighs 6.6 pounds. Withdrawing 10 mL of blood represents what percentage of the neonate's blood volume?
    a   1-2%
    b   2-4%
    c   5-10%
    d   10-15%

334. The blood volume of a neonate may be calculated using the neonate's:
    a   age
    b   Apgar score
    c   length
    d   weight

335. What information must be monitored to minimize iatrogenic blood loss in pediatric patients?
    a   amount of blood to be drawn at one time and neonate length
    b   amount of blood to be drawn at one time and cumulative amount of blood collected over one hospital admission
    c   cumulative amount of blood collected over one hospital admission and neonate age
    d   neonate length and weight

336. One strategy to minimize iatrogenic blood loss in neonates includes:
    a   collecting extra specimen volumes to limit redraws for additional tests ordered
    b   drawing small amounts frequently throughout the day
    c   strict adherence to quality assurance protocols for specimen collection
    d   using the maximum length lancet available to ensure good blood flow

337. Which of the following patient populations may be monitored closely to prevent iatrogenic anemia?
    a   oncology patient admitted for chemotherapy
    b   orthopedic patient admitted for hip replacement
    c   psychiatric patient admitted for depression
    d   renal patient admitted with kidney stones

338. Which of the following collection containers should be used to collect capillary blood gases from a neonate?
    a   heparinized glass capillary tube
    b   plain glass capillary tube
    c   heparinized plastic capillary tube
    d   plain plastic capillary tube

339. Which of the following specimens requires warming a collection tube to 37°C?
    a   blood culture
    b   cold agglutinin titers
    c   glucose tolerance testing
    d   type and screen

340. Which of the following analytes routinely included in an electrolyte panel is also used to manufacture EDTA evacuated tubes?
    a   ammonium
    b   calcium
    c   chloride
    d   potassium

Questions

Specimen Collection

341. Introducing bacteria from a patient's skin into a specimen for blood culture analysis may cause:
    a false-negative results
    b false-positive results
    c hemoconcentration
    d hemolysis

342. Introducing iodine into a specimen for blood culture analysis may cause:
    a false-negative results
    b false-positive results
    c hemoconcentration
    d hemolysis

343. Repalpating a site prior to venipuncture for blood culture analysis, may cause:
    a false-negative results
    b false-positive results
    c hemoconcentration
    d lipemia

344. Introducing air into an anaerobic blood culture collection container may cause:
    a false-negative results
    b false-positive results
    c hemoconcentration
    d hemolysis

345. Specimens for home glucose monitoring are routinely collected by:
    a accessing indwelling lines
    b arterial puncture
    c skin puncture
    d venipuncture

346. Which of the following tests is most commonly performed on skin puncture samples?
    a PCV
    b pH
    c PKU
    d PTT

347. Which of the following test procedures cannot be performed on specimens collected by skin puncture?
    a bilirubin
    b blood cultures
    c calcium
    d T3

Specimen Collection   **Questions**

348. Which of the following test procedures cannot be performed on specimens collected by skin puncture?

    a bilirubin
    b calcium
    c erythrocyte sedimentation rate
    d T3

349. Which of the following test procedures cannot be performed on specimens collected by skin puncture?

    a bilirubin
    b calcium
    c partial thromboplastin time (PTT)
    d T3

350. An inherited condition that is caused by the body's inability to metabolize phenylalanine is called:

    a packed cell volume (PCV)
    b pelvic inflammatory disease (PID)
    c phenylketonuria (PKU)
    d pleuropneumonialike organisms (PPLO)

351. Which of the following constituents is present in higher concentrations in blood collected by skin puncture than in blood collected by venipuncture?

    a calcium
    b glucose
    c potassium
    d total protein

352. The rationale for the sequence of multiple specimen collection following venipuncture is to primarily prevent:

    a additive carryover
    b glycolysis
    c hemolysis
    d platelet clumping

353. The following evacuated tubes are to be collected during routine venipuncture: SST (serum tube with clot activator and serum separator gel), yellow (SPS), light blue (sodium citrate), green (heparin). According to CLSI guidelines, which evacuated tube should be collected first?

    a green
    b light blue
    c SPS
    d SST

Questions

Specimen Collection

354. The following evacuated tubes are to be collected during routine venipuncture: SST (serum tube with clot activator and serum separator gel), yellow (SPS), light blue (sodium citrate), green (heparin). According to CLSI guidelines, which evacuated tube should be collected last?

   a green
   b light blue
   c SPS
   d SST

355. The following evacuated tubes are to be collected during routine venipuncture: SST (serum tube with clot activator and serum separator gel), yellow (SPS), light blue (sodium citrate), green (heparin). According to CLSI guidelines, in what sequence should the tubes be collected, following venipuncture?

   a SST, light blue, green, yellow (SPS)
   b SST, yellow (SPS), light blue, green
   c yellow (SPS), light blue, SST, green
   d yellow (SPS), SST, green, light blue

356. The following evacuated tubes with conventional stoppers are to be collected during routine venipuncture: gray (sodium fluoride), red (serum tube), light blue (sodium citrate), lavender (EDTA). According to CLSI guidelines, which evacuated tubes should be collected second?

   a gray
   b lavender
   c light blue
   d red

357. The following evacuated tubes with conventional stoppers are to be collected during routine venipuncture: gray (sodium fluoride), red (serum tube), light blue (sodium citrate), lavender (EDTA). According to CLSI guidelines, which evacuated tubes should be collected third?

   a gray
   b lavender
   c light blue
   d red

358. The following evacuated tubes with conventional stoppers are to be collected during routine venipuncture: gray (sodium fluoride), SST (serum tube with clot activator and serum separator gel), light blue (sodium citrate), lavender (EDTA). According to CLSI guidelines, which evacuated tubes should be collected first?

   a gray
   b lavender
   c light blue
   d SST

Specimen Collection   **Questions**

359. The following evacuated tubes with conventional stoppers are to be collected during routine venipuncture: gray (sodium fluoride), SST (serum tube with clot activator and serum separator gel), light blue (sodium citrate), lavender (EDTA). According to CLSI guidelines, which evacuated tubes should be collected last?

    a   gray
    b   lavender
    c   light blue
    d   SST

360. The following evacuated tubes with conventional stoppers are to be collected during routine venipuncture: gray (sodium fluoride), SST (serum tube with clot activator and serum separator gel), light blue (sodium citrate), lavender (EDTA). According to CLSI guidelines, in what sequence should the evacuated tubes be collected, following venipuncture?

    a   light blue, gray, lavender, SST
    b   light blue, lavender, gray, SST
    c   light blue, SST, lavender, gray
    d   SST, gray, light blue, lavender

361. The following evacuated tubes are to be collected during routine venipuncture: lavender (EDTA), SST (serum tube with clot activator and serum separator gel), light blue (sodium citrate), yellow (SPS). According to CLSI guidelines, which tube stopper color should be collected first?

    a   lavender
    b   light blue
    c   SST
    d   yellow (SPS)

362. The following evacuated tubes are to be collected during routine venipuncture: lavender (EDTA), SST (serum tube with clot activator and serum separator gel), light blue (sodium citrate), yellow (SPS). According to CLSI guidelines, which evacuated tube should be collected last?

    a   lavender
    b   light blue
    c   SST
    d   yellow (SPS)

363. The following evacuated tubes are to be collected during routine venipuncture: lavender (EDTA), SST (serum tube with clot activator and serum separator gel), light blue (sodium citrate), yellow (SPS). According to CLSI guidelines, in what sequence should the evacuated tubes be collected, following venipuncture?

    a   lavender, SST, yellow (SPS), light blue
    b   SST, yellow (SPS), lavender, light blue
    c   yellow (SPS), light blue, SST, lavender
    d   yellow (SPS), SST, light blue, lavender

Questions

Specimen Collection

364. The following evacuated tubes with conventional stoppers are to be collected during routine venipuncture: green (heparin), gray (sodium fluoride), SST (serum tube with clot activator and serum separator gel), light blue (sodium citrate). According to CLSI guidelines, which tube should be collected second?

   a   gray
   b   green
   c   light blue
   d   SST

365. The following evacuated tubes with conventional stoppers are to be collected during routine venipuncture: green (heparin), gray (sodium fluoride), SST (serum tube with clot activator and serum separator gel), light blue (sodium citrate). According to CLSI guidelines, which tube should be collected third?

   a   gray
   b   green
   c   light blue
   d   SST

366. The following evacuated tubes with conventional stoppers are to be collected during routine venipuncture: green (heparin), gray (sodium fluoride), SST (serum tube with clot activator and serum separator gel), light blue (sodium citrate). According to CLSI guidelines, in what sequence should the evacuated tubes be collected, following venipuncture?

   a   green, gray, light blue, SST
   b   light blue, green, SST, gray
   c   light blue, SST, green, gray
   d   SST, green, gray, light blue

367. A phlebotomist is to collect a specimen for an activated PTT and prothrombin time from a patient using an evacuated tube system. According to CLSI guidelines, what evacuated tube stopper color should the phlebotomist collect first?

   a   discard tube
   b   green
   c   light blue
   d   yellow

368. The following evacuated tubes with stoppers are to be collected during routine venipuncture: SST (serum tube with clot activator and serum separator gel), green (heparin), gray (sodium fluoride), lavender (EDTA). According to CLSI guidelines, which tube should be collected first?

   a   gray
   b   green
   c   lavender
   d   SST

Specimen Collection — **Questions**

369. The following evacuated tubes with stoppers are to be collected during routine venipuncture: SST (serum tube with clot activator and serum separator gel), green (heparin), gray (sodium fluoride), lavender (EDTA). According to CLSI guidelines, which tube should be collected last?

    a   gray
    b   green
    c   lavender
    d   SST

370. The following evacuated tubes with stoppers are to be collected during routine venipuncture: SST (serum tube with clot activator and serum separator gel), green (heparin), gray (sodium fluoride), lavender (EDTA). According to CLSI guidelines, in what sequence should the evacuated tubes be collected, following venipuncture?

    a   gray, green, lavender, SST
    b   gray, lavender, green, SST
    c   SST, green, lavender, gray
    d   SST, lavender, gray, green

371. The following evacuated tubes with stoppers are to be collected during routine venipuncture: red (serum), light blue (sodium citrate), green (heparin), gray (sodium fluoride), lavender (EDTA). According to CLSI guidelines, which tube should be collected third?

    a   gray
    b   green
    c   lavender
    d   light blue

372. The following evacuated tubes with stoppers are to be collected during routine venipuncture: red (serum), light blue (sodium citrate), green (heparin), gray (sodium fluoride), lavender (EDTA). According to CLSI guidelines, which tube should be collected fourth?

    a   gray
    b   green
    c   lavender
    d   light blue

373. The following evacuated tubes with stoppers are to be collected during routine venipuncture: red (serum), light blue (sodium citrate), green (heparin), gray (sodium fluoride), lavender (EDTA). According to CLSI guidelines, in what sequence should the evacuated tubes be collected, following venipuncture?

    a   gray, green, lavender, light blue, red
    b   gray, green, lavender, red, light blue
    c   light blue, lavender, red, gray, green
    d   light blue, red, green, lavender, gray

Questions
Specimen Collection

374. The rationale for the order of draw for syringes is to minimize:
    a   additive transfer to a subsequent tube
    b   clotting in anticoagulant tubes
    c   hemolysis of the specimen
    d   platelet clumping

375. Following venipuncture by syringe, blood must be aliquoted into the following evacuated tubes: red (clot activator), light blue (sodium citrate), green (heparin). In what order should blood be transferred to the evacuated tubes?
    a   green, red, light blue
    b   light blue, red, green
    c   red, green, light blue
    d   red, light blue, green

376. The following evacuated tubes with conventional stoppers are to be collected during routine venipuncture using a syringe: green (heparin), lavender (EDTA), SST (serum tube with clot activator and serum separator gel), light blue (sodium citrate). According to CLSI guidelines, blood should be transferred to which evacuated tube first?
    a   green
    b   lavender
    c   light blue
    d   SST

377. The following evacuated tubes with conventional stoppers are to be collected during routine venipuncture using a syringe: green (heparin), lavender (EDTA), SST (serum tube with clot activator and serum separator gel), light blue (sodium citrate). According to CLSI guidelines, which tube should be collected last?
    a   green
    b   lavender
    c   light blue
    d   SST

378. The following evacuated tubes with conventional stoppers are to be collected during routine venipuncture using a syringe: green (heparin), gray (sodium fluoride), SST (serum tube with clot activator), light blue (sodium citrate). According to CLSI guidelines, in what sequence should the evacuated tubes be collected, following venipuncture?
    a   green, gray, light blue, SST
    b   light blue, green, SST, gray
    c   light blue, SST, green, gray
    d   SST, green, gray, light blue

Specimen Collection   **Questions**

379. A phlebotomist must collect the following evacuated tubes with conventional stoppers during routine venipuncture using a winged infusion needle: SST (serum tube with clot activator and serum separator gel), green (heparin), and light blue (sodium citrate). According to CLSI guidelines, which tube should be collected first?

   a   discard tube
   b   green
   c   light blue
   d   SST

380. The following evacuated tubes with conventional stoppers are to be collected during routine venipuncture using a winged infusion needle: SST (serum tube with clot activator and serum separator gel), green (heparin), gray (sodium fluoride), lavender (EDTA). According to CLSI guidelines, which tube should be collected last?

   a   gray
   b   green
   c   lavender
   d   SST

381. A phlebotomist is to collect a specimen for an activated partial thromboplastin time (PTT) and prothrombin time (PT) from a patient using a winged infusion needle. According to CLSI guidelines, what evacuated tube stopper color should the phlebotomist collect first?

   a   discard tube
   b   green
   c   light blue
   d   yellow

382. The order of draw for the collection of multiple specimens following skin puncture was established to minimize:

   a   contamination
   b   hemoconcentration
   c   hemolysis
   d   platelet clumping

383. The following tests were to be collected from a patient following skin puncture: platelet count (lavender top microcollection container), bilirubin (red top microcollection container), electrolytes (green top microcollection container). In what order should these tests be collected?

   a   bilirubin, electrolytes, platelet count
   b   bilirubin, platelet count, electrolytes
   c   electrolytes, bilirubin, platelet count
   d   platelet count, electrolytes, bilirubin

Questions
Specimen Collection

384. The following microcollection containers were to be collected following skin puncture: lavender, green, red SST. In what order should the microtainers be collected?
    a   green, lavender, red
    b   green, red, lavender
    c   lavender, green, red
    d   red, lavender, green

385. Which of the following tests would most likely be affected if citrate is carried over from a previous evacuated tube during a multiple evacuated tube collection?
    a   acid phosphatase
    b   alkaline phosphatase
    c   amylase
    d   potassium

386. Which of the following tests would most likely be affected if citrate is carried over from a previous evacuated tube during a multiple evacuated tube collection?
    a   calcium
    b   creatine kinase
    c   potassium
    d   sodium

387. Which of the following tests would most likely be affected if citrate is carried over from a previous evacuated tube during a multiple evacuated tube collection?
    a   creatine kinase
    b   phosphorous
    c   potassium
    d   sodium

388. Which of the following tests would most likely be affected if EDTA is carried over from a previous evacuated tube during a multiple evacuated tube collection?
    a   calcium
    b   lithium
    c   phosphorous
    d   red cell morphology

389. Which of the following tests would most likely be affected if EDTA is carried over from a previous evacuated tube during a multiple evacuated tube collection?
    a   acid phosphatase
    b   alkaline phosphatase
    c   amylase
    d   phosphorous

390. Which of the following tests would most likely be affected if EDTA is carried over from a previous evacuated tube during a multiple evacuated tube collection?
    a   acid phosphatase
    b   amylase
    c   creatine kinase
    d   lactate dehydrogenase

391. Which of the following tests would most likely be affected if EDTA is carried over from a previous evacuated tube during a multiple evacuated tube collection?
    a   lithium
    b   phosphorous
    c   potassium
    d   red cell morphology

392. Which of the following tests would most likely be affected if EDTA is carried over from a previous evacuated tube during a multiple evacuated tube collection?
    a   lactate dehydrogenase
    b   lithium
    c   phosphorous
    d   sodium

393. Which of the following tests would most likely be affected if heparin is carried over from a previous evacuated tube during a multiple evacuated tube collection?
    a   acid phosphatase
    b   alkaline phosphatase
    c   amylase
    d   creatine kinase

394. Which of the following tests would most likely be affected if heparin is carried over from a previous evacuated tube during a multiple evacuated tube collection?
    a   calcium
    b   creatine kinase
    c   phosphorous
    d   red cell morphology

395. Which of the following tests would most likely be affected if heparin is carried over from a previous evacuated tube during a multiple evacuated tube collection?
    a   alkaline phosphatase
    b   creatine kinase
    c   phosphorous
    d   partial thromboplastin time

| Questions | Specimen Collection |

396. Which evacuated tube additive is most likely to adversely affect test results if carried over to a subsequent evacuated tube?
    a   citrate
    b   EDTA
    c   heparin
    d   oxalate

397. Which of the following evacuated tubes may be collected separately to eliminate carryover contamination?
    a   red
    b   lavender
    c   light blue
    d   royal blue

398. What order of draw should be used when transferring blood from a syringe to multiple evacuated tubes?
    a   reverse order as collecting specimens by skin puncture
    b   same order as collecting specimens by skin puncture
    c   reverse order as collecting specimens by skin puncture
    d   same order as collecting specimens by venipuncture

399. After venipuncture, the patient is diaphoretic and pale. The phlebotomist should:
    a   apply ice to the venipuncture site
    b   call a code
    c   disregard these symptoms because they are normal after a venipuncture
    d   lower the patient's head and instruct her to breathe deeply

400. Once a patient who has experienced syncope regains consciousness, he should remain at the draw station for at least:
    a   5 minutes
    b   10 minutes
    c   15 minutes
    d   20 minutes

401. During a venipuncture, the patient vomits. The phlebotomist should:
    a   complete the procedure and notify housekeeping
    b   discontinue the venipuncture immediately
    c   hand the patient an emesis basin and complete the venipuncture
    d   hand the patient a tissue and complete the venipuncture

402. What response may some patients have at the sight of his/her blood being drawn?
    a   hematoma
    b   hemolysis
    c   syncope
    d   synergy

Specimen Collection — **Questions**

403. If a specimen is hemolyzed, what color is the serum?
    a   green
    b   pink
    c   white
    d   yellow

404. A phlebotomist approaches a patient who has an intravenous line inserted in his right antecubital area (antecubital fossa). What site should the phlebotomist consider for venipuncture?
    a   right arm above the IV
    b   right arm below the IV
    c   left antecubital area (antecubital fossa)
    d   skin puncture

405. A phlebotomist approaches a patient who has an intravenous line inserted in his right wrist. What site should the phlebotomist *first* consider for venipuncture?
    a   right arm above the IV
    b   right hand below the IV
    c   left antecubital area (antecubital fossa)
    d   skin puncture

406. A phlebotomist approaches a patient who has an intravenous line inserted in his right antecubital area (antecubital fossa). What site should the phlebotomist consider *first* for venipuncture?
    a   right arm above the IV
    b   right arm below the IV
    c   left hand
    d   skin puncture

407. A phlebotomist approaches a patient who has an intravenous line inserted in his right antecubital area (antecubital fossa). What site should the phlebotomist consider *last* to secure the specimen?
    a   right arm above the IV
    b   right hand below the IV
    c   left arm
    d   left hand

408. A patient has a fistula in his left forearm. What area should the phlebotomist examine first for a suitable vein for venipuncture?
    a   left antecubital area (antecubital fossa)
    b   left wrist
    c   right antecubital area (antecubital fossa)
    d   right wrist

Questions

Specimen Collection

409. A phlebotomist performs a puncture in the antecubital area (antecubital fossa) using the basilic vein. The blood entering the tube is a bright orange red. The phlebotomist should:
    a apply heat to the puncture site
    b complete the venipuncture following standard procedures
    c immediately discontinue the procedure
    d leave the tourniquet tied throughout the procedure and complete the draw

410. The phlebotomist approaches a patient and realizes both arms are in plaster casts from fingers to above the elbows. What procedure and site should be used for blood collection, assuming physician's permission?
    a arterial puncture on the patient's brachial artery
    b patient finger tips
    c venipuncture on the basilic vein
    d venipuncture on the patient's great saphenous vein

411. The phlebotomist approaches a patient and realizes the patient has intravenous lines running in the antecubital area (antecubital fossa) of both arms. What procedure and site should be used for blood collection, assuming physician's permission?
    a arterial puncture using the patient's brachial artery
    b cephalic vein in the antecubital area (antecubital fossa)
    c venipuncture using the palmar venous network on the anterior side of the hand
    d venipuncture using the patient's dorsal hand veins

412. A phlebotomist inserts a needle into a site selected for venipuncture in a patient who has pronounced edema in both arms. The phlebotomist was unsuccessful and, contrary to institutional policy, began to probe the venipuncture site with the needle. The patient cried out, complaining of intense pain, describing it as a shooting electrical sensation. What is the likely cause?
    a the patient has a high pain tolerance
    b the patient has a low pain tolerance
    c the phlebotomist may have damaged a nerve
    d the specimen was hemolyzed

413. Positioning the evacuated tube incorrectly during venipuncture may result in:
    a additive carryover
    b hemoconcentration
    c hemolysis
    d nothing—it is a nonissue

414. After needle withdrawal, pressure should be applied to the puncture site for at least:
    a   0-3 minutes
    b   3-5 minutes
    c   5-7 minutes
    d   7-9 minutes

415. After 3 minutes of applying pressure, a phlebotomist examines the venipuncture site and recognizes that the bleeding has not stopped. The phlebotomist should:
    a   bandage the patient's arm and move to the next patient
    b   call a code
    c   notify the patient's doctor
    d   notify the patient's nurse

416. After inspecting a patient's venipuncture site, the phlebotomist determines that the patient has stopped bleeding and applies a bandage. The patient should be instructed to keep the bandage on for at least:
    a   5 minutes
    b   10 minutes
    c   15 minutes
    d   20 minutes

417. Using a needle that is too small to accommodate the force of the vacuum of an evacuated tube may cause which of the following in a patient's specimen?
    a   hemoconcentration
    b   hemolysis
    c   hemostasis
    d   hematoma

418. Which of the following conditions may be caused by a needle penetrating all the way through the vein during venipuncture?
    a   hematoma
    b   hemolysis
    c   syncope
    d   synergy

419. During pregnancy, the increase of body fluids may cause a patient's red blood cell count (RBC) to:
    a   decrease
    b   increase
    c   remain unchanged
    d   show no difference due to gender

Questions

Specimen Collection

420. Hemoconcentration of the specimen may be caused by:
    a   drawing from a hematoma
    b   residual alcohol on the site
    c   shaking additive tubes
    d   prolonged tourniquet application

421. Hemoconcentration of the specimen may be caused by:
    a   drawing from a hematoma
    b   residual alcohol on the site
    c   shaking additive tubes
    d   vigorous hand pumping

422. A phlebotomist transfixes a vein during venipuncture. Which of the following specimen characteristics may result?
    a   clotting in plasma tubes
    b   hemolyzed specimen
    c   hemoconcentration of specimen
    d   short draw

423. A phlebotomist collects a sodium citrate tube from a patient for a prothrombin time and an activated partial thromboplastin time. It was a very difficult draw and she was only able to obtain half a tube. She attempted a second venipuncture and again was only able to obtain half a tube. What is the appropriate course of action?
    a   ask a colleague to recollect the specimen
    b   pour the contents from the second tube into the first tube and submit a full tube
    c   submit the first tube collected for analysis
    d   submit the second tube collected for analysis

424. A patient has undergone a left radical mastectomy. Which site should the phlebotomist use for venipuncture?
    a   either right or left cephalic hand vein
    b   either right or left arm
    c   left arm
    d   right arm

425. What condition sometimes occurs following mastectomy that becomes a factor in venipuncture site selection?
    a   hemostasis
    b   homeostasis
    c   lymphostasis
    d   venous stasis

Specimen Collection   **Questions**

426. After the needle is inserted and the evacuated tube engaged, the phlebotomist notices a purple swelling around the puncture site. The phlebotomist should:
    a. discontinue the procedure
    b. proceed, using the site selected
    c. select another site
    d. write "Can't get" on the requisition

427. What may result if a phlebotomist performs a venipuncture through a hematoma?
    a. erroneous test results
    b. hemostasis
    c. homeostasis
    d. quality specimen collection

428. If a phlebotomist notes that the arm selected for venipuncture is edematous, she should:
    a. perform the venipuncture
    b. notify the patient's nurse
    c. select another site
    d. write "Can't get" on the requisition

429. A phlebotomist collects a blood specimen from a patient's arm with marked edema. Which of the following may occur as a result?
    a. contamination with tissue fluid
    b. contamination with skin bacteria
    c. destruction of platelets
    d. destruction of red blood cells

430. Drawing blood through a hematoma may cause which of the following in a patient's specimen?
    a. hemoconcentration
    b. hemolysis
    c. hemostasis
    d. hematoma

431. A patient suffers a transfusion reaction. What may this condition cause in the patient's specimen?
    a. hemoconcentration
    b. hemolysis
    c. hemostasis
    d. hematoma

432. If a phlebotomist palpates a vein and determines that it is sclerosed, the phlebotomist should:
    a. draw above the sclerosed area
    b. notify the patient's physician
    c. select another site
    d. turn off the IV and perform the draw

Questions
Specimen Collection

433. Which of the following is a cause of sclerosed veins?
    a   numerous venipunctures
    b   prolonged tourniquet application
    c   radical mastectomy
    d   residual alcohol

434. While performing a venipuncture with a syringe, a phlebotomist notices blood frothing between the hub of the needle and the syringe. As a result, the specimen may be:
    a   activated
    b   contaminated
    c   hemolyzed
    d   iontophoretic

435. A lavender evacuated tube (EDTA) must be redrawn because of clots in the tube. What collection error causes this?
    a   improper patient preparation
    b   insufficient mixing of additive with specimen
    c   transfixed vein
    d   traumatized specimen

436. During a first attempt to secure a blood specimen via venipuncture, the phlebotomist engages the evacuated tube, but no blood appears in the tube. The phlebotomist attempted to rescue the draw but determined the venipuncture was unsuccessful. What should the phlebotomist do FIRST to end the procedure?
    a   call the nurse
    b   tighten the tourniquet
    c   untie the tourniquet
    d   withdraw the needle

437. During venipuncture, the phlebotomist inserts the needle into the patient's vein. No blood appears in the evacuated tube. The phlebotomist should first:
    a   completely withdraw the needle
    b   establish the location of the vein relative to the needle
    c   pull back and reinsert the needle toward the lateral aspect of the patient's arm
    d   pull back and reinsert the needle toward the medial aspect of the patient's arm

438. Which of the following may cause petechiae on a patient's skin?
    a   allergy to the iodine
    b   blood leaking into the tissues
    c   patient platelet abnormalities
    d   the sight of blood

Specimen Collection — Questions

439. During venipuncture, a phlebotomist moves the tube gently up and down in the holder, moving the contents back and forth. What may this cause?
    a   hematoma
    b   hemolysis
    c   petechiae
    d   reflux

440. Shaking an evacuated tube containing an additive too forcefully to mix the contents may cause which of the following in a patient's specimen?
    a   hemoconcentration
    b   hemolysis
    c   hemostasis
    d   hematoma

441. Drawing blood through a hematoma may cause:
    a   hemoconcentration
    b   hemolysis
    c   hemostasis
    d   hematoma

442. A specimen for ABG analysis would be rejected if the specimen:
    a   contained air bubbles
    b   was collected in EDTA
    c   was collected in heparin
    d   was transported on ice

443. Clinically significant changes will occur in a specimen collected for ABG analysis if the specimen is left at room temperature (22°C) for more than:
    a   5 minutes
    b   10 minutes
    c   15 minutes
    d   30 minutes

444. Which of the following actions may result in a hemolyzed skin puncture specimen?
    a   anemic condition of the patient
    b   contamination with iodine
    c   failure to wipe away the first drop of blood
    d   insufficient puncture

445. A potential complication of accidentally puncturing the calcaneus bone during skin puncture, characterized by inflammation of the bone and bone marrow, is called:
    a   osteocarcinoma
    b   osteochondritis
    c   osteomyelitis
    d   osteoporosis

Questions

Specimen Collection

446. A potential complication of accidentally puncturing the calcaneus bone during skin puncture, characterized by inflammation of the bone and cartilage, is called:
    a   osteocarcinoma
    b   osteochondritis
    c   osteomyelitis
    d   osteoporosis

447. A significant risk of injuring a bone during finger puncture is very likely in patients who are less than:
    a   1 year old
    b   2 years old
    c   3 years old
    d   4 years old

448. Which of the following values is higher in newborns than in adults?
    a   electrolyte levels
    b   red cell counts
    c   heterophile titer levels
    d   varicella zoster virus

449. Which of the following blood constituents will increase as the oxygen content of the air decreases?
    a   red blood cell counts
    b   white blood cell counts
    c   CK levels
    d   LDH levels

450. Which of the following patient conditions may cause a transient elevation in WBC count results?
    a   altitude change
    b   gender
    c   pregnancy
    d   stress

451. Which of the following could cause hemolysis of a specimen obtained by skin puncture?
    a   collecting specimens in an incorrect order
    b   residual alcohol left on the site
    c   using povidone iodine to clean the site
    d   warming the site

452. Which of the following could cause hemolysis of a specimen collected by skin puncture?
    a   excessive squeezing of the puncture site to secure the specimen
    b   incorrect order of draw
    c   using povidone iodine to prepare the site
    d   warming the site

Specimen Collection **Questions**

453. Which of the following blood constituents may be falsely elevated if the skin puncture site is prepared with povidone iodine?
    a   hemoglobin
    b   hepatitis B surface antigen
    c   platelet count
    d   potassium

454. If a tourniquet is properly applied, it will:
    a   restrict all blood flow
    b   restrict arterial blood flow, but not venous blood flow
    c   restrict venous blood flow, but not arterial blood flow
    d   be tied like a shoelace

455. Which of the following may be used if a tourniquet is not available?
    a   glove
    b   rubber tubing
    c   sphygmomanometer
    d   splint

456. If a blood pressure cuff is used in place of a tourniquet, the gauge should be set no higher than:
    a   180 mm Hg
    b   200 mm Hg
    c   the patient's diastolic pressure
    d   the patient's systolic pressure

457. The purpose of tourniquet application is to:
    a   decrease venous filling
    b   increase venous filling
    c   distract the patient from the phlebotomy procedure
    d   stop all blood flow

458. Which of the following may serve as a mechanism for transmitting infection?
    a   evacuated tube
    b   evacuated tube holder
    c   heel warmer
    d   tourniquet

459. If a tourniquet transmits infection, what is the most likely source?
    a   patient's arms
    b   patient's beds
    c   phlebotomist's hands
    d   methicillin resistant *Staphylococcus aureus* (MRSA)

Questions
Specimen Collection

460. A patient confirms he has a latex allergy. The phlebotomist should use a tourniquet made of:
   a elastic
   b latex
   c nitrile
   d rubber

461. A patient confirms he has a latex allergy. The phlebotomist should use a tourniquet made of:
   a elastic
   b paper
   c rubber
   d vinyl

462. Where should the needle be discarded once the safety feature is activated?
   a at the nurse's station
   b biohazardous waste bag
   c patient's bedside trash receptacle
   d sharps container

463. Where should the packaging from gauze and alcohol prep pads be discarded?
   a at the nurse's station
   b biohazardous waste bag
   c sharps container
   d wastebasket

464. Where should gauze used to apply pressure following venipuncture be discarded?
   a at the nurse's station
   b biohazardous waste bag
   c patient's bedside trash receptacle
   d sharps container

465. Which of the following needle gauges is used most often to collect units of blood from blood donors?
   a 16 & 18
   b 19 & 20
   c 21 & 22
   d 32 & 24

466. The closed system that is composed of a needle, a holder, and a tube containing a premeasured amount of vacuum is the:
   a evacuated blood collection system
   b nonevacuated blood collection system
   c Microtainer
   d Unopette

Specimen Collection

467. Which of the following needle lengths is most commonly used for adult venipuncture?
    a   ½ & 1 inch needles
    b   1 & 1½ inch needles
    c   1½ & 2 inch needles
    d   2 & 2½ inch needles

468. Evacuated tubes are manufactured in a range of sizes. Which of the volume ranges below most accurately reflects evacuated tubes typically used during venipuncture?
    a   1.8-18 mL
    b   1.0-10 mL
    c   4-10 mL
    d   4-20 mL

469. Which of the following blood collection devices is manufactured with a rubber sheath?
    a   single sample needle
    b   multisample needle
    c   evacuated tube
    d   nonevacuated tube

470. The standard for measuring the diameter of the lumen of a needle is the needle:
    a   bore
    b   brand
    c   gauge
    d   length

471. The internal space of a needle is the:
    a   bevel
    b   brand
    c   gauge
    d   lumen

472. Which of the following needle gauges represents the largest interior diameter?
    a   18
    b   19
    c   20
    d   21

473. Which of the following needle gauges represents the smallest interior diameter?
    a   20
    b   21
    c   22
    d   23

Questions

Specimen Collection

474. Which of the following needle gauges is used most often to perform routine venipuncture?
    a 16 & 18
    b 19 & 20
    c 21 & 22
    d 23 & 24

475. Where should needle caps be discarded?
    a at the nurse's station
    b biohazardous waste bag
    c wastebasket
    d sharps container

476. Needle safety features must:
    a be an accessory to the phlebotomist's equipment roster
    b be provided if requested
    c create barrier between the needle and the phlebotomist's hands
    d provide at least temporary shielding from a contaminated needle

477. An example of a needle shield activated by pressing the shield on a hard surface is the:
    a Becton-Dickinson Eclipse™
    b safety transfer device
    c Venipuncture Needle-Pro®
    d VanishPoint®

478. An example of a needle shield activated by phlebotomist using his thumb to move the shield over the needle is the:
    a BD Microtainer® Quikheel™ safety lancet
    b safety transfer device
    c Vacuette™ Quickshield
    d A phlebotomist's fingers should never be that close to a contaminated needle

479. An example of a needle shield activated by a retraction mechanism is the:
    a Becton-Dickinson Eclipse™
    b safety transfer device
    c Venipuncture Needle-Pro®
    d VanishPoint®

480. What color is most commonly used for puncture resistant, leakproof containers suitable for discarding used sharps?
    a black
    b blue
    c green
    d red

Specimen Collection

481. A phlebotomist prepares to discard a used needle in a sharps container, which is overflowing with contaminated needles and holders. The phlebotomist should:
    a   locate a sharps container that is not full and discard the contaminated needle there
    b   shake the sharps container until the contents settle out near the bottom making room for her needle
    c   use the lid of the sharps container to push the materials down to make room for the needle she needs to dispose
    d   use the needle she must dispose of to move items around and create a spot for the contaminated needle she needs to dispose

482. A phlebotomist selects a needle to use for venipuncture and notices that the seal surrounding the needle cap is broken. She should:
    a   call security
    b   discard the needle in a sharps container
    c   discard the needle in the patient's wastebasket
    d   use the needle because it came from the supply room

483. Which of the following equipment is used for a routine venipuncture?
    a   heel warmer, safety lancet, microcollection container
    b   heel warmer, needle, microcollection container
    c   multisample needle, evacuated tube, holder
    d   syringe, evacuated tube

484. Which of the following equipment is used for site selection and preparation during routine skin puncture?
    a   betadine
    b   heel warmer
    c   povidone iodine
    d   tourniquet

485. Which of the following conventional stopper colors corresponds to the evacuated tube suitable for blood culture specimen collection?
    a   lavender
    b   light blue
    c   royal blue
    d   yellow

486. Which of the following evacuated tube additives inhibits complement?
    a   sodium citrate
    b   sodium fluoride
    c   sodium heparin
    d   sodium polyanethol sulfonate (SPS)

Questions
Specimen Collection

487. Which of the following blood culture specimen collection containers incorporates an aerobic bottle and an anaerobic bottle?
    a   Bactec system
    b   gas impermeable syringe
    c   sodium polyanethol sulfonate (SPS) evacuated tube/conventional stopper
    d   sodium polyanethol sulfonate (SPS) evacuated tube/Hemogard closure

488. An evacuated tube manufactured by Becton-Dickinson contains clot activator and serum separator gel. What color is the Hemogard closure?
    a   gold
    b   green
    c   light green
    d   royal blue

489. An evacuated tube manufactured by Becton-Dickinson contains thrombin. What color is the Hemogard closure?
    a   gold
    b   green
    c   orange
    d   royal blue

490. If an evacuated tube contains heparin and plasma separator gel, what color is the Hemogard closure?
    a   gold
    b   light green
    c   orange
    d   royal blue

491. Which of the following additives is found in a plastic evacuated tube with a red stopper?
    a   clot activator
    b   EDTA
    c   sodium heparin
    d   sodium polyanethol sulfonate (SPS)

492. What is the ratio of blood to anticoagulant in sodium citrate tubes?
    a   1:1
    b   3:1
    c   6:1
    d   9:1

493. Which of the following additives is found in an evacuated tube with a green conventional stopper?
    a   EDTA
    b   none
    c   sodium heparin
    d   sodium polyanethol sulfonate (SPS)

Specimen Collection — Questions

494. Which of the following additives is found in an evacuated tube with a gray conventional stopper?
   a EDTA
   b sodium citrate
   c sodium fluoride
   d sodium polyanethol sulfonate (SPS)

495. Which of the following additives is found in an evacuated tube with a yellow conventional stopper?
   a EDTA
   b sodium citrate
   c sodium fluoride
   d sodium polyanethol sulfonate (SPS)

496. Which of the following anticoagulants inhibits glycolysis?
   a EDTA
   b potassium oxalate
   c sodium fluoride
   d sodium heparin

497. Which of the following additives in evacuated tubes neutralizes thrombin?
   a acid citrate dextrose (ACD)
   b EDTA
   c sodium citrate
   d sodium heparin

498. Which of the following evacuated tube stoppers is manufactured with the lowest verified levels of trace elements available?
   a lavender
   b light blue
   c royal blue
   d sodium polyanethol sulfonate (SPS)

499. Which of the following evacuated tube stoppers is manufactured with very low levels of lead?
   a lavender
   b red
   c red/gray serum separator tube (SST)
   d tan

500. Which of the following additives is found in evacuated tubes with lavender stoppers?
   a acid citrate dextrose (ACD)
   b citrate phosphate dextrose-adenine (CPDA)
   c ethylenediamine tetraacetic acid (EDTA)
   d sodium polyanethol sulfonate (SPS)

Questions — Specimen Collection

501. Which of the following additives is found in an evacuated tube with a yellow conventional stopper?
- a acid citrate dextrose (ACD)
- b ethylenediamine tetraacetic acid (EDTA)
- c lithium heparin
- d sodium citrate

502. Which of the following additives is found in an evacuated tube with a light blue conventional stopper?
- a acid citrate dextrose (ACD)
- b ethylenediamine tetraacetic acid (EDTA)
- c lithium heparin
- d sodium citrate

503. Which of the following additives in evacuated tubes is an antiglycolytic agent?
- a ethylenediamine tetraacetic acid (EDTA)
- b potassium oxalate
- c sodium fluoride
- d sodium heparin

504. Which of the following additives in evacuated tubes promotes clotting?
- a acid citrate dextrose (ACD)
- b EDTA
- c lithium heparin
- d thrombin

505. Listed below are conventional stopper colors of evacuated tubes. Which stopper color should be used when collecting specimens for analyses that require both a patient's cells and serum?
- a green
- b green PST
- c red
- d red SST

506. What angle should a phlebotomist use to invert evacuated tubes in order to ensure adequate mixing of the specimen with the anticoagulant?
- a 30°
- b 45°
- c 90°
- d 180°

507. A phlebotomist delivered a lavender top evacuated tube to the hematology department for analysis. The tube was approximately 60% filled. What effect will this have on the results?
- a falsely decreased size of the red blood cells
- b falsely increased size of the red blood cells
- c no effect—the specimen is suitable for analysis
- d the specimen will be hemolyzed, but suitable for analysis

Specimen Collection — Questions

508. Which of the following additives in evacuated tubes prevents platelet aggregation?
     a ethylenediamine tetraacetic acid (EDTA)
     b sodium polyanethol sulfonate (SPS)
     c potassium oxalate
     d sodium citrate

509. Which of the following additives in evacuated tubes preserves labile coagulation factors?
     a sodium fluoride
     b sodium polyanethol sulfonate (SPS)
     c sodium citrate
     d sodium heparin

510. Which of the following additives in evacuated tubes produces artifact residue on blood smears stained with Wright stain?
     a ethylenediamine tetraacetic acid (EDTA)
     b fibrin
     c sodium heparin
     d thrombin

511. A winged infusion needle is commonly referred to as a(n):
     a butterfly needle
     b engineering control
     c luer-lock needle
     d safety hazard

512. Which of the following needles pose the greatest risk to phlebotomists for accidental self puncture?
     a BD Microtainer® Quikheel™ safety lancet
     b single draw needles
     c syringe needles
     d winged infusion needles

513. The most common lengths of winged infusion needles are:
     a ½ or ¾ inch
     b 1 or 1½ inches
     c 1½ or 2 mm
     d 2 or 3 mm

514. Safety features for winged infusion needles include which of the following mechanisms?
     a bending
     b cutting
     c locking shields
     d resheathing

Questions

Specimen Collection

515. When is a syringe most commonly employed to collect a blood specimen?
    a blood culture specimen collection
    b type and crossmatch specimen collection
    c when a patient has very thin, fragile veins
    d when drawing a donor for a unit of blood

516. Syringe use should be limited because they increase the risk of:
    a accidental needlestick
    b additive carryover
    c hemoconcentration
    d lipemia

517. Syringes used for venous blood collection must always be used with a:
    a heparin lock
    b lancet
    c evacuated tube
    d transfer device

518. What equipment does the phlebotomist need for site preparation prior to skin puncture?
    a heel warmer, alcohol, sterile gauze
    b heel warmer, povidone iodine, sterile gauze
    c lancet, Unopette, sharps, gloves
    d gown, gloves, sharps, biohazard bag

519. Which of the following equipment would a phlebotomist carry on his or her tray for a skin puncture procedure?
    a holder, needle, evacuated tube
    b safety lancet, microcollection container, sterile gauze
    c Simplate, filter paper, stopwatch
    d syringe, heparin, ice

520. Heel warmers should not exceed what temperature?
    a 39°C
    b 40°C
    c 41°C
    d 42°C

521. The depth of a heel puncture should never exceed:
    a 2.0 mm
    b 3.0 mm
    c 2.0 cm
    d 3.0 cm

522. A sharp device used to puncture the skin prior to capillary blood collection is called a:
    a   bleeding time device
    b   lancet
    c   multisample needle
    d   syringe

523. What engineering control is prescribed by OSHA to reduce accidental sharps injury when using lancets?
    a   lasers
    b   retractable blades
    c   reusable blades
    d   standardized incision

524. Which of the following should never be used to perform a skin puncture?
    a   1.75 mm safety lancets
    b   1.85 mm safety lancets
    c   1.90 mm safety lancets
    d   surgical blades

525. Obese patients have a body mass index (BMI) in excess of:
    a   15 kg/m^2
    b   20 kg/m^2
    c   25 kg/m^2
    d   30 kg/m^2

526. Veins that are blocked and prevent blood flow are termed:
    a   occipital
    b   occluded
    c   scleriasis
    d   sclerosed

527. Veins that are hardened are termed:
    a   occipital
    b   occluded
    c   scleriasis
    d   sclerosed

528. Fluctuations in the body's function or fluids during the daytime hours are called:
    a   abnormal
    b   diurnal rhythms
    c   nocturnal rhythms
    d   reference ranges

Questions

Specimen Collection

529. Small, non-raised bruises the size of a pinpoint are called:
    a patella
    b pedicel
    c petechiae
    d pellicle

530. The liberation of hemoglobin into the plasma following destruction of red blood cells is called:
    a hemagglutination
    b hemoconcentration
    c hemolysis
    d hemostasis

531. What is the medical term for the following symptoms: dizziness, pallor, sweating, clammy skin, unconsciousness?
    a emesis
    b hematoma
    c syncope
    d tetany

532. The angle formed between the patient's arm and the needle is called the angle of:
    a indwelling line
    b incision
    c insertion
    d input

533. Swelling caused by an abnormal accumulation of fluid is called:
    a edema
    b emesis
    c hemostasis
    d hematoma

534. A substance that prevents the breakdown of glucose by red blood cells is:
    a glucagon
    b glycolytic inhibitor
    c insulin resistant
    d International Normalized Ratio

535. What value represents a comparison of a patient's prothrombin time result to a reference range result?
    a blood-to-anticoagulant ratio
    b International Classification of Diseases
    c international normalized ratio
    d lecithin-to-sphingomyelin ratio

Specimen Collection — **Questions**

536. Which of the following medical specialties focuses on the care and treatment of the elderly?
    a   gastroenterology
    b   geriatrics
    c   pediatrics
    d   psychiatry

537. The state of being freely open (the opposite of occluded) is called:
    a   aggregated
    b   parenteral
    c   patency
    d   sclerosed

538. A method of medication administration which involves piercing the skin or mucous membranes is:
    a   parenteral
    b   patency
    c   pathogenesis
    d   pre-evacuation

539. The antecubital area (antecubital fossa) is located:
    a   anterior to the elbow on the arm
    b   dorsal side of the hand
    c   palmer surface of the hand
    d   posterior to the elbow on the arm

540. A return flow of blood from an evacuated tube into a patient's arm during a venipuncture procedure is called:
    a   reagent
    b   reflex
    c   reflux
    d   refractile

541. The phlebotomist inspects the antecubital area (antecubital fossa) of a patient and notes that the area surrounding the puncture site is purple, accompanied by swelling of the puncture site. What is the name of this condition?
    a   hematoma
    b   hemangioma
    c   lipoma
    d   lymphoma

542. A substance being analyzed is a(n):
    a   analyte
    b   biorhythm
    c   circadian rhythm
    d   diurnal variation

Questions
Specimen Collection

543. The term meaning breakdown of glucose is:
    a glucagon
    b glycogenesis
    c glycolysis
    d hypoglycemia

544. Daily changes that occur during daytime hours in the body and reflected in test results are called:
    a abnormal
    b diurnal rhythms
    c critical (panic) values
    d reference ranges

545. The condition in which the plasma portion of the blood filters into the tissues is called:
    a hematoma
    b hemoconcentration
    c hemolysis
    d hemostasis

546. A physician would most likely order a blood culture on a patient who has:
    a AML
    b CABG
    c COPD
    d FUO

547. The presence of bacteria and their toxins in the bloodstream is called:
    a bacteremia
    b basophilia
    c hyperemia
    d septicemia

548. The term that means "without air" is:
    a aerobic
    b anaerobic
    c afebrile
    d antimicrobial

549. The term that means "with air" is:
    a aerobic
    b anaerobic
    c afebrile
    d antimicrobial

Specimen Collection — Questions

550. Which of the following agencies is responsible for developing standards of practice in clinical laboratory testing?
    a   American Society for Clinical Pathology
    b   Clinical Laboratory Standards Institute
    c   Food & Drug Administration
    d   National Accrediting Agency for Clinical Laboratory Sciences

551. Extreme, deep, sideways redirection of the needle is:
    a   consistent with CLSI standards
    b   necessary
    c   probing
    d   standard protocol

552. If a skin puncture site is warmed prior to blood collection, the specimen is said to be:
    a   arterialized
    b   concentrated
    c   hemolyzed
    d   ischemic

553. Preexamination replaces which of the following terms related to laboratory testing?
    a   preanalytical
    b   preemptive
    c   premature
    d   postanalytical

554. The preexamination/preanalytical process includes practices beginning with:
    a   appropriate test methodologies for the analysis requested
    b   completing all STAT requests first
    c   reporting the final result
    d   requisition by the patient's physician

555. The preexamination/preanalytical process ends when the specimen has been:
    a   delegated to a phlebotomist
    b   entered into the computer
    c   ordered by the patient's physician
    d   received in the lab

556. A range of values compiled from data based on results obtained from healthy individuals including high and low limits are:
    a   abnormal results
    b   compromised
    c   quality control parameters
    d   reference ranges

Questions

Specimen Collection

557. Early in the morning, when a patient is resting, fasting for approximately 12 hours and in a supine position is:

   a   a coma
   b   anatomic position
   c   asleep
   d   basal state

558. Once a specimen arrives in the laboratory, it is issued a unique number used to correlate the patient's specimen and all procedures conducted. That number is called a(n):

   a   accession number
   b   derivative number
   c   integer number
   d   standard number

559. The term describing adverse effects of medical treatment is:

   a   idiopathic
   b   iatrogenic
   c   iatrology
   d   incompetence

560. Extensive loss of blood resulting in death is:

   a   anaphylactic
   b   exsanguination
   c   exothermic
   d   urticaria

561. Any ingredient added to an evacuated tube to perform a specific function, such as prevention or promotion of coagulation is called a(n):

   a   additive
   b   anticoagulant
   c   clot activator
   d   glycolytic inhibitor

Specimen Collection — Explanations

The following items have been identified as appropriate for those preparing for both PBT & QDP examinations.

1. **a** Accession is the process required to ensure a patient specimen and corresponding documentation absolutely correlate to the same patient.
   [McCall 7e, p218]

2. **c** The preexamination/preanalytical process of testing begins with generation of a requisition following a physician's order for a laboratory analysis.
   [Garza 10e, p8]

3. **c** Multipart manual requisition forms may serve both as a requisition and report forms. Multipart manual requisition forms often serve as a back-up system for requisitioning laboratory tests and reporting results when a laboratory information system is off-line.
   [Garza 10e, p68]

Please consult the diagram below for questions 4-10 regarding laboratory requisition interpretation.

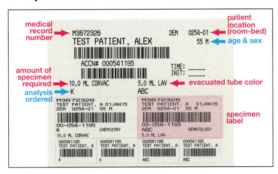

4. **b** Phlebotomists are required to interpret information presented on laboratory requisitions. The item at the arrow in the figure indicates the patient's medical record number. The medical record number is a unique number assigned to each patient.
   [McCall 7e, p217-219]

5. **d** Phlebotomists are required to interpret information presented on laboratory requisitions. The item labeled "B" in the diagram indicates the amount of specimen required to perform the analysis, in this case, 10 mL.
   [McCall 7e, p217-219]

6. **a** Phlebotomists are required to interpret information presented on laboratory requisitions. The item at the arrow in the figure indicates the analysis ordered by the patient's physician, in this case, K, which is the abbreviation for potassium.
   [McCall 7e, p217-219]

Explanations

Specimen Collection

7. **d** Phlebotomists are required to interpret information presented on laboratory requisitions. The item at the arrow in the figure indicates the patient's location, including room (0254) and bed number (01).
[McCall 7e, p217-219]

8. **b** Phlebotomists are required to interpret information presented on laboratory requisitions. The item at the arrow in the figure indicates the patient's age (55) and sex (male).
[McCall 7e, p217-219]

9. **d** Phlebotomists are required to interpret information presented on laboratory requisitions. The item at the arrow in the figure indicates the evacuated tube stopper color (lavender) required for the analysis requested by the physician, automated blood count (ABC).
[McCall 7e, p217-219]

10. **d** Phlebotomists are required to interpret information presented on laboratory requisitions. The light and dark bands are bar codes. Barcodes relate to specific alphanumeric symbols and may code for information including but not limited to patient name, medical number or test requested. The item within the highlighted area in the figure indicates the label that may be affixed to the patient's specimen following collection and before leaving the patient.
[Garza 10e, p68-69]

11. **d** Requisitions may be generated manually or using the health care facility's computer system. Computer generated requisitions that include a barcode feature are most accurate and error-free.
[McCall 7e, p217-219]

12. **c** Once generated, requisitions for laboratory analysis become part of the patient's medical record.
[McCall 7e, p217-218]

13. **d** Requisitions for laboratory analysis are typically initiated by the patient's physician.
[McCall 7e, p217-218]

14. **d** Outpatient requisition forms requesting laboratory analysis often include billing and coding information. Billing and coding information is not typically included on an inpatient requisition form.
[McCall 7e, p217-218]

15. **c** Requisitions for laboratory analysis are typically initiated by the patient's physician and may be generated manually or by the health care facility's computer system.
[McCall 7e, p217-218]

Specimen Collection — Explanations

16. **c** Bar codes and radio frequency identification (RFID) systems are dependent upon the health care facility's computerized network. If the computer system is offline, requisitions must be submitted manually, using the multipart manual requisition form.
[McCall 7e, p218, 379]

17. **c** Computer generated requisitions, including bar codes and radio frequency identification (RFID) systems are dependent upon the health care facility's computerized network and characteristically include specimen requirements as part of the requisition generated. Multipart manual requisition form characteristically do not include specimen requirements.
[McCall 7e, p218, 379]

18. **a** Bar codes include a series of stripes and white spaces corresponding to letters and numbers. Bar codes are used to document patient name and identification numbers.
[McCall 7e, p217-219]

19. **d** Following specimen collection and specimen labeling, the phlebotomist must manually write the date and time of collection and also her initials on the specimen tube before leaving the patient.
[CLSI Standard GP41, p29]

20. **a** Patients have the right to know the name of the person collecting his/her blood, the department he represents and if the phlebotomist is a student. Phlebotomists should never attempt to provide an explanation of the purpose of the test ordered.
[McCall 7e, p220-221]

21. **b** Most of the specimens collected from inpatients are collected very early in the morning, so oftentimes the patients are sleeping when the phlebotomist arrives to collect the blood specimen. Patients cannot participate in the identification process if they are sleeping, so the phlebotomist should gently wake the patients, taking care not to startle them.
[McCall 7e, p220-221]

22. **b** Patients cannot participate in the identification process if they are unconscious, so the phlebotomist should ask a nurse or family member to verify the patient's identity and record the name of the person making the identification. Once the patient has been identified, the phlebotomist should speak to the patient as though he were awake.
[McCall 7e, p223]

23. **a** If a patient is not in is/her room when the phlebotomist arrives, the phlebotomist should first ask the patient's designated healthcare proveder (often a nurse) for the patient's location. If the patient is not available, the phlebotomist should follow the institution's policies for documenting this information, including the time and why the patient was not available.
[McCall 7e, p220-221]

Explanations

Specimen Collection

24. **b** Once the phlebotomist has located the patient, the phlebotomist should introduce himself and tell the patient he is there to collect a blood specimen for a test ordered by the patient's physician.
[McCall 7e, p220-221]

25. **b** Most patients have never seen the internal workings of a clinical laboratory or the professionals who work there. The only laboratory professional patients regularly encounter is the phlebotomist. Therefore, the phlebotomist serves as the patient's window to the laboratory and has the greatest public relations responsibility.
[McCall 7e, p4, 7]

26. **a** First impressions count. Most people form opinions of a person within the first 3 seconds of meeting them so the first 3 seconds of a patient encounter will set the tone.
[McCall 7e, p7-8]

27. **b** Oftentimes, if a patient is hard-of-hearing or deaf the patient's limitation will be noted on the sign over the patient's bed. However, the phlebotomist should also assess the patient to ensure understanding of the procedure by asking questions such as, "Have you ever had your blood drawn before?" If the patient is hearing impaired, the phlebotomist should look directly at the patient and speak slowly and slightly louder than normal directly to the patient.
[Garza 10e, p48]

28. **a** Pace is the term used to describe the rate and urgency of a person's speech.
[Garza 10e, p50]

29. **d** Tone is the term used to describe the pitch, including high and low tones, of a person's speech.
[Garza 10e, p50]

30. **b** Oftentimes, if a patient is blind, the patient's limitation will be noted on the sign over the patient's bed. However, the phlebotomist should also assess the patient to ensure understanding of the procedure by asking questions such as, "Have you ever had your blood drawn before?" If the patient is blind, the phlebotomist should look directly at the patient and speak slowly in a normal tone of voice directly to the patient.
[Garza 10e, p48-50]

31. **a** It is acceptable and appropriate to say to a person who is visually impaired, "It was nice to see you."
[Garza 10e, p50]

32. **d** The appropriate way to offer assistance to a visually impaired patient is to offer the patient an arm and lead him/her into the draw station, advising the patient of items that may be in the way.
[Garza 10e, p50]

Specimen Collection — Explanations

33. **d**   80-90% of communication is nonverbal.
[Garza 10e, p54]

34. **b**   A pregnancy test on a 16-year-old patient could be ordered for a variety of reasons, so the phlebotomist should answer the question as truthfully as possible, but without provoking alarm in the patient. In circumstances such as these, it is always best to refer the patients to their physicians while reassuring them this is a commonly ordered test.
[Garza 10e, p62]

35. **c**   The phlebotomist should always respond truthfully when a patient asks if a venipuncture procedure will hurt even if the patient is a child and reassure the patient that the procedure will be over quickly.
[Garza 10e, p62]

36. **c**   Informed consent is a legal term documenting a patient's voluntary and competent consent to examination, touching, and treatment by a qualified health care provider.
[Garza 10e, p92, 631]

37. **a**   Implied consent occurs when a physician determines that medical intervention is required to save the patient's life or to prevent permanent medical damage.
[Garza 10e, p93]

38. **c**   Parents or legal guardians may legally provide informed consent on behalf of their minor children.
[Garza 10e, p91]

39. **a**   The intentional touching of another person without consent is the legal definition of battery. Battery always occurs with an assault. The patient clearly asked the phlebotomist to refrain from taking blood. The phlebotomist could be charged with assault and battery for collecting the patient's blood without consent.
[Garza 10e, p88]

40. **b**   The intentional touching of another person without consent is the legal definition of battery. The patient clearly asked the phlebotomist to refrain from taking blood. The phlebotomist should inform the patient's designated healthcare provider (often a nurse) of the patient's refusal and document the patient's refusal to have blood drawn per the institution's policy.
[McCall 7e, p226-227]

41. **b**   The phlebotomist must take a patient's a history of fainting following a blood collection procedure very seriously. The appropriate course of action is to move the patient to a reclining chair or to a bed to ensure the patient's safety in the event of fainting (syncope) following the procedure.
[McCall 7e, p286]

Explanations   Specimen Collection

42. **d**   Patients should not have any foreign objects in their mouth during the venipuncture procedure. In this instance, the patient should be asked to discard their gum prior to the procedure to eliminate a choking hazard.
[CLSI Standard GP41, p13]

43. **d**   Once the venipuncture procedure is completed, the specimen tubes are labeled and the trash appropriately discarded, the phlebotomist should thank the patient and quietly exit the room.
[McCall 7e, p244]

44. **a**   Gloves should be removed following completion of the venipuncture procedure. Gowns, safety goggles, and N95 fit-tested masks are not routinely used for routine venipuncture procedures.
[McCall 7e, p244]

45. **d**   Gloves should be removed aseptically (in a pathogen free manner) following completion of a procedure.
[McCall 7e, p70-71]

46. **a**   To aseptically remove gloves following a venipuncture procedure, the cuff of the first glove should be grasped and pulled over the hand, inside out and into the palm of the second hand. The second glove should be removed by slipping the fingers into the cuff of the second glove and removing that glove pulling it so the contaminated surface is over the first glove and all contaminated surfaces are contained with the second glove once removed.
[McCall 7e, p71]

47. **c**   Immediately after gloves are removed, the phlebotomist should sanitize his/her hands.
[McCall 7e, p244]

48. **b**   The Joint Commission (TJC) requires confirmation of at least 2 patient identifiers, starting with the patient's first and last names. Additionally, CLSI Standard GP41 requires patients to state and spell their first and last names. A second identifier such as the patient's date of birth or medical record number is also required. The phlebotomist must verify that information with the requisition and the patient's identification band. The specimen must be labeled after collecting the specimen and while in the patient's presence. The third identifier required by CLSI Standard GP41 is the verification of specimen labeling information. Before leaving the patient, the phlebotomist must verify the patient identification information on the specimen labels with the patient's wristband or present the labeled specimens to the patient for confirmation.
[CLSI Standard GP41, p10, 28-29; Garza 10e, p63]

49. **a**   CLSI Standard GP41 requires patients to state and spell their first and last names as the first step in patient identification.
[CLSI Standard GP41, p10]

Specimen Collection — Explanations

50. **d** CLSI Standard GP41 requires patients to state and spell their first and last names as the first step in patient identification.
[CLSI Standard GP41, p10]

51. **d** CLSI Standard GP41 requires patients to state and spell their first and last names. The phlebotomist must verify that information with the requisition and the patient's wristband, when applicable. The specimen must be labeled after collecting the specimen and while in the patient's presence. Before leaving the patient, the phlebotomist must verify the patient identification information on the specimen labels with the patient's wristband or present the labeled specimens to the patient for confirmation.
[CLSI Standard GP41, p10, 28-29]

52. **d** The phlebotomist correctly completed the initial steps of patient identification. Step 1: The mother stated and spelled the baby's first and last names. Step 2: The identification bracelet was appropriately attached to the baby. The information provided by the mother, posted on the baby's identification bracelet and included on the requisition matched, so the phlebotomist may proceed with the blood collection procedure. The phlebotomist must document the name of the mother as verifier of the baby's identity, following institutional policies.
[CLSI Standard GP41, p11, 234]

53. **a** The emergency department of the hospital is the area of patient care at highest risk for patient identification errors. Within the context of the commotion often associated with treating trauma patients, sometimes blood specimens must be collected before a patient can be absolutely identified making this area of the hospital at highest risk for patient identification errors.
[McCall 7e, p223-224]

54. **d** The medical record number is the one identifier on a patient's wristband unique to each patient and that will remain constant throughout the patient's hospital stay.
[McCall 7e, p215, 222]

55. **c** The patient's name, medical record number, and date of birth or age on the requisition must match the patient's wristband exactly. If discrepancies are noted, they must be resolved with the patient's nurse or caregiver as specified by the facility's policy before the specimen may be obtained.
[CLSI Standard GP41]

56. **a** The patient's identification bracelet must be attached to the patient, usually the wrist, but an ankle is also acceptable. In this instance, the identification bracelet is on the patient's nightstand, so the phlebotomist must ask the patient's designated healthcare provider (often a nurse) to affix the wristband to the correct patient before drawing the specimen.
[McCall 7e, p223]

Explanations
Specimen Collection

57. d Type and crossmatch tests are ordered prior to the transfusion of certain blood products. Although not mandated by regulatory agencies, some facilities may require the use of an additional identification bracelet and labeling system when specimens are being drawn for type and crossmatch.
[McCall 7e, p221-223]

58. b The most important step in specimen collection is accurate patient identification and its corollary, specimen labeling.
[Garza 10e, p324-325]

59. c There are 2 agencies prescribing standards for patient identification procedures. The agencies are The Joint Commission (TJC) and CLSI Standard GP41. There is overlap between the two standards of practice, with CLSI Standard being the most stringent, requiring a 3-step process for patient identification. The 3-step process for patient identification prescribed by CLSI Standard GP41 is as follows:
1. Ask the patient to state *and spell* their first and last names. Verify the information provided by the patient with the requisition, labels, and the patient's wristband, if available.
2. Confirm the patient's identity with a second identifier, such as a birthdate. Verify the information provided by the patient with the requisition, labels, and the patient's wristband, if available.
3. After collecting and labeling the specimen, confirm the information on the labels with the patient's wristband or if there is no wristband, invite the patent to verify the label information.
[CLSI Standard GP41, p10, 28-29; Garza 10e, p323-324]

60. b The toddler cannot identify himself so a parent, guardian, or health care worker must identify the patient and spell the toddler's first and last names. The name of the person providing the information must be documented. Also, the patient's wristband is attached to the crib and not the toddler so the phlebotomist must not collect the blood specimen until the wristband is properly affixed to the patient. The phlebotomist must verify identification information with the requisition and the patient's wristband and document the person providing the patient's name. The specimen must be labeled after collecting the specimen and while in the patient's presence. Before leaving the patient, the phlebotomist must verify the patient identification information on the specimen labels using the patient's wristband or by presenting the labeled specimens to the patient's representative for confirmation.
[CLSI Standard GP41, p10-11 & 28-29]

61. **a** The comatose patient cannot identify himself so a family member, guardian, or health care worker must identify the patient. Additionally, CLSI Standard GP41 requires the patient's representative to state and spell the patient's first and last names and document the person providing the information. The phlebotomist must verify that information with the requisition and the patient's wristband. The specimen must be labeled after collecting the specimen and while in the patient's presence. Before leaving the patient, the phlebotomist must verify the patient identification information on the specimen labels using the patient's wristband or by presenting the labeled specimens to the patient's representative for confirmation.
[CLSI Standard GP41, p10, 28-29]

62. **c** The patient's name, medical record number, and date of birth or age on the requisition must match the patient's wristband exactly. In this case, the middle initials do not match, which is a discrepancy. If discrepancies are noted, they must be resolved with the patient's patient's designated healthcare provider (often a nurse) before the specimen may be obtained.
[CLSI Standard GP41, p9]

63. **c** In the absence of identification, a mechanism for positively identifying the patient must be employed. In this case, the jogger should be assigned a temporary master identification number, following the institution's procedure. Once the patient's identity is confirmed and a permanent identification number is assigned, all test results assigned to the temporary identification number must be cross-referenced to the permanent number.
[CLSI Standard GP41, p11, 235]

64. **c** The patient's identification bracelet must be attached to the patient, usually the wrist, but an ankle is also acceptable. In this instance, the identification bracelet is on the railing of the patient's cart, so the phlebotomist must ask the patient's designated healthcare provider (often a nurse) to affix the correct wristband to the patient before drawing the specimen.
[CLSI Standard GP41, p9]

65. **c** The patient's name, medical record number, and date of birth or age on the requisition must match the patient's wristband exactly. In this case, the patient's age printed on the requisition does not match the physical characteristics of the patient, which is a discrepancy. If discrepancies are noted, they must be resolved with the patient's designated healthcare provider (often a nurse) before the specimen may be obtained.
[CLSI Standard GP41, p9]

66. **d** All inpatients must have identification bracelets attached to their person. However, facility policy may exempt this practice. Examples may include long term care facilities and psychiatric units. The phlebotomist must follow the facility's policy for patient identification in these unique circumstances.
[CLSI Standard GP41, p9-11]

Explanations

Specimen Collection

67. **c** Outpatients typically provide photo identification at the time of registration, which is often verified by the registration staff. Outpatients may not be issued identification bracelets so after calling the patient to the draw station, the phlebotomist must ask the patient to state and spell their first and last name and provide confirmation of a third identifier, such as a driver's license or other photo ID.
[CLSI Standard GP41, p9-10; Garza 10e, p325-327]

68. **a** The use of bar code technology is accurate and efficient, reducing the number of transcription errors and increasing the speed associated with specimen processing.
[Garza 10e, p68-69]

69. **a** Bar codes are light and dark bands that correlate to numbers and letters. The band sequence corresponds to patient names, identification numbers, and other information. Bar codes may be scanned using light or laser technology to enter information into the laboratory information system.
[Garza 10e, p68]

70. **b** Radio frequency identification employs silicon chips and wireless receivers to remotely enter information into the laboratory information system. This system also eliminates the need for a laser or light source to scan a patient's label.
[Garza 10e, p71]

71. **b** Patients scheduled for a test that requires fasting should be instructed not to eat any food or drink any beverages, except water unless contraindicated, for at least 8-12 hours prior to specimen collection. Fasting does not include abstinence from water, unless the patient is NPO for a different procedure. Drinking water while fasting prior to a blood test will allow the patient to remain hydrated which will facilitate blood collection.
[Garza 10e, 289]

72. **c** Triglyceride analysis requires at least a 12-14 hour fast instead of the standard 8-12 hour fast. However, fasting longer than 14 hours prior to collecting a specimen for triglyceride analysis will falsely elevate triglyceride levels in the patient's blood.
[McCall 7e, p460]

73. **c** Patients scheduled for a test that requires fasting should be instructed not to eat any food or drink any beverages, except water unless contraindicated, for at least 8-12 hours prior to specimen collection. Fasting does not include abstinence from water, unless the patient is NPO for a different procedure. Drinking water while fasting prior to a blood test will allow the patient to remain hydrated which will facilitate blood collection and will more accurately reflect the patient's basal state.
[Garza 10e, p289]

Specimen Collection — Explanations

74. **d** Patients should never fast longer than 14 hours prior to blood collection. Fasting longer than 14 hours can create health issues for the patient, such as electrolyte imbalance and cardiac dysrhythmias. Blood specimens collected after a patient has fasted longer than 14 hours may result in false elevations of the following analytes: amino acids, bilirubin, fatty acids, glucagon, growth hormone, ketones, lactate, and triglycerides.
[McCall 7e, p406-407]

75. **a** Patients should never fast longer than 14 hours prior to blood collection. Fasting longer than 14 hours can create health issues for the patient, such as electrolyte imbalance and cardiac dysrhythmias. Blood specimens collected after a patient has fasted longer than 14 hours may result in false elevations of the following analytes: amino acids, bilirubin, fatty acids, glucagon, growth hormone, ketones, lactate, and triglycerides.
[McCall 7e, p406-407]

76. **a** Patients should never fast longer than 14 hours prior to blood collection. Fasting longer than 14 hours can create health issues for the patient, such as electrolyte imbalance and cardiac dysrhythmias. Blood specimens collected after a patient has fasted longer than 14 hours may result in false elevations of the following analytes: amino acids, bilirubin, fatty acids, glucagon, growth hormone, ketones, lactate, and triglycerides.
[McCall 7e, p406-407]

77. **c** Patients should never fast longer than 14 hours prior to blood collection. Fasting longer than 14 hours can create health issues for the patient, such as electrolyte imbalance and cardiac dysrhythmias. Blood specimens collected after a patient has fasted longer than 14 hours may result in false decreases of the following analytes: glucose, HDL cholesterol, insulin, lactic dehydrogenase, T3.
[McCall 7e, p406-407]

78. **c** Patients should never fast longer than 14 hours prior to blood collection. Fasting longer than 14 hours can create health issues for the patient, such as electrolyte imbalance and cardiac dysrhythmias. Blood specimens collected after a patient has fasted longer than 14 hours may result in false decreases of the following analytes: glucose, HDL cholesterol, insulin, lactic dehydrogenase, T3.
[McCall 7e, p406-407]

79. **d** Patients should never fast longer than 14 hours prior to blood collection. Fasting longer than 14 hours can create health issues for the patient, such as electrolyte imbalance and cardiac dysrhythmias. Blood specimens collected after a patient has fasted longer than 14 hours may result in false decreases of the following analytes: glucose, HDL cholesterol, insulin, lactic dehydrogenase, T3.
[McCall 7e, p406-407]

Explanations
Specimen Collection

80. **c** A plasma or serum specimen may appear cloudy or turbid (lipemic) if a patient has ingested fatty substances such as butter, cheese, cream, and meat. Nutritional supplements high in fat content may also cause lipemic plasma or serum.
[Garza 10e, p290]

81. **c** A plasma or serum specimen may appear cloudy or turbid (lipemic) if a patient has ingested fatty substances such as butter, cheese, cream, and meat. Nutritional supplements high in fat content may also cause lipemic plasma or serum.
[Garza 10e, p290]

82. **d** Obese patients may present challenges for the phlebotomist, specifically during site selection as part of a venipuncture procedure, because their veins are not readily apparent either visually or through palpation. A phlebotomist is experiencing difficulty locating a suitable vein on an obese patient may want to first ask the patient, "Where have you been drawn successfully before?" Oftentimes, the patient can provide a strong recommendation for site selection.
[Garza 10e, p290]

83. **c** Sclerosed or hardened, veins are often the result of frequent, multiple venipuncture procedures and the resulting inflammatory response.
[Garza 10e, p290]

84. **a** Areas of the skin that have been recently burned should be avoided during phlebotomy procedures because the skin is very sensitive and prone to infection.
[Garza 10e, p291]

85. **c** Scarred areas of the skin resulting from burn injuries should be avoided during phlebotomy procedures because veins are very difficult to palpate through scar tissue and have impaired circulation, which may falsely alter test results.
[Garza 10e, p291]

86. **d** The area should be avoided when selecting a site for venipuncture because it is prone to infection, may have impaired circulation, and the dye from the tattoo could interfere with laboratory results.
[Garza 10e, p291]

87. **c** After running a marathon, the following analytes will be elevated 24 hours after the race: alanine aminotransferase (ALT), aspartate aminotransferase (AST), bilirubin, blood urea nitrogen (BUN), creatinine, and uric acid.
[Garza 10e, p292]

88. **c** If a patient experiences high anxiety associated with a phlebotomy procedure, certain analytes will be temporarily affected. White cell counts may be temporarily elevated as a result of the patient's emotional stress.
[Garza 10e, p292]

Specimen Collection — Explanations

89. **b** If a patient experiences high anxiety associated with a phlebotomy procedure, certain analytes will be temporarily affected. Some may be temporarily decreased as a result of the patient's emotional stress, including serum iron levels.
[Garza 10e, p292]

90. **c** If a patient experiences high anxiety associated with a phlebotomy procedure, certain analytes will be temporarily affected. Studies have documented marked increases in white cell counts in infants who are violently crying in response to a heelstick procedure. One report documents increases over baseline WBC of 140% as a result of the baby's emotional stress.
[Garza 10e, p292]

91. **b** Certain blood component levels may fluctuate throughout the day (diurnal) or over a 24-hour cycle (circadian). The analyte category most susceptible to diurnal variation includes hormones, such as adrenocorticotropic hormone (ACTH), cortisol, and thyroid stimulating hormone.
[Garza 10e, p292]

92. **c** Some analytes susceptible to diurnal variations are higher in the afternoon, including creatinine, glucose, and eosinophil counts.
[McCall 7e, p275, 277]

93. **c** When a person's position changes from supine to standing, water molecules shift from the bloodstream to the tissues and may decrease plasma volume up to 10%.
[McCall 7e, p275, 277]

94. **a** Travel over several time zones may upset a patient's diurnal rhythm and may take several days to return to baseline levels.
[Garza 10e, p293]

95. **c** Laboratory test results can vary considerably across the life span. For example, estrogen levels will be higher in a 20-year-old female than in an 85-year-old female.
[Garza 10e, p293]

96. **d** Laboratory test results can vary considerably across the life span. For example, triglyceride levels will typically be higher in a 85-year-old female than in an 20-year-old female.
[Garza 10e, p293]

97. **c** Patients in renal failure often display edema. Edematous areas should be avoided for venipuncture because site selection will be very challenging and the specimen may be contaminated with excess tissue fluid. The phlebotomist should first determine if another non-edematous site is available for venipuncture site selection. If a non-edematous venipuncture site is not available, the patient's physician should be consulted before collecting the blood specimen.
[Garza 10e, p293]

Explanations
Specimen Collection

98. c Patients in renal failure often display edema. In this case, both arms were edematous. Edematous areas should be avoided for venipuncture because site selection will be very challenging and the specimen may be contaminated with excess tissue fluid and therefore diluted. The phlebotomist should first determine if another non-edematous site is available for venipuncture site selection. If a non-edematous venipuncture site is not available, the patient's physician should be consulted before collecting the blood specimen.
[Garza 10e, p293]

99. d Winged infusion needles are typically used on the veins of patients who have small veins and are difficult to draw such as burn, very young pediatric, geriatric, and oncology patients.
[Garza 10e, p273, 350]

100. d A heparin lock is an indwelling catheter with a stopcock attached providing easy access to a patient's vein for medication administration or blood specimen collection. A syringe may be used by specifically trained personnel to collect blood specimens from a heparin lock. Following collection, the blood must be transferred to an evacuated tube using a safety transfer device.
[Garza 10e, p446-447]

101. c The lumen size of the vein selected for venipuncture is used by the phlebotomist to select the best needle gauge size for a venipuncture procedure.
[McCall 7e, p191-192]

102. d Creatine kinase levels may remain elevated for up to 24 hours following exercise.
[McCall 7e, p276]

103. d Thiazide diuretics may impact the levels of certain analytes, such as enzymes. It is ultimately the physician's responsibility to monitor the impact of medications on patient laboratory results.
[McCall 7e, p275-276]

104. b There are three instructions patients receive to prepare for a 3-hour glucose tolerance test: 1) ingest approximately 150 g of carbohydrates for 3 days prior to the test; 2) fast for 8-12 hours before the test, but do not fast more than 12 hours before the test; 3) refrain from strenuous exercise for at least 12 hours prior to the test.
[Garza 10e, p485]

105. c There are three instructions patients receive to prepare for a 3-hour glucose tolerance test: 1) ingest approximately 150 g of carbohydrates for 3 days prior to the test; 2) fast for 8-12 hours before the test, but do not fast more than 12 hours before the test; 3) refrain from strenuous exercise for at least 12 hours prior to the test.
[Garza 10e, p485]

106. c There are three instructions patients receive to prepare for a 3-hour glucose tolerance test: 1) ingest approximately 150 g of carbohydrates for 3 days prior to the test; 2) fast for 8-12 hours before the test, but do not fast more than 12 hours before the test; 3) refrain from strenuous exercise for at least 12 hours prior to the test.
[Garza 10e, p485]

107. b NPO is the abbreviation that means nil per os or nothing by mouth. The phlebotomist should confirm the patient is fasting.
[Garza 10e, p364]

108. a "Stat" means the test results are urgently needed and must be collected immediately. However, the patient's privacy must be respected, so the phlebotomist should announce herself and wait a moment before pulling back the curtain to approach the bedside.
[Garza 10e, p364]

109. c "Stat" means the test results are urgently needed and must be collected immediately. However, the patient's privacy while in conversation with her priest must be respected, so the phlebotomist should announce herself, explain she has a stat specimen to obtain and wait to be invited to the bedside.
[McCall 7e, p220-221]

110. d Syringes should not be used routinely for blood collection. Control over the amount of pressure exerted on a patient's vein is the advantage of using a syringe instead of an evacuated tube system to collect a blood specimen. This advantage may be most useful when collecting blood specimens from patients with thin, fragile veins.
[CLSI Standard GP41, p25-27; Garza 10e, p351]

111. a Health care providers must be trained and authorized to access central venous access devices (CVAD) for specimen collection. Phlebotomists may assist in this procedure by transferring the specimen into the correct evacuated tubes.
[McCall 7e, p283]

112. c "Stat" means the test results are urgently needed and must be collected immediately. However, the patient's privacy while in conversation with his physician must be respected, so the phlebotomist should announce herself, explain she has a stat specimen to obtain and wait to be invited to the bedside.
[McCall 7e, p220-221]

113. c When a person's position changes from supine to standing, water molecules shift from the bloodstream to the tissues and may cause certain analytes to increase.
[Garza 10e, p292]

Explanations
Specimen Collection

114. d The extended family may gather to support the patient during his/her illness. The phlebotomist should politely knock on the door, introduce himself, indicate that he is there to collect a blood specimen, and politely ask the family to wait outside the room.
[McCall 7e, p220]

115. c Triglyceride analysis requires a fasting specimen. The patient is eating breakfast (not fasting) so the patient's designated healthcare provider (often a nurse) should be consulted about the appropriate course of action. If the nurse directs the phlebotomist to collect the specimen, the phlebotomist should document the name of the healthcare provider giving that instruction and write "nonfasting" on the requisition.
[Garza 10e, p289, 591]

116. c Glucose analysis requires an 8-12 hour fast. The patient is eating breakfast (not fasting) so the patient's designated healthcare provider (often a nurse) should be consulted about the appropriate course of action. If the nurse directs the phlebotomist to collect the specimen, the phlebotomist should document the name of the healthcare provider giving that instruction and write "nonfasting" on the requisition.
[Garza 10e, p289, 590]

117. d If a patient's allergy is noted, as in this case, the phlebotomist must make every effort to use an alternative product so the patient is not exposed to the allergen. In this case, the patient is allergic to the adhesive on the bandage, so a self-adhesive gauze, such as Coban should be used.
[Garza 10e, p291]

118. c OSHA's blood-borne pathogen standard mandates gloves must be worn during blood collection procedures.
[CLSI Standard GP41, p22; Garza 10e, p110, 121]

119. b Petechiae are small, pinpoint bruises in the skin indicative of a coagulation abnormality. If a phlebotomist notes petechiae on a patient's skin, she should anticipate the patient will bleed longer than usual following venipuncture.
[Garza 10e, p634]

120. d A patient with active tuberculosis will likely be housed in an airborne infection isolation room (AIIR). Anytime a health care worker enters an AIIR, he must wear a National Institute for Occupational Safety & Health (NIOSH) approved N95 fit-tested mask.
[McCall 7e, p67]

121. d As part of a mastectomy surgical procedure, lymph nodes adjacent to the breast may be removed in addition to the breast tissue. If the lymph nodes are removed, lymph fluid may abnormally accumulate in the proximal arm, a condition called lymphedema.
[Garza 10e, p293]

Specimen Collection — Explanations

122. b According to the Healthcare Infection Control Practices Advisory Committee (HICPAC), droplet precautions are required if the patient is transmitting infectious droplets larger than 5 μm and includes infectious diseases such as diphtheria, pertussis, and meningitis. Healthcare workers working within 3 feet of the patient are required to wear masks in addition to gloves required by universal precautions.
[Garza 10e, p118-120]

123. a According to the Healthcare Infection Control Practices Advisory Committee (HICPAC), contact precautions are required if the patient is known or suspected to be infected or colonized with epidemiologically significant microorganisms transmitted by direct or indirect skin-to-skin contact, such as diptheria, herpes simplex, and *Staphylococcus*. Healthcare workers administering to patients in contact isolation are required to wear gowns in addition to gloves as a universal precaution.
[Garza 10e, p119-121]

124. a Certain blood component levels may fluctuate throughout the day (diurnal), including cortisol. Peak cortisol levels characteristically occur around 8:00 AM.
[Garza 10e, p292, 364]

125. b A plasma or serum specimen may appear cloudy or turbid (lipemic) if a patient has ingested fatty substances such as butter, cheese, cream, and meat. Nutritional supplements high in fat content may also cause lipemic plasma or serum.
[Garza 10e, p290]

126. a Cortisol levels may be falsely elevated if the specimen is collected after the patient ingests caffeine.
[McCall 7e, p274]

127. a The phlebotomist should collect the blood specimen, per the nurse's directive and document the nurse's name and that the patient was nonfasting, per institutional policy.
[McCall 7e, p222-273]

128. a Hyperemesis (excessive vomiting) may cause dehydration in a patient. Dehydration may lead to hemoconcentration of the specimen.
[McCall 7e, p274]

129. c Skin puncture procedures yield capillary blood specimens in small quantities. This procedure is preferred for neonates so iatrogenic blood loss is minimized and the risk of complications resulting from blood loss is also minimized.
[Garza 10e, p231, 372-373, 596-597, 631]

Explanations

Specimen Collection

130. d Skin puncture procedures yield capillary blood specimens in small quantities. This procedure may be preferred for oncology patients so their veins may be reserved for administration of therapeutic agents, *e.g.*, chemotherapy and also to minimize iatrogenic blood loss.
[Garza 10e, p372-373, 631]

131. c Skin puncture procedures yield capillary blood specimens in small quantities. This procedure is preferred for neonates so iatrogenic blood loss is minimized and the risk of complications, including anemia, resulting from blood loss is also minimized.
[Garza 10e, p231, 372-373, 596-597, 631]

132. c "Antecubital" means in front of, or anterior to, the elbow when the patient is in anatomic position.
[Garza 10e, p173, 277, 626]

133. c "Fossa" means shallow depression. The antecubital fossa is the shallow depression located in the antecubital area in front of or anterior to the elbow when the patient is in anatomic position.
[CLSI Standard GP41, p19]

134. d The antecubital fossa is the shallow depression located in front of or anterior to the elbow when the patient is in anatomic position.
[Garza 10e, p173, 277, 626]

135. b The venous distribution patterns of the antecubital area (antecubital fossa) resemble the large case letters H and M.
[CLSI Standard GP41, p19]

136. b The venous distribution patterns of the antecubital area (antecubital fossa) resemble the large case letters H and M. The H-shaped venous pattern is found in approximately 70% of the population and includes the median cubital, cephalic, and basilic veins.
[CLSI Standard GP41, p19]

137. b The venous distribution patterns of the antecubital area (antecubital fossa) resemble the letters they are named after, ie, large case H and M. The H-shaped venous pattern is found in approximately 70% of the population and includes the median cubital, cephalic, and basilic veins.
[CLSI Standard GP41, p19]

Specimen Collection — Explanations

Please consult the diagram below for questions 138-145 regarding the H-shaped antecubital fossa anatomy.

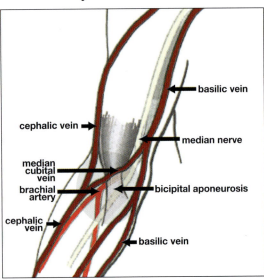

138. **c** The structure indicated by the arrow is the cephalic vein. The cephalic vein is a large, full vein appearing on the lateral side of the antecubital area (antecubital fossa). The order of vein selection in the H-shaped venous pattern is: 1) median cubital vein; 2) cephalic vein; 3) basilic vein, making the cephalic vein the second choice when selecting a site for venipuncture.
    [CLSI Standard GP41, p19-21; Garza 10e, p330-333]

139. **d** The structure indicated by the arrow is the median cubital vein. The median cubital vein is a large, full, surface vein appearing near the center of the antecubital area (antecubital fossa). The order of vein selection in the H-shaped venous pattern is: 1) median cubital vein; 2) cephalic vein; 3) basilic vein, making the median cubital vein the first choice when selecting a site for venipuncture. CLSI Standard GP41 requires a phlebotomist to look for a median cubital vein in both arms before selecting an alternative site for venipuncture.
    [CLSI Standard GP41, p19-21; Garza 10e, p330-333]

140. **b** The structure indicated by the arrow is the brachial artery. Accidental puncture of the brachial artery represents one of the risks associated with venipuncture, especially if the basilic vein is selected as a site for venipuncture.
    [CLSI Standard GP41, p19-21; Garza 10e, p331, 489-490]

141. **c** The structure indicated by the arrow is the cephalic vein. The cephalic vein continues distally after the juncture with the median cubital vein. The cephalic vein is a large, full vein appearing on the lateral side of the antecubital area (antecubital fossa). The order of vein selection in the H-shaped venous pattern is: 1) median cubital vein; 2) cephalic vein; 3) basilic vein, making the cephalic vein the second choice when selecting a site for venipuncture.
    [CLSI Standard GP41, p19-21; Garza 10e, p330-333]

Explanations

Specimen Collection

142. a The structure indicated by the arrow is the basilic vein. The basilic vein is a smaller vein appearing on the medial side of the antecubital area (antecubital fossa). The order of vein selection in the H-shaped venous pattern is: 1) median cubital vein; 2) cephalic vein; 3) basilic vein, making the basilic vein the third choice when selecting a site for venipuncture. Additionally, the basilic vein is located in proximity to the brachial artery and median nerve so other vein choices are preferred as venipuncture sites.
[CLSI Standard GP41, p19-21; Garza 10e, p330-333]

143. d The structure indicated by the arrow is the median nerve. Accidental puncture of the median nerve represents one of the risks associated with venipuncture, especially if the basilic vein is selected as a site for venipuncture.
[CLSI Standard GP41, p19-21; Garza 10e, p335]

144. b The structure indicated by the arrow is the bicipital aponeurosis, which is characteristically located beneath the median cubital and median veins. The bicipital aponeurosis is a fibrous membrane which offers some protection to underlying arteries and nerves.
[CLSI Standard GP41, p19]

145. a The structure indicated by the arrow is the basilic vein, which continues distally on the medial part of the forearm after the juncture with the median cubital vein in the H-shaped configuration. The basilic vein is a smaller vein appearing on the medial side of the antecubital area (antecubital fossa). The order of vein selection in the H-shaped venous pattern is: 1) median cubital vein; 2) cephalic vein; 3) basilic vein, making the basilic vein the third choice when selecting a site for venipuncture. Additionally, the basilic vein is located in proximity to the brachial artery and median nerve so other vein choices are preferred as venipuncture sites.
[CLSI Standard GP41, p19-21; Garza 10e, p330-335]

Please consult the diagram below for questions 146-151 regarding the M-shaped antecubital fossa anatomy.

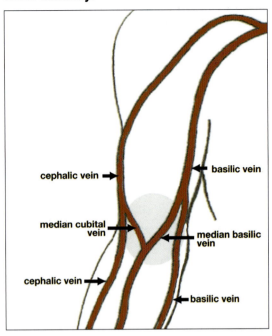

146. **c** The structure indicated by the arrow is the cephalic vein. The cephalic vein is a large, full vein appearing on the lateral side of the antecubital area (antecubital fossa). The order of vein selection is: 1) median veins; 2) cephalic vein; 3) basilic vein, making the cephalic vein the second choice when selecting a site for venipuncture.
[CLSI Standard GP41, p19-21; Garza 10e, p330-333]

147. **d** The structure indicated by the arrow is the median cephalic vein. The median cephalic vein is a large, full, surface vein appearing near the center of the antecubital area (antecubital fossa). The order of vein selection in the M-shaped venous pattern is: 1) median vein; 2) median cephalic vein; 3) median basilic vein, making the median cephalic vein the second choice when selecting a site for venipuncture. CLSI Standard GP41 requires a phlebotomist to look for a median cubital vein in both arms before selecting an alternative site for venipuncture.
[CLSI Standard GP41, p19-21; Garza 10e, p330-333]

148. **b** The structure indicated by the arrow is the cephalic vein. The cephalic vein continues distally after the juncture with the median cubital vein. The cephalic vein is a large, full vein appearing on the lateral side of the antecubital area (antecubital fossa). The order of vein selection is: 1) median vein; 2) cephalic vein; 3) basilic vein, making the cephalic vein the second choice when selecting a site for venipuncture.
[CLSI Standard GP41, p19-21; Garza 10e, p330-333]

Explanations

Specimen Collection

149. a The structure indicated by the arrow is the basilic vein. The basilic vein is a smaller vein appearing on the medial side of the antecubital area (antecubital fossa). The order of vein selection is: 1) median cubital vein; 2) cephalic vein; 3) basilic vein, making the basilic vein the third choice when selecting a site for venipuncture. Additionally, the basilic vein is located in proximity to the brachial artery and median nerve so other choices are typically preferred.
[CLSI Standard GP41, p19-21; Garza 10e, p330-333, 335]

150. c The structure indicated by the arrow is the median basilic vein. The median basilic vein is located near the center of the antecubital area (antecubital fossa). The order of vein selection in the M-shaped venous pattern is: 1) median vein; 2) median cephalic vein 3) median basilic vein, making the median basilic vein the third choice when selecting a site for venipuncture. CLSI Standard GP41 requires a phlebotomist to look for a median cubital vein in both arms before selecting an alternative site for venipuncture.
[CLSI Standard GP41, p15, 19-21; Garza 10e, p330-333, 335]

151. a The structure indicated by the arrow is the basilic vein, which continues distally on the medial part of the forearm after the juncture with the median cubital vein. The basilic vein is a smaller vein appearing on the medial side of the antecubital area (antecubital fossa). The order of vein selection is: 1) median cubital vein; 2) cephalic vein; 3) basilic vein, making the basilic vein the third choice when selecting a site for venipuncture. Additionally, the basilic vein is located in proximity to the brachial artery and median nerve so other choices are typically preferred.
[CLSI Standard GP41, p19-21; Garza 10e, p330-333, 335]

Please consult the diagram below for questions 152-154 regarding the venous anatomy on the dorsal aspect of the hand.

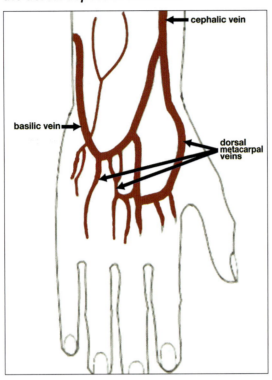

152. **a** The structure indicated by the arrow is the basilic vein. The basilic vein is a smaller vein appearing on the medial side of the antecubital area (antecubital fossa) and the dorsal side of the hand. CLSI Standard GP41 acknowledges that the larger, fuller median, median cubital, cephalic, and accessory cephalic veins of the antecubital area (antecubital fossa) are used most frequently for venipuncture, but dorsal hand veins are also acceptable. Veins on the underside of the wrist must never be used.
[CLSI Standard GP41, p15, 19-21; Garza 10e, p333-334]

153. **b** The structures indicated by the arrows represent the dorsal metacarpal veins. CLSI Standard GP41 acknowledges that the larger, fuller median, median cubital, cephalic, and accessory cephalic veins of the antecubital area (antecubital fossa) are used most frequently for venipuncture, but dorsal hand veins are also acceptable. Veins on the underside of the wrist must never be used.
[CLSI Standard GP41, p15; Garza 10e, p333-334]

Explanations

Specimen Collection

154. c The structure indicated by the arrow is the cephalic vein. The cephalic vein appears on the lateral side of the antecubital area (antecubital fossa) and the dorsal side of the hand. CLSI Standard GP41 acknowledges that the larger, fuller median, median cubital, cephalic, and accessory cephalic veins of the antecubital area are used most frequently for venipuncture, but dorsal hand veins are also acceptable. Veins on the underside of the wrist must never be used.
[CLSI Standard GP41, p15; Garza 10e, p333-334]

155. a The site should be cleansed by applying a 70% isopropyl alcohol solution using a back-and-forth friction motion which has been found to be more effective than the concentric circular motion typically used.
[CLSI Standard GP41, p22]

156. b To examine by touch or feel is to palpate (verb).
[CLSI Standard GP41, p17]

157. c The cephalic vein is often the easiest vein to palpate in obese patients.
[McCall 7e, p160]

158. b If a patient is receiving IV fluids in one arm, the phlebotomist should first try to use the alternate arm to perform venipuncture. If a vein in the alternate arm is not suitable and a capillary puncture does not meet specimen requirements, the phlebotomist may draw from below an IV following institutional policy for this procedure.
[CLSI Standard GP41, p44; Garza 10e, p301]

159. d The median cubital vein is a large, full, surface vein appearing near the center of the antecubital area (antecubital fossa). The order of vein selection is: 1) median cubital vein; 2) cephalic vein, and 3) basilic vein, making the median cubital vein the first choice when selecting a site for venipuncture. CLSI Standard GP41 requires a phlebotomist to look for a median cubital vein in both arms before selecting an alternative site for venipuncture.
[CLSI Standard GP41, p19-21; Garza 10e, p330-333]

160. a The basilic vein is a smaller vein appearing on the medial side of the antecubital area (antecubital fossa). The order of vein selection is: 1) median cubital vein, 2) cephalic vein, and 3) basilic vein, making the basilic vein the least suitable choice when selecting a site for venipuncture. Additionally, the basilic vein is located in proximity to the brachial artery and median nerve so other choices are typically preferred.
[CLSI Standard GP41, p19-21; Garza 10e, p330-333, 335]

161. b The phlebotomist should next examine the right antecubital area (antecubital fossa). CLSI Standard GP41 requires a phlebotomist to look for a median cubital vein in both arms before selecting an alternative site for venipuncture.
[CLSI Standard GP41, p15, 19-21; Garza 10e, p330-333]

Specimen Collection — Explanations

162. a The phlebotomist should next examine the left antecubital area (antecubital fossa). CLSI Standard GP41 requires a phlebotomist to look for a median cubital vein in both arms before selecting an alternative site for venipuncture.
[CLSI Standard GP41, p15, 19-21; Garza 10e, p330-333]

163. d The phlebotomist should next examine the right hand. CLSI Standard GP41 acknowledges that the larger, fuller median, median cubital, cephalic, and accessory cephalic veins of the antecubital area (antecubital fossa) are used most frequently, but dorsal hand veins are also acceptable. Veins on the underside of the wrist must never be used.
[CLSI Standard GP41, p15, 19-21; Garza 10e, p330-333]

164. a The phlebotomist should examine the left antecubital area (antecubital fossa) for a suitable vein. A fistula results when an artery and a vein have been surgically and permanently fused in preparation for ongoing kidney dialysis. An arm with a fistula should never be considered as a potential venipuncture site. Moreover, tourniquets should never be applied to an arm containing a fistula. In these circumstances, phlebotomists should strictly adhere to institutional policy.
[CLSI Standard GP41, p15-17; Garza 10e, p499]

165. c A vein that feels hard and cordlike is sclerosed, often the result of frequent, multiple venipuncture procedures and the resulting inflammatory response.
[Garza 10e, p290-291]

166. a Tourniquets should be applied approximately 3-4 inches above the venipuncture site and away from any skin lesions.
[CLSI Standard GP41, p17]

167. a Tourniquets should be applied approximately 3-4 inches above the venipuncture site and away from any skin lesions.
[CLSI Standard GP41, p17]

168. a The purpose of tourniquet administration is to diminish venous blood flow, and make the veins more turgid, allowing for easier venipuncture site selection through palpation.
[CLSI Standard GP41, p17; Garza 10e, p275-276, 337]

169. d Tourniquets should never be applied over an area of skin with open sores.
[McCall 7e, p231-233]

170. d Health care workers responsible for performing venipuncture rely most heavily on their sense of touch to locate a vein.
[Garza 10e, p330]

171. a Phlebotomists should use the index fingers to palpate for a vein prior to venipuncture.
[CLSI Standard GP41, p17; Garza 10e, p330, 338]

172. c When examining a site for venipuncture, a phlebotomist uses the index finger to palpate the vein and determine its size, depth, and direction.
[Garza 10e, p330, 338]

Explanations   Specimen Collection

173. d CLSI Standard GP41 requires a phlebotomist to look for a median cubital vein in both arms before selecting an alternative site for venipuncture.
[CLSI Standard GP41, p20; Garza 10e, p330]

174. d The median cubital vein, a large, full, surface vein appearing near the center of the antecubital area (antecubital fossa), is located over the bicipital aponeurosis, which provides natural support and anchoring for the vein during venipuncture. (The phlebotomist must also always anchor the vein.) The bicipital aponeurosis is a fibrous membrane which also offers some protection to underlying arteries and nerves. CLSI Standard GP41 requires a phlebotomist to look for a median cubital vein in both arms before selecting an alternative site for venipuncture.
[CLSI Standard GP41, p19-21]

175. d In the M-shaped venous pattern, the median cephalic vein is a large, full, surface vein appearing near the center of the antecubital area (antecubital fossa) and is located over the bicipital aponeurosis, providing additional natural anchoring and support for the vein during venipuncture. (The phlebotomist must also always anchor the vein). The bicipital aponeurosis is a fibrous membrane which also offers some protection to underlying arteries and nerves. CLSI Standard GP41 requires a phlebotomist to look for a median vein in both arms before selecting an alternative site for venipuncture.
[CLSI Standard GP41, p15, 19-21]

176. d In the M-shaped venous pattern, the median cephalic vein is a large, full, surface vein appearing near the center of the antecubital area (antecubital fossa) and is located over the bicipital aponeurosis, providing additional natural anchoring for the vein during venipuncture. (The phlebotomist must also always anchor the vein). The bicipital aponeurosis is a fibrous membrane that also offers some protection to underlying arteries and nerves. CLSI Standard GP41 requires a phlebotomist to look for a median cubital vein in both arms before selecting an alternative site for venipuncture. The median veins are also typically the least painful during needle insertion.
[CLSI Standard GP41, p15, 19-21]

177. a The bicipital aponeurosis, characteristically located beneath the median cubital vein, is a fibrous membrane which offers some protection to underlying arteries and nerves as well as some support to the median cubital vein during venipuncture.
[CLSI Standard GP41, p19]

178. b The cephalic vein appears on the lateral side of the antecubital area (antecubital fossa) and the dorsal side of the hand. CLSI Standard GP41 acknowledges that the larger, fuller median, median cubital, cephalic, and accessory cephalic veins of the antecubital area are used most frequently for venipuncture, but dorsal hand veins are also acceptable. Veins on the underside of the wrist must never be used.
[CLSI Standard GP41, p15, 19; Garza 10e, p173, 330-334]

Specimen Collection — Explanations

179. a The basilic vein is a smaller vein appearing on the medial side of the antecubital area (antecubital fossa) and the dorsal side of the hand. Additionally, the basilic vein is located in proximity to the brachial artery and median nerve so other choices are typically preferred. CLSI Standard GP41 acknowledges that the larger, fuller median, median cubital, cephalic, and accessory cephalic veins of the antecubital area are used most frequently, but dorsal hand veins are also acceptable. Veins on the underside of the wrist must never be used.
[CLSI Standard GP41, p15, 19; Garza 10e, p173, 330-334]

180. a The basilic vein is a smaller vein appearing on the medial side of the antecubital area (antecubital fossa) and the dorsal side of the hand. Additionally, the basilic vein is located in proximity to the brachial artery and median nerve so other venous choices are preferred.
[CLSI Standard GP41, p15, 19-21; Garza 10e, p173, 330-334]

181. a The basilic vein is a smaller vein appearing on the medial side of the antecubital area (antecubital fossa) and the dorsal side of the hand. Additionally, the basilic vein is located in proximity to the brachial artery and median nerve so other venous choices are preferred.
[CLSI Standard GP41, p15, 19-21; Garza 10e, p173, 330-334]

182. d The median cubital vein, a large, full, surface vein appearing near the center of the antecubital area (antecubital fossa), is the vein least prone to damage. Also, it is located over the bicipital aponeurosis, which provides additional natural anchoring for the vein during venipuncture. The bicipital aponeurosis is a fibrous membrane which also offers some protection to underlying arteries and nerves. CLSI Standard GP41 requires a phlebotomist to look for a median cubital vein in both arms before selecting an alternative site for venipuncture.
[CLSI Standard GP41, p15, 19-21; Garza 10e, p173, 330-333]

183. a The basilic vein is a smaller vein appearing on the medial side of the antecubital area (antecubital fossa) and the dorsal side of the hand. Additionally, the basilic vein is located in proximity to the brachial artery and median nerve so other venous choices are preferred to minimize the risk of injury to surrounding structures.
[CLSI Standard GP41, p15, 19-21; Garza 10e, p173, 330-335]

184. a The basilic vein is a smaller vein appearing on the medial side of the antecubital area (antecubital fossa) and the dorsal side of the hand. It is often easy to see and palpate, but is not well supported by surrounding musculature and tissue so it tends to roll easily, increasing the risk of accidental puncture of the brachial artery and median cutaneous nerve. Other choices are preferred.
[CLSI Standard GP41, p15, 19-21; Garza 10e, p173, 330-334]

Explanations

Specimen Collection

185. d CLSI Standard GP41 acknowledges that the larger, fuller median, median cubital, cephalic, and accessory cephalic veins of the antecubital area (antecubital fossa) are used most frequently for venipuncture, but dorsal hand veins are also acceptable. Veins on the underside or palmar surface of the wrist must never be used for venipuncture.
[CLSI Standard GP41, p15, 19-21; Garza 10e, p173, 330-334]

186. c Skin punctures for heelstick procedures must be performed on the most medial or lateral aspects of the plantar surface of the infant's heel. Phlebotomists should perform a skin puncture on the plantar surface of the infant's heel lateral to an imaginary line starting between the fourth and fifth toes and extending to the infant's heel.
[Garza 10e, p380, 432, 435]

187. d Skin punctures for heelstick procedures must be performed on the most medial or lateral aspects of the plantar surface of the infant's heel. Phlebotomists should perform a skin puncture on the plantar surface of the infant's heel medial to an imaginary line starting at the middle of the infant's great toe and extending to the infant's heel.
[Garza 10e, p380, 432, 435]

188. b Skin punctures are performed on the plantar surface of a baby's heel until the child is 12 months old. After a child reaches 1 year of age, a fingerstick procedure may be used.
[Garza 10e, p380, 432, 435]

189. a The following sites should never be selected for heelstick procedures on infants: central area of the infant's heel, the arch area of the foot, or the toes. If skin puncture is performed in these sites, injury to bone, cartilage, nerves, and tendons may result.
[Garza 10e, p380, 432, 435]

190. a Complications resulting from neonatal heelsticks include cellulitis and osteochondritis and osteomyelitis.
[Garza 10e, p380, 436]

191. b Capillary beds at the dermal-subcutaneous junction are typically located 0.35-1.6 mm below the skin surface of an infant's heel.
[Garza 10e, p432]

192. c Skin punctures, or fingerstick procedures, should be performed on the palmar surface and distal segment of the index, ring, or middle fingers. The middle or ring fingers are best to use since the index finger has an increased number of nerve endings and is more sensitive to pain. The sides and the tips of the distal segment should not be used because the tissue is only half as thick as the palmar surface of the finger. The fifth finger should not be used because the tissue of the fifth finger is considerably thinner than the other fingers. The thumb should never be used because it has a pulse.
[Garza 10e, p378-380, 382]

Specimen Collection — Explanations

193. **c** Skin punctures, or fingerstick procedures, should be performed on the palmar surface and distal segment of the index, ring, or middle fingers. The middle or ring fingers are best to use since the index finger has an increased number of nerve endings and is more sensitive to pain. The sides and the tips of the distal segment should not be used because the tissue is only half as thick as the palmar surface of the finger. The fifth finger should not be used because the tissue of the fifth finger is considerably thinner than the other fingers. The thumb should never be used because it has a pulse.
[Garza 10e, p378-380, 382]

194. **d** Skin punctures, or fingerstick procedures, should be performed on the palmar surface and distal segment of the index, ring, or middle fingers. The middle or ring fingers are best to use since the index finger has an increased number of nerve endings and is more sensitive to pain. The sides and the tips of the distal segment should not be used because the tissue is only half as thick as the palmar surface of the finger. The fifth finger should not be used because the tissue of the fifth finger is considerably thinner than the other fingers. The thumb should never be used because it has a pulse.
[Garza 10e, p378-380, 382]

195. **d** Skin punctures should be made perpendicular to the fingerprint grooves. If the puncture is made parallel to the fingerprint grooves, the blood will channel down the patient's finger instead of forming a collectable drop at the puncture site, making specimen collection much more difficult.
[Garza 10e, p379, 382]

196. **c** The fifth finger should not be used because the tissue of the fifth finger is considerably thinner than the other fingers and the risk of accidentally puncturing the bone is greater.
[Garza 10e, p378-380, 382]

197. **b** The index finger has an increased number of nerve endings and is more sensitive to pain so it should be avoided whenever possible to lessen the patient's discomfort during and following skin puncture.
[Garza 10e, p378-380, 382]

198. **c** The correct sequence is: 1) locate a suitable vein in the patient's right antecubital area (antecubital fossa); 2) untie the tourniquet; 3) use isopropyl alcohol to prepare the site. Ethyl alcohol is not an appropriate antiseptic solution to use for site preparation. CLSI Standard GP41 requires a phlebotomist to look for a median cubital vein in both arms before selecting an alternative site for venipuncture.
[CLSI Standard GP41, p15, 19-22; Garza 10e, p337-339, 342-346]

Explanations
Specimen Collection

199. b The correct sequence is: 1) tie the tourniquet; 2) locate a suitable vein; 3) untie the tourniquet; 4) prepare the site. Tourniquets should not be applied longer than 1 minute. By releasing the tourniquet during site preparation, tourniquet application time is diminished.
[CLSI Standard GP41, p18; Garza 10e, p337-339, 342-346]

200. d The correct sequence is: 1) release the tourniquet; 2) put on gloves; 3) prepare the site; 4) reapply the tourniquet. Once a site has been prepared prior to venipuncture, it should not be repalpated. If a site is repalpated, it must be cleansed again. Tourniquets should not be applied longer than 1 minute. By releasing the tourniquet during site preparation, tourniquet application time is diminished.
[CLSI Standard GP41, p18; Garza 10e, p337-339, 342-346]

201. a The correct sequence is: 1) put on gloves; 2) prepare the site; 3) reapply the tourniquet; 4) uncap the needle. The phlebotomist should put on gloves before cleansing the site. The needle is uncapped after the tourniquet is applied.
[CLSI Standard GP41, p17-18, 22; Garza 10e, p341-342]

202. b The correct sequence is: 1) apply tourniquet; 2) palpate site; 3) release tourniquet. Tourniquets should not be applied longer than 1 minute. By releasing the tourniquet during site preparation, tourniquet application time is diminished.
[CLSI Standard GP41, p17-18; Garza 10e, p337-338]

203. c The correct sequence is: 1) uncap the needle; 2) anchor the vein; 3) insert the needle. The needle assembly should be held in one hand while the phlebotomist uses the other hand to anchor the vein. According to CLSI Standard GP41, the phlebotomist should anchor the vein by positioning the thumb about 1 to 2 inches below the intended puncture site and slightly to the side. Use the thumb to pull the skin toward the wrist and use the remaining fingers to hold the patient's arm away from the intended puncture site.
[CLSI Standard GP41, p17-18, 23-24; Garza 10e, p342-343]

204. c The correct sequence is: 1) release vein; 2) engage tube; 3) release tourniquet. Once the needle has been inserted into the patient's vein, the thumb anchoring the vein may be moved. The hand used to anchor the vein and hold the patient's arm still may be used to engage the evacuated tube. Once blood flow is established in the evacuated tube, the tourniquet may be released.
[CLSI Standard GP41, p23-25; Garza 10e, p343]

205. c The correct sequence is: 1) engage the first evacuated tube; 2) confirm blood flow is established; 3) release the tourniquet; 4) fill subsequent evacuated tubes. The first evacuated tube must be engaged to confirm the needle is in the vein. Once blood flow is established, the tourniquet is released. The phlebotomist must hold the needle absolutely still, and use a gentle twist and pull motion to remove the first evacuated tube and replace with other evacuated tubes following the order of draw.
[CLSI Standard GP41, p23-25; Garza 10e, p343-344]

Specimen Collection — Explanations

206. **a** Immediately after the last evacuated tube is filled the safety mechanism must be activated following manufacturer's directions. Some safety mechanisms will allow activation in the patient's vein prior to needle withdrawal and others require activation immediately after the vein is withdrawn from the patient's arm.
[CLSI Standard GP41, p28; Garza 10e, p344-345]

207. **a** Systemic venous blood is typically dark purple-red in color. The color of the blood in the tube confirms that the phlebotomist is drawing blood from the basilic vein and the evacuated tube should be allowed to fill, following standard procedures.
[Garza 10e, p230]

208. **c** The specimen should be recollected because evacuated tubes containing sodium citrate must be filled to capacity to ensure accurate blood:anticoagulant ratio. Underfilled sodium citrate tubes will result in an excess of anticoagulant, inaccurately prolonging clotting times. Visibly underfilled sodium citrate tubes will not be accepted by most coagulation laboratories. No more than 2 attempts to successfully complete a venipuncture procedure may be attempted by a phlebotomist.
[CLSI Standard GP41, p32-33; Garza 10e, p264, 356]

209. **d** Using a blood pressure cuff set with the gauge set below the patient's diastolic pressure as a tourniquet would generate the best quality specimen. A 10 mL evacuated tube used with either a butterfly needle or a syringe would likely create a hemolyzed specimen particularly if used with a very small 25 gauge needle because the strength of the vacuum could cause the red cells to rupture as they are pulled by the vacuum through the small needle. If a vein in another arm is not suitable and a capillary puncture does not meet specimen requirements, the phlebotomist may draw from below an IV and always following institutional policy for this procedure. Blood specimens must never be collected from above an IV.
[CLSI Standard GP41, p17-18, 44-46; Garza 10e, p269, 275, 301, 329-330, 338]

210. **a** Phlebotomists should always check the expiration of each evacuated tube before using it in a venipuncture procedure. Outdated evacuated tubes should be discarded.
[McCall 7e, p198, 236-237, 295]

211. **c** Reflux, or the backwash of contents from an evacuated tube into a patient's vein, may be prevented if a patient's arm is positioned downward during venipuncture.
[McCall 7e, p229, 291]

212. **d** The patient's arm should be positioned in a straight line from the shoulder to wrist.
[McCall 7e, p229]

Explanations

Specimen Collection

213. **b** Positioning the patient's arm in a straight line from the shoulder to wrist during venipuncture in the antecubital area (antecubital fossa) will help to anchor the veins during venipuncture.
[McCall 7e, p229]

214. **c** Patients should be directed to open their fist after the needle is inserted and blood appears in the first evacuated tube.
[McCall 7e, p296-297, 344]

215. **a** Tourniquets should be applied for only 1 minute. If tourniquet application exceeds 1 minute, the tourniquet should be removed and reapplied after 2 minutes have elapsed.
[CLSI Standard GP41, p18; McCall 7e, p296-297, 338, 340]

216. **d** The tourniquet should be applied above and proximal (near) to the wrist if the venipuncture is going to be performed on a hand vein.
[McCall 7e, p230-231]

217. **a** Once the tourniquet has been applied, the patient should be instructed to close his/her fist.
[Garza 10e, p342]

218. **b** Hemoconcentration is a decrease in the fluid portion of the blood resulting in an increased concentration of cells and large molecules. Prolonged tourniquet application can cause hemoconcentration.
[Garza 10e, p296-297, 300, 340]

219. **c** The tourniquet should be released after the needle is inserted into the vein selected and blood flow into the first evacuated tube is established.
[CLSI Standard GP41, p25; Garza 10e, p338, 340, 342]

220. **c** Prolonged tourniquet application can result in hemoconcentration, including an increase in cholesterol levels by as much as 5% after 2 minutes of tourniquet application.
[McCall 7e, p292]

221. **c** The compound most commonly used to prepare a site prior to venipuncture is 70% isopropyl alcohol.
[CLSI Standard GP41, p22]

222. **c** Venipuncture sites must be cleansed with an antiseptic prior to puncture to minimize contamination of the needle with microorganisms on the skin. If the needle becomes contaminated the microorganisms can be introduced into the patient's vein, potentially causing an infection or into the specimen tube, contaminating the specimen.
[CLSI Standard GP41, p22; Garza 10e, p339-340]

223. **a** Following decontamination of a venipuncture site with alcohol, the phlebotomist should allow the site to air dry.
[CLSI Standard GP41, p22; Garza 10e, p339-340, 342]

Specimen Collection — Explanations

224. c Approximately 30-60 seconds is required for a venipuncture site to air dry following alcohol application.
[McCall 7e, p236]

225. b When anchoring a vein in the antecubital area (antecubital fossa) prior to venipuncture, the phlebotomist should place the thumb approximately 2 inches below the puncture site.
[CLSI Standard GP41, p15, 23; Garza 10e, p342]

226. d When anchoring a vein in the antecubital area (antecubital fossa) prior to venipuncture, the phlebotomist should place the thumb approximately 2 inches below the puncture site and pull the skin taut by stretching the skin toward the patient's wrist.
[CLSI Standard GP41, p23; Garza 10e, p342]

227. d When anchoring a hand vein prior to venipuncture, the phlebotomist may use his/her thumb to pull the patient's skin taut over the knuckles.
[McCall 7e, p253-254]

228. b During routine venipuncture, the needle should be inserted with the bevel up.
[CLSI Standard GP41, p24; Garza 10e, p343]

229. c During venipuncture, the needle should be inserted at a 30-degree angle or less. Shallow veins may require a smaller angle 15 degrees while deeper veins may require a larger angle (30 degrees).
[CLSI Standard GP41, p24; Garza 10e, p343]

230. d The needle must be positioned in the same direction as the vein and at an angle of 15-30 degrees to the patient's arm.
[Garza 10e, p343]

231. c During routine venipuncture, the needle should be inserted until a decrease in resistance is felt.
[Garza 10e, p343]

232. d The needle posing the greatest risk to phlebotomists is the winged infusion needle because failure to activate the safety feature according to manufacturer's recommendations may result in a higher incidence of needlestick injuries.
[CLSI Standards GP41, p54-55; Garza 10e, p110-111, 272-274, 317, 318, 350]

233. d During a venipuncture procedure after the needle is uncapped the phlebotomist should visually inspect the needle for any defects. If defects are observed, the needle should be discarded and another selected.
[McCall 7e, p237]

234. c During a venipuncture procedure, the phlebotomist should visually inspect the needle after the needle is uncapped. The needles should be discarded if imperfections, including burrs, are noted and another needle selected for use.
[McCall 7e, p237]

Explanations

Specimen Collection

235. d The phlebotomist's thumb should be positioned on the top of the evacuated tube holder to insert the needle during a venipuncture procedure.
[CLSI Standard GP41, p23-24, 249]

236. d The phlebotomist gently inverted the blood specimen collected in an EDTA tube 8 times. This is consistent with manufacturer's recommendations so the specimen will not be adversely affected.
[McCall 7e, p241]

237. c Evacuated tubes containing additives should be mixed with the patient's blood by gentle inversion immediately upon removal from the evacuated tube holder.
[Garza 10e, p344, 355]

238. b Evacuated tubes containing additives should be mixed with the patient's blood by gentle inversion immediately upon removal from the evacuated tube holder.
[Garza 10e, p344, 355]

239. d Most evacuated tubes containing anticoagulants should be mixed with the patient's blood by gently inverting the tube at least 8 times. One exception is the sodium citrate tube which only requires 3-4 inversions.
[McCall 7e, p241]

240. b Evacuated tubes containing additives should be mixed with the patient's blood by gentle inversion immediately upon removal from the evacuated tube holder. If an evacuated tube with additive is vigorously shaken, the specimen may become hemolyzed.
[Garza 10e, p302, 361]

241. d The phlebotomist may adjust the needle following venipuncture if no blood appears in the evacuated tube. Adjustments to needle placement may be made only after establishing vein location relative to the needle. Acceptable adjustments include slightly rotating the needle, slightly advancing the needle if needle insertion is too shallow relative to the vein or withdrawing the needle if initial placement is too deep relative to the vein. The phlebotomist may also remove the evacuated tube and replace it with another to rule out a defective evacuated tube as the source of the issue. Under no circumstances should lateral needle relocation be attempted to access the basilic vein because the risk of accidentally puncturing the median nerve or the brachial artery is too great.
[CLSI Standard GP41, p32-33; Garza 10e, p344, 353]

Specimen Collection — Explanations

242. **c** The phlebotomist may adjust the needle following venipuncture if no blood appears in the evacuated tube. Adjustments to needle placement may be made only after establishing vein location relative to the needle. Acceptable adjustments include slightly rotating the needle, slightly advancing the needle if needle insertion is too shallow relative to the vein or withdrawing the needle if initial placement is too deep relative to the vein. The phlebotomist may also remove the evacuated tube and replace it with another to rule out a defective evacuated tube as the source of the issue. Under no circumstances should lateral needle relocation be attempted to access the basilic vein because the risk of accidentally puncturing the median nerve or the brachial artery is too great.
[CLSI Standard GP41, p32-33; Garza 10e, p344, 353]

243. **d** The phlebotomist may adjust the needle following venipuncture if no blood appears in the evacuated tube. Adjustments to needle placement may be made only after establishing vein location relative to the needle. Acceptable adjustments include slightly rotating the needle, slightly advancing the needle if needle insertion is too shallow relative to the vein or withdrawing the needle if initial placement is too deep relative to the vein. The phlebotomist may also remove the evacuated tube and replace it with another to rule out a defective evacuated tube as the source of the issue. Under no circumstances should lateral needle relocation be attempted to access the basilic vein because the risk of accidentally puncturing the median nerve or the brachial artery is too great.
[CLSI Standard GP41, p32-33; Garza 10e, p344, 353]

244. **b** Two is the maximum number of attempts a phlebotomist should make to secure a blood specimen.
[CLSI Standard GP41, p33; Garza 10e, p354]

245. **b** Two is the maximum number of attempts a phlebotomist should make to secure a blood specimen. However, phlebotomists should always adhere to the institution's policy for securing a blood specimen after an unsuccessful collection attempt.
[CLSI Standard GP41, p33; Garza 10e, p354]

246. **d** After the last evacuated tube to be collected is filled, the phlebotomist should disengage the tube from the back of the needle by using the flange as a brace.
[McCall 7e, p195, 242]

247. **c** Withdraw the needle from the patient's arm, place a clean gauze pad over the puncture site, and activate the needle safety feature. Cotton or rayon balls are not acceptable because they could dislodge the platelet plug at the puncture site.
[CLSI Standard GP41, p28; Garza 10e, p345, 358]

Explanations
Specimen Collection

248. c Withdraw the needle from the patient's arm, place a clean gauze pad over the puncture site, and activate the needle safety feature. Cotton or rayon balls are not acceptable because they could dislodge the platelet plug at the puncture site.
[CLSI Standard GP41, p28; Garza 10e, p345, 358]

249. b The appropriate procedural sequence is: withdraw the needle from the patient's arm, place a clean gauze pad over the puncture site, and activate the needle safety feature. In this case, the phlebotomist likely placed the gauze over the puncture site while withdrawing the needle and pushed down on the gauze before the needle was completely withdrawn resulting in the scratch.
[CLSI Standard GP41, p28; Garza 10e, p345, 358]

250. c After the needle is withdrawn, the patient should be instructed to use the gauze pad to apply pressure to the site while keeping the arm straight. Patients should not be instructed to hold the gauze in place while bending their arm up. Studies have shown this procedure actually increases the chance of bruising at the venipuncture site.
[CLSI Standard GP41, p28; Garza 10e, p346, 358-359]

251. c Specimen labels should be affixed to evacuated tubes after specimen collection is completed and before leaving the patient's bedside or outpatient draw station.
[CLSI Standard GP41, p28; Garza 10e, p346, 357-358]

252. d All specimen labels must include 1) the patient's first and last names; 2) the patient's identification number; 3) the date and time of specimen collection; and 4) the identity of the person collecting the specimen. The physician's name is an optional component of a specimen label and may be included as a function of the Laboratory Information System (LIS) or institutional policy.
[CLSI Standard GP41, p7, 28; Garza 10e, p346, 357-358]

253. b All specimen labels must include 1) the patient's first and last names; 2) the patient's identification number; 3) the date and time of specimen collection; and 4) the identity of the person collecting the specimen. In order to comply with HIPAA guidelines, the patient's diagnosis would never be included on a specimen label.
[CLSI Standard GP41, p7, 28; Garza 10e, p346, 357-358]

254. c Specimen labels must be affixed to evacuated tubes in a very specific manner so the analyzer performing the test can detect the label. Computer generated requisitions, including bar codes, are often read by the analyzer using a light source. If labels are not affixed properly, the light source cannot detect and read the label information.
[Garza 10e, p68-71, 346, 357-358]

255. c The 3-step identification procedure requires the phlebotomist to confirm specimen label information with the patient's wristband.
[CLSI Standard GP41, p28; Garza 10e, p324-328, 346, 357-358]

Specimen Collection — Explanations

256. d After the needle is withdrawn, the patient should be instructed to use the gauze pad to apply pressure to the site while keeping the arm straight. Patients should not be instructed to hold the gauze in place while bending their arm up. Studies have shown this procedure actually increases the chance of bruising at the venipuncture site.
[CLSI Standard GP41, p28; Garza 10e, p346, 358-359]

257. d If a venipuncture site is not allowed to adequately air dry prior to needle insertion, the alcohol may contaminate the specimen and cause hemolysis.
[Garza 10e, p302, 340]

258. a If a venipuncture site is not allowed to adequately air dry prior to needle insertion, the patient may experience a burning sensation due to residual alcohol on the site.
[Garza 10e, p340]

259. c Veins located in the hands and wrist are not well supported by surrounding musculature and have a tendency to roll or move during needle insertion. Phlebotomists selecting these sites for venipuncture must exercise care to adequately anchor the vein prior to venipuncture to ensure a successful blood collection procedure.
[Garza 10e, p333-334]

260. d Because of the increased risk of thrombosis associated with the use of leg or ankle veins for venipuncture, phlebotomists should not use leg or ankle veins as venipuncture sites without the permission of the patient's physician and consistent with institutional policy.
[Garza 10e, p336]

261. c During venipuncture, the evacuated tube should be positioned so the non-stoppered end of the tube is below the puncture site to prevent reflux.
[McCall 7e, p291]

262. b EDTA is the evacuated tube additive most commonly associated with adverse patient experiences due to reflux.
[McCall 7e, p291]

263. a Veins located in the hands and wrist are not well supported by surrounding musculature and have a tendency to roll or move during needle insertion. Phlebotomists selecting these sites for venipuncture must exercise care to adequately anchor the vein prior to venipuncture to ensure a successful blood collection procedure.
[Garza 10e, p333-334]

264. d Specimens transported to the laboratory using a pneumatic tube system should be placed in plastic bags labeled with the biohazard symbol and placed in the pneumatic tube car surrounded by shock absorbent material such as foam rubber.
[McCall 7e, p384-385]

Explanations
Specimen Collection

265. a Blood culture specimens must be collected by sterile technique to minimize contamination of the specimen with skin flora.
[CLSI Standard GP41, p42; Garza 10e, p474-475]

266. c Venipuncture site preparation prior to collection of a blood culture specimen typically includes using two cleansing agents, characteristically 70% isopropyl alcohol with a 30-second friction scrub followed by an iodine compound. If tincture of iodine is used, it must remain on the site for at least 30 seconds; an iodophor compound must remain on the site for 1.5-2 minutes, with time allowed between cleansing agents for the site to air dry. Chlorhexidine gluconate may be applied instead of iodine and also requires 30 second application. Chlorhexidine gluconate may *not* be used on premature infants or infants < 2 months of age.
[CLSI Standard GP41, p42; Garza 10e, p474-476]

267. d If a phlebotomist repalpates a venipuncture site after it was prepared for blood culture collection, the site is contaminated. Skin flora may be introduced into the specimen collection bottles, causing a false-positive result.
[CLSI Standard GP41, p42; Garza 10e, p339, 475-476]

268. c To minimize the risk of specimen contamination with skin flora, the venipuncture site must be cleansed for a minimum of 30 seconds using a friction scrub technique and an appropriate disinfectant.
[CLSI Standard GP41, p42; Garza 10e, p339, 475]

269. c Adequate blood specimen volume is critical to quality blood culture results. The American Society for Microbiology (ASM) recommends a 20-30 mL specimen volume for quality blood culture results on adult patients.
[McCall 7e, p343]

270. b Because of the increased number of patients with sensitivity to iodine, some facilities have opted to use a 1-step site preparation compound of chlorhexidine gluconate and isopropyl alcohol. Chlorhexidine gluconate may be used instead of iodine if the patient is allergic to iodine and is also safe for use on infants older than 2 months of age.
[CLSI Standard GP41, p42; Garza 10e, p339, 475-476]

271. c The volume will be decreased by 0.5 mL because the tubing attached to the winged infusion needle contains air in that volume. The vacuum in the evacuated tube will remove the air from the tubing first and then collect the blood specimen. When using a winged infusion needle to collect a specimen, it is recommended that a small red top discard tube be drawn first and discarded to ensure that an adequate amount of specimen is collected and that accurate blood:anticoagulant ratios in subsequent additive tubes are achieved.
[Garza 10e, p349]

Specimen Collection — Explanations

272. c It is recommended that small volume evacuated tubes be used with winged infusion needles to prevent hemolysis of the specimen collected and also vein collapse during the venipuncture procedure.
[Garza 10e, p349]

273. a The needle posing the greatest risk to phlebotomists is the winged infusion needle because failure to activate the safety feature according to manufacturer's recommendations may result in a higher incidence of needlestick injuries. Phlebotomists should carefully comply with the manufacturer's directions to minimize risk to the phlebotomist.
[Garza 10e, p110-112, 272-274, 317-318, 350]

274. b Because dorsal metacarpal veins are typically shallow, the winged infusion needle should be inserted at a 10-15° angle to the patient's hand.
[McCall 7e, p239]

275. c When using a winged infusion needle for blood collection, often the first indication the needle is successfully inserted in the vein is a small amount of blood in the tubing, sometimes referred to as a "flash" of blood.
[McCall 7e, p239]

276. b The volume will be decreased by 0.5 mL because the tubing attached to the winged infusion needle contains air in that volume. The vacuum in the evacuated tube will remove the air from the tubing first and then collect the blood specimen. When using a winged infusion needle to collect a specimen, it is recommended that a small red top discard tube be drawn first and discarded to ensure that an adequate amount of specimen is collected and that accurate blood:anticoagulant ratios in subsequent additive tubes are achieved.
[Garza 10e, p349]

277. d The volume will be decreased by 0.5 mL because the tubing attached to the winged infusion needle contains air in that volume. The vacuum in the evacuated tube will remove the air from the tubing first and then collect the blood specimen. When using a winged infusion needle to collect a specimen, it is recommended that a small red top discard tube be drawn first and discarded to ensure that an adequate amount of specimen is collected and that accurate blood:anticoagulant ratios in subsequent additive tubes are achieved. This is critically important in sodium citrate tubes, which must be completely filled to ensure the correct 9:1 blood:anticoagulant ratio.
[Garza 10e, p264, 349]

278. a The blood specimen will be discarded because the blood:anticoagulant ratio will be inaccurate. When using a winged infusion needle to collect a specimen, a small red top discard tube must be drawn first and discarded to ensure that an adequate amount of specimen is collected and that accurate blood:anticoagulant ratios in the APTT specimen tube are achieved.
[CLSI Standard GP41, p28; Garza 10e, p264, 349]

Explanations
Specimen Collection

279. a If a winged infusion needle is used to collect a specimen for coagulation studies, including a PT/APTT, or if the coagulation tube is the first tube needed in a multiple specimen collection, a discard tube must be used to prime the tubing connected to the needle to ensure proper blood:anticoagulant ratio in the sodium citrate (blue top) tube. The discard tube may be either a red top or a tube containing additive.
[CLSI Standard GP41, p28; Garza 10e, p349]

280. a The evacuated tube should be held so the blood enters the tube filling it from the bottom up. The blood should not be allowed to contact the needle or be moved in the holder during specimen collection because this may cause transfer of additives. Tubes should be held horizontally or slightly downward to facilitate filling the tube from the bottom up.
[Garza 10e, p344]

281. c Syringes should not be used routinely for venipuncture. However, sometimes syringes provide the phlebotomist with the ability to limit the force on fragile veins that collapse easily. Safety transfer devices must be used to transfer blood from syringes to evacuated tubes.
[CLSI Standard GP41, p27; Garza 10e, p268-269, 351-353]

282. c The safety transfer device is equipped with a permanent needle inside the transfer device. By using this device, the syringe needle is not required to aliquot specimen from the syringe into evacuated tubes and must be used every time blood is transferred from a syringe to an evacuated tube. The vacuum from the evacuated tube will withdraw the specimen from the syringe.
[CLSI Standard GP41, p27; Garza 10e, p268-269, 351-353]

283. c Syringes should not be routinely used to collect blood specimens because of multiple safety and specimen quality concerns. However, sometimes syringes provide the phlebotomist with the ability to limit the force on fragile veins that collapse easily. To comply with OSHA standards, syringes used for blood collection must be equipped with a resheathing device.
[CLSI Standard GP41, p27; Garza 10e, p268-269, 351-353]

284. b When using a syringe for blood collection, often the first indication that the needle is successfully inserted in the vein is a small amount of blood in the hub of the syringe needle sometimes referred to as a "flash" of blood.
[McCall 7e, p239]

285. c Blood collection occurs when the phlebotomist sees a small amount of blood in the hub of the needle and slowly pulls back on the plunger allowing blood to flow into the syringe.
[McCall 7e, p239]

Specimen Collection — Explanations

286. d The 75-year-old oncology patient is the most suitable candidate for blood specimen collection by skin puncture. If she is an oncology patient, she is likely receiving chemotherapy and her veins must be preserved for administering the chemotherapy medications. Blood cultures and erythrocyte sedimentation rates may not be collected by skin puncture for a variety of reasons, including that a sufficient sample cannot be obtained by skin puncture for these analyses.
[Garza 10e, p372-373]

287. a The 8-month-old toddler is the most suitable candidate for blood specimen collection by skin puncture. Skin puncture is the preferred blood collection method for infants and very young children to eliminate risks and complications associated with excessive blood loss.
[Garza 10e, p373, 431-432]

288. c The car crash victim with IVs in both the right and left hands and casts on both legs is the most suitable candidate for skin puncture. The patient's left and right antecubital area (antecubital fossa) and hands are not suitable for venipuncture because there are IVs in both hands and blood specimens may not be obtained above an IV. Both legs are in casts and also unavailable for venipuncture.
[Garza 10e, p373-374]

289. b Specimens for point-of-care testing may be collected by skin puncture. Specimens for blood culture, erythrocyte sedimentation rate, and coagulation studies requiring plasma samples may not be collected by skin puncture.
[Garza 10e, p373-374]

290. a Capillary blood obtained by skin puncture is the preferred specimen for neonatal screening tests, including phenylketonuria (PKU).
[Garza 10e, p439-441]

291. c The correct sequence in the skin puncture procedure for an infant is to: 1) identify the patient; 2) sanitize hands; 3) apply a heel warmer; 4) select appropriate safety lancet.
[Garza 10e, p433-434]

292. d The correct sequence in the skin puncture procedure for an infant is to: 1) sanitize hands; 2) apply a heel warmer; 3) cleanse the skin puncture site with alcohol; 4) allow the site to air dry.
[Garza 10e, p433]

293. b The correct sequence in the skin puncture procedure for an infant is to: 1) cleanse the site with 70% isopropyl alcohol; 2) allow the site to air dry; 3) verify sterility of the safety lancet; 4) wipe away the first drop of blood using a dry sterile gauze pad.
[Garza 10e, p433-435]

Explanations

Specimen Collection

294. a The correct way to hold an infant's foot during heelstick is to use the phlebotomist's nondominant hand and place the thumb around the bottom of the foot, the index finger across the arch of the foot, and the remaining fingers across the top of the foot.
[McCall 7e, p313]

295. a The correct sequence in the skin puncture procedure for an infant is to deploy the safety lancet, gently squeeze the baby's foot to generate the first drop of blood. Wipe away the first drop of blood using a sterile gauze pad and gently squeeze the baby's foot again to generate the specimen for collection.
[Garza 10e, p434-436]

296. c Skin puncture collects blood specimens from the capillary beds underneath the skin. Capillaries connect the arterial and venous sides of blood circulation so blood collected from capillaries by skin puncture is a mixture of arterial, capillary, and venous blood.
[Garza 10e, p230, 373-374]

297. b The electrolyte panel from the neonate would be most significantly affected by excessive squeezing of the puncture site. Excessive squeezing, sometimes called "milking," can cause hemolysis of the blood specimen. One element measured in an electrolyte panel is potassium, which is falsely elevated in hemolyzed specimens.
[Garza 10e, p302, 435]

298. b Excessive squeezing, sometimes called "milking," can cause hemolysis of the blood specimen. Additionally, the specimen may be contaminated with interstitial and intracellular fluid.
[Garza 10e, p435]

299. d Excessive squeezing, sometimes called "milking," can cause hemolysis of the blood specimen. Additionally, the specimen may be contaminated with interstitial and intracellular fluid.
[Garza 10e, p435]

300. c Hemolyzed specimens submitted for bilirubin analysis must be recollected. Hemolysis can falsely decrease bilirubin results. The patient is an infant so skin puncture is the appropriate specimen collection technique to use.
[McCall 7e, p323-324]

301. b Reference ranges are different for certain analytes when collected by skin puncture instead of venipuncture. Glucose levels in specimens collected by skin puncture will be higher than glucose specimens collected by venipuncture. For this reason, it must be noted that specimens in adult patients were collected by skin puncture so the physician may interpret the result within that context.
[McCall 7e, p308]

Specimen Collection — Explanations

302. a Reference ranges are different for certain analytes when collected by skin puncture instead of venipuncture. Calcium levels in specimens collected by skin puncture will be lower than calcium specimens collected by venipuncture. For this reason, it must be noted that specimens in adult patients were collected by skin puncture so the physician may interpret the result within that context.
[McCall 7e, p308]

303. b Excessive squeezing, sometimes called "milking," can cause hemolysis of the blood specimen. Potassium is falsely elevated in hemolyzed specimens.
[Garza 10e, p435]

304. b The skin puncture specimen for bilirubin analysis should be collected in an amber microcollection container with a red stopper. Bilirubin is performed on serum samples so the red stopper container is correct to use for serum samples. Additionally, bilirubin is light sensitive so must be transported shielded from the light. The amber container will protect the specimen from the light. If a specimen for bilirubin analysis is exposed to the light, up to 50% of the bilirubin in the specimen may be destroyed in an hour.
[McCall 7e, p342, 323-324]

305. b The specimen should be rejected for testing. Specimens for coagulation studies requiring plasma samples may not be collected by skin puncture. Some manufacturers supply light blue top microcollection containers but these are intended for use following a syringe draw not following skin puncture.
[Garza 10e, p374]

306. b Prior to performing a heelstick, the infant's foot should be positioned lower than his torso so gravity can assist blood flow following skin puncture.
[Garza 10e, p433]

307. c Prior to performing a fingerstick, the patient's arm should be extended with the palm facing up.
[Garza 10e, p382]

308. b Warming the site prior to skin puncture increases blood flow to the site, making blood collection following puncture easier and reducing the need to squeeze the site to generate the blood specimen. Warming the site prior to skin puncture arterializes the specimen and can increase blood flow to the site by as much as 7 times.
[McCall 7e, p307]

309. d Warming the site prior to skin puncture increases blood flow to the site, making blood collection following puncture easier and reducing the need to squeeze the site to generate the blood specimen. Warming the site prior to skin puncture arterializes the specimen and can increase blood flow to the site by as much as 7 times.
[McCall 7e, p307]

Explanations

Specimen Collection

310. **a** Warming the site prior to skin puncture increases blood flow to the site, making blood collection following puncture easier and reducing the need to squeeze the site to generate the blood specimen. Warming the site prior to skin puncture arterializes the specimen and can increase blood flow to the site by as much as 7 times.
[McCall 7e, p307]

311. **c** If the phlebotomist determines warming a skin puncture site is necessary, the warmer should be applied for 3-5 minutes before making the puncture.
[Garza 10e, p434]

312. **c** It is critically important that the skin puncture site be warmed prior to the collection of capillary blood gases. Warming the site prior to skin puncture arterializes the specimen and can increase blood flow to the site by as much as 7 times.
[McCall 7e, p307]

313. **c** The temperature of commercial heel warmers should not exceed 42°C. Temperatures exceeding 42°C can burn an infant's sensitive skin.
[Garza 10e, p434]

314. **a** Skin puncture sites should be cleaned with 70% isopropyl alcohol prior to puncture.
[Garza 10e, p381-382, 433]

315. **a** Povidone-iodine should never be used to cleanse skin puncture sites prior to puncture. Povidone-iodine can significantly interfere with a number of test results including bilirubin, phosphorous, potassium, and uric acid.
[McCall 7e, p313]

316. **d** Povidone-iodine should never be used to cleanse skin puncture sites prior to puncture. Povidone-iodine can significantly interfere with a number of test results including bilirubin, phosphorous, potassium, and uric acid.
[McCall 7e, p313]

317. **c** Povidone-iodine should never be used to cleanse skin puncture sites prior to puncture. Povidone-iodine can significantly interfere with a number of test results including bilirubin, phosphorous, potassium, and uric acid.
[McCall 7e, p313]

318. **b** Povidone-iodine should never be used to cleanse skin puncture sites prior to puncture. Povidone-iodine can significantly interfere with a number of test results including bilirubin, phosphorous, potassium, and uric acid.
[McCall 7e, p313]

319. **a** The correct procedure for collecting a specimen following skin puncture is to apply gentle pressure near (proximal) to the site (without touching the site) while holding the puncture site in a downward position.
[Garza 10e, p382]

Specimen Collection — Explanations

320. d The phlebotomist activates the safety lancet and blood appears at the puncture site. The phlebotomist should first wipe away the first drop of blood using a dry gauze pad.
[Garza 10e, p382, 435]

321. c A phlebotomist is performing a heelstick using an automated heel incision device. Most manufacturers recommend positioning the device at an angle of 90° to the length of the infant's foot.
[McCall 7e, p313]

322. b A phlebotomist can stimulate platelet clumping, requiring a redraw of the specimen if she employs a scooping method to collect the specimen from the infant by repeatedly scraping the scoop along the infant's skin.
[McCall 7e, p314]

323. d Microcollection specimen tubes containing additives should be inverted at least 8-10× after filling to ensure adequate mixing of the specimen with the tube additive.
[McCall 7e, p314]

324. b An infant's heel should not be punctured more than twice in an attempt to secure a specimen, and never twice at the same point.
[McCall 7e, p314]

325. d Specimen labels are affixed after collecting the specimen and before leaving the patient. Labeling a specimen ahead of time increases the risk of selecting an incorrectly labeled tube for a venipuncture procedure. Labeling a tube after leaving a patient's bedside increases the risk of applying a label to an incorrect patient specimen.
[Garza 10e, p72, 357-358]

326. c The phlebotomist's initials are required on every specimen label in case there are questions regarding the specimen during the pre-, post- or examination processes.
[Garza 10e, p357]

327. b The phlebotomist should remove the stopper from a red evacuated tube, place the 6 capillary tubes in the evacuated tube and label the evacuated tube, following standard labeling procedures.
[Garza 10e, p383]

328. d The phlebotomist should apply pressure to the puncture site using a dry, clean gauze pad to stop bleeding following specimen collection.
[Garza 10e, p383, 435]

329. d The phlebotomist should apply pressure to the puncture site using a dry, sterile gauze pad to stop bleeding following specimen collection.
[Garza 10e, p383, 435]

Explanations

Specimen Collection

330. d The phlebotomist should notify the baby's healthcare provider (often a nurse) immediately if a skin puncture site bleeds longer than 5 minutes after the puncture is completed.
[McCall 7e, p285, 317]

331. a One of the most common reasons for neonatal blood transfusion is iatrogenic blood loss. Iatrogenic is a term referring to an adverse effect caused by medical treatment.
[Garza 10e, p33, 373, 431-432, 596-597, 631]

332. d A patient's life may be threatened if 10% of the patient's blood volume is removed at once or over a short period of time.
[Garza 10e, p33, 373, 431-432, 596-597, 631]

333. c Withdrawing 10 mL of blood from a premature or newborn infant equates to 5-10% of the infant's total blood volume.
[Garza 10e, p33, 373, 431-432, 596-597, 631]

334. d Blood volume calculation is based on the patient's weight. Adult blood volume may also be calculated using the patient's weight.
[Garza 10e, p33, 431-432, 596-597, 631]

335. b The amount of blood drawn at one time as well as the cumulative amount of blood collected over one hospital admission of 1 month or less may be used to monitor and minimize iatrogenic blood loss in pediatric patients.
[Garza 10e, p596-597]

336. c Strict adherence to quality assurance protocols for blood collection procedures minimizes the number of redraws required and the amount of blood collected for laboratory testing, which may limit iatrogenic blood loss.
[McCall 7e, p261]

337. a Most adult patients tolerate blood loss as a result of venipuncture for routine testing very well. However, patients who are very ill may require close monitoring and frequent blood specimen collection and these patients must be closely monitored to limit iatrogenic anemia. Of the patients listed, the oncology patient for chemotherapy is most critically ill and therefore the patient most at risk for iatrogenic anemia due to blood specimen collection.
[Garza 10e, p33, 373, 431-432, 596-597, 631]

338. c Specimens for capillary blood gases from neonates should be collected in heparinized plastic capillary tubes. Capillary blood gas specimens must be collected in heparinized capillary tubes. The capillary tubes used to collect the specimen should be plastic to reduce the risk of breakage and injury to the health care worker.
[Garza 10e, p280, 282, 381, 437]

Specimen Collection — Explanations

339. b Specimens for cold agglutinin titer testing must be collected in an evacuated tube prewarmed, transported, and stored at 37°C until the serum is separated from the cells. The antibody detected in a cold agglutinin titer is indicative of primary atypical pneumonia, caused by the pathogen *Mycoplasma pneumoniae*.
[Garza 10e, p401]

340. d Electrolyte panels characteristically include sodium, potassium, chloride, and carbon dioxide (Na, K, Cl, CO_2) analysis. Lavender top evacuated tubes include a di- or tripotassium salt of EDTA.
[Garza 10e, p266, 590]

341. b Blood cultures are used to confirm the presence of microorganisms and/or toxins in the patient's bloodstream, a very serious condition often manifested in patients as fevers of unknown origin (FUO). Blood is normally sterile, and therefore the reference range for blood culture analysis is negative. Bacteria normally exist on the skin surface. Introducing bacteria from the patient's skin into the blood culture specimen can result in a false positive, indicating a patient has bacteremia or septicemia when he/she does not. This can result in significant extensions of hospital stays (up to 4.5 days) and an increased treatment cost of $5,000.00.
[CLSI Standard GP41, p42; Garza 10e, p474-476]

342. a Blood cultures are used to confirm the presence of microorganisms and/or toxins in the patient's bloodstream, a very serious condition often manifested in patients as fevers of unknown origin (FUO). Introducing iodine, an antiseptic used to remove bacteria from the skin surface, into the specimen may result in a negative blood culture, when the patient does in fact have bacteremia or septicemia leading to life-threatening delays in treatment.
[Garza 10e, p474-476]

343. b Blood cultures are used to confirm the presence of microorganisms and/or toxins in the patient's bloodstream, a very serious condition often manifested in patients as fevers of unknown origin (FUO). Blood is normally sterile, and therefore the reference range for blood culture analysis is negative. Bacteria normally exist on the skin surface and on the phlebotomist's gloves. Repalpating the site prior to venipuncture introduces bacteria from the phlebotomist's glove into the blood culture specimen and can result in a false positive, indicating a patient has bacteremia or septicemia when he/she does not. This can result in significant extensions of hospital stays (up to 4.5 days) and an increased treatment cost of $5,000.00.
[CLSI Standard GP41, p42; Garza 10e, p474-476, 483]

Explanations

Specimen Collection

344. a Blood culture collections often involve inoculation into 2 culture bottles for 2 different types of bacteria. Anaerobic bacteria survive best in environments without oxygen and aerobic bacteria survive best in environments rich in oxygen. Introducing air into an anaerobic collection container may result in a false-negative result because anaerobic bacteria typically cannot survive in oxygen-rich environments. For this reason, anaerobic blood culture bottles should be inoculated first for all collection techniques except for the winged infusion needle. When less than the recommended amount of blood is collected for blood culture, the aerobic bottle should be filled first.
[CLSI Standard GP41, p42; Garza 10e, p482]

345. c Specimens for home glucose monitoring are routinely collected by skin puncture.
[Garza 10e, p460, 464]

346. c Newborn screening may detect a variety of genetic, infectious, and metabolic diseases using specimens collected on filter paper circles included on newborn screening cards. Phenylketonuria (PKU) is one of the most commonly ordered tests on newborns and screens for a genetic defect preventing the enzymatic breakdown of phenylalanine, which may ultimately accumulate in toxic levels leading to brain damage and mental retardation.
[Garza 10e, p439-441]

347. b Blood cultures and erythrocyte sedimentation rates may not be collected by skin puncture for a variety of reasons, including that a sufficient sample cannot be obtained by skin puncture for these analyses.
[Garza 10e, p374]

348. c Blood cultures and erythrocyte sedimentation rates may not be collected by skin puncture for a variety of reasons, including that a sufficient sample cannot be obtained by skin puncture for these analyses.
[Garza 10e, p374]

349. c Partial thromboplastin times (PTT) are characteristically performed on plasma specimens collected by venipuncture. Specimens for coagulation studies requiring plasma samples may not be collected by skin puncture. Some manufacturers supply light blue top microcollection containers but these are intended for use following a syringe draw, not following skin puncture.
[Garza 10e, p374]

350. c Newborn screening may detect a variety of genetic conditions, infections, and metabolic diseases using specimens collected on filter paper circles included on newborn screening cards. Phenylketonuria (PKU) is one of the most commonly ordered tests on newborns and screens for a genetic defect preventing the enzymatic breakdown of phenylalanine, which may ultimately accumulate in toxic levels leading to brain damage and mental retardation.
[Garza 10e, p439-441]

Specimen Collection — Explanations

351. **b** Reference ranges are different for certain analytes when collected by skin puncture instead of venipuncture. Glucose levels in specimens collected by skin puncture will be higher than glucose specimens collected by venipuncture. For this reason, it must be noted that specimens in adult patients were collected by skin puncture so the physician may interpret the result within that context.
[McCall 7e, p308]

352. **a** According to CLSI Standard GP41, a specific order of draw must be followed when collecting multiple specimen evacuated tubes following venipuncture. Sodium polyanethol sulfonate (yellow stopper) tubes must be collected first to minimize the risk of blood culture specimen contamination. After specimens for blood culture are collected, additional order-of-draw procedures are in place to prevent additive carryover from one tube to the next. Additive carryover may cause erroneous laboratory results. The order of draw recommended by CLSI is: 1) sodium polyanethol sulfonate (yellow stopper); 2) sodium citrate (light blue stopper); 3) serum tube (red or serum separator gel stopper); 4) heparin tubes with or without plasma separator gel (green stoppers); 5) EDTA (lavender); 6) sodium fluoride (gray stopper). Blood collection equipment may contaminate specimens collected for trace metal analysis. Consult manufacturer recommendations and facility policy for trace metal evacuated tube order-of-draw procedures.
[CLSI Standard GP41, p26-27; Garza 10e, p354-356; McCall 7e, p209]

Please consult the explanation below for questions 353-376 regarding the sequence of filling evacuated tubes following venipuncture.

According to CLSI Standard GP41, a specific order of draw must be followed when collecting multiple evacuated tubes following venipuncture. Sodium polyanethol sulfonate (yellow stopper) tubes must be collected first to minimize the risk of blood culture specimen contamination. After specimens for blood culture are collected, additional order-of-draw procedures are in place to prevent additive carryover from one tube to the next. Additive carryover may cause erroneous laboratory results. The order of draw recommended by CLSI is:

1) sodium polyanethol sulfonate (yellow stopper)

2) sodium citrate (light blue stopper)

3) serum tube (red or serum separator gel stopper)

4) heparin tubes with or without plasma separator gel (green stoppers)

5) EDTA (lavender stopper)

6) sodium fluoride (gray stopper)

Explanations

Specimen Collection

Blood collection equipment may contaminate specimens collected for trace metal analysis. Consult manufacturer recommendations and facility policy for trace metal evacuated tube order-of-draw procedures.
[CLSI Standard GP41, p26-27; Garza 10e, p354-356; McCall 7e, p209]

353. **c** The SPS evacuated tube should be collected first.
[CLSI Standard GP41, p26-27; Garza 10e, p354-356; McCall 7e, p209]

354. **a** The green stopper evacuated tube should be collected last.
[CLSI Standard GP41, p26-27; Garza 10e, p354-356; McCall 7e, p209]

355. **c** The tubes required for specimen collection should be collected in the following order: yellow (SPS), light blue, SST, green.
[CLSI Standard GP41, p26-27; Garza 10e, p354-356; McCall 7e, p209]

356. **d** The red stopper evacuated tube should be collected second.
[CLSI Standard GP41, p26-27; Garza 10e, p354-356; McCall 7e, p209]

357. **b** The lavender stopper evacuated tube should be collected third.
[CLSI Standard GP41, p26-27; Garza 10e, p354-356; McCall 7e, p209]

358. **c** The light blue stopper evacuated tube should be collected first.
[CLSI Standard GP41, p26-27; Garza 10e, p354-356; McCall 7e, p209]

359. **a** The gray stopper evacuated tube should be collected last.
[CLSI Standard GP41, p26-27; Garza 10e, p354-356; McCall 7e, p209]

360. **c** The tubes required for specimen collection should be collected in the following order: light blue, SST, lavender, gray.
[CLSI Standard GP41, p26-27; Garza 10e, p354-356; McCall 7e, p209]

361. **d** The yellow (SPS) evacuated tube should be collected first.
[CLSI Standard GP41, p26-27; Garza 10e, p354-356; McCall 7e, p209]

362. **a** The lavender stopper evacuated tube should be collected last.
[CLSI Standard GP41, p26-27; Garza 10e, p354-356; McCall 7e, p209]

363. **c** The tubes required for specimen collection should be collected in the following order: yellow (SPS), light blue, SST, lavender.
[CLSI Standard GP41, p26-27; Garza 10e, p354-356; McCall 7e, p209]

364. **d** The serum separator tube (SST) should be collected second.
[CLSI Standard GP41, p26-27; Garza 10e, p354-356; McCall 7e, p209]

365. **b** The green top tube containing heparin should be collected third.
[CLSI Standard GP41, p26-27; Garza 10e, p354-356; McCall 7e, p209]

366. **c** The tubes required for specimen collection should be collected in the following order: light blue, SST, green, gray.
[CLSI Standard GP41, p26-27; Garza 10e, p354-356, McCall 7e, p209]

Specimen Collection — Explanations

367. **c** Coagulation specimens may be collected directly into light blue top (sodium citrate) evacuated tubes.
[CLSI Standard GP41, p26-27; Garza 10e, p354-356; McCall 7e, p209-210]

368. **d** The serum tube with clot activator and serum separator gel (SST) evacuated tube should be collected first.
[CLSI Standard GP41, p26-27; Garza 10e, p354-356; McCall 7e, p209]

369. **a** The gray stopper evacuated tube should be collected last.
[CLSI Standard GP41, p26-27; Garza 10e, p354-356; McCall 7e, p209]

370. **c** The tubes required for specimen collection should be collected in the following order: SST, green, lavender, gray.
[CLSI Standard GP41, p26-27; Garza 10e, p354-356; McCall 7e, p209]

371. **b** The green top tube containing heparin should be collected third.
[CLSI Standard GP41, p26-27; Garza 10e, p354-356; McCall 7e, p209]

372. **c** The lavender top tube containing EDTA should be collected fourth.
[CLSI Standard GP41, p26-27; Garza 10e, p354-356; McCall 7e, p209]

373. **d** The tubes required for specimen collection should be collected in the following order: light blue, red, green, lavender, gray.
[CLSI Standard GP41, p26-27; Garza 10e, p354-356; McCall 7e, p209]

374. **a** According to CLSI Standard GP41, filling evacuated tubes from a syringe using a transfer device follows the same order of draw used for blood specimen collection using an evacuated tube system to prevent additive carryover.
[CLSI Standard GP41, p26-27; Garza 10e, p351-356; McCall 7e, p209]

375. **b** Evacuated tubes are filled in the same sequence following blood specimen collection using a syringe as evacuated tube order of draw. Therefore, the sequence the evacuated tubes should be filled following blood collection using a syringe and safety transfer device is: light blue, red, green.
[CLSI Standard GP41, p27; Garza 10e, p352-356]

376. **c** The light blue (sodium citrate tube) should be filled first using a transfer device following blood specimen collection in a syringe. According to CLSI Standard GP41, filling evacuated tubes from a syringe using a transfer device follows the same order of draw used for blood specimen collection using an evacuated tube system.
[CLSI Standard GP41, p26-27; Garza 10e, p352-356; McCall 7e, p209]

Explanations

Specimen Collection

Please consult the explanation below for questions 377-380 regarding the sequence of filling evacuated tubes following venipuncture.

According to CLSI Standard GP41, a specific order of draw must be followed when collecting multiple evacuated tubes following venipuncture. Sodium polyanethol sulfonate (yellow stopper) tubes must be collected first to minimize the risk of blood culture specimen contamination. After specimens for blood culture are collected, additional order-of-draw procedures are in place to prevent additive carryover from one tube to the next. Additive carryover may cause erroneous laboratory results. The order of draw recommended by CLSI is:

1) sodium polyanethol sulfonate (yellow stopper)

2) sodium citrate (light blue stopper)

3) serum tube (red or serum separator gel stopper)

4) heparin tubes with or without plasma separator gel (green stoppers)

5) EDTA (lavender stopper)

6) sodium fluoride (gray stopper)

Blood collection equipment may contaminate specimens collected for trace metal analysis. Consult manufacturer recommendations and facility policy for trace metal evacuated tube order-of-draw procedures.

[CLSI Standard GP41, p26-27; Garza 10e, p354-356; McCall 7e, p209]

377. **b** The lavender (EDTA) tube should be filled last using a transfer device following blood specimen collection in a syringe. According to CLSI Standard GP41, filling evacuated tubes from a syringe using a transfer device follows the same order of draw used for blood specimen collection using an evacuated tube system.
[CLSI Standard GP41, p26-27; Garza 10e, p352-356; McCall 7e, p209]

378. **c** The tubes required for specimen collection should be filled in the following order: light blue, SST, green, gray. According to CLSI Standard GP41, filling evacuated tubes from a syringe using a transfer device follows the same order of draw used for blood specimen collection using an evacuated tube system.
[CLSI Standard GP41, p26-27; Garza 10e, p352-356; McCall 7e, p209]

Specimen Collection — Explanations

379. a When using a winged infusion needle to collect a coagulation specimen first, it is recommended that a small red top discard tube be drawn first and discarded to ensure that an adequate amount of specimen is collected and that accurate blood:anticoagulant ratios in the light blue (sodium citrate) evacuated tube is achieved. The volume of the first evacuated tube collected will be decreased by 0.5 mL because the tubing attached to the winged infusion needle contains air in that volume. The vacuum in the discard evacuated tube will remove the air from the tubing first and then collect the blood specimen. The order of draw recommended by CLSI Standard GP41 should be followed after collection of a discard tube.
[CLSI Standard GP41, p26, 28; Garza 10e, p349, 354]

380. a The gray stopper evacuated tube should be collected last.
[CLSI Standard GP41, p26-27; Garza 10e, p349, 354-356; McCall 7e, p209]

381. a When using a winged infusion needle to collect a coagulation specimen first, it is recommended that a small red top discard tube be drawn first and discarded to ensure that an adequate amount of specimen is collected and that accurate blood:anticoagulant ratios in subsequent additive tubes are achieved. The volume of the first evacuated tube collected will be decreased by 0.5 mL because the tubing attached to the winged infusion needle contains air in that volume. The vacuum in the evacuated tube will remove the air from the tubing first and then collect the blood specimen. The order of draw recommended by CLSI Standard GP41 should be followed after collection of a discard tube.
[CLSI Standard GP41, p26, 28; Garza 10e, p349, 354]

382. d The order of draw following skin puncture is different from the order of draw following venipuncture. The rationale for the order of draw following skin puncture is to minimize platelet clumping of hematology specimens and clotting in specimens collected in anticoagulant. Order of draw following skin puncture is: 1) hematology specimens collected first; 2) other anticoagulant microcollection containers; 3) serum specimens.
[Garza 10e, p385-386]

383. d The tests ordered should be collected in the following order: platelet count, electrolytes, bilirubin. The rationale for the order of draw following skin puncture is to minimize platelet clumping of hematology specimens and clotting in specimens collected in anticoagulant. Order of draw following skin puncture is: 1) hematology specimens collected first; 2) other anticoagulant microcollection containers; 3) serum specimens.
[Garza 10e, p385-386]

Explanations
Specimen Collection

384. c The specimens should be collected in the following order: lavender, green, red. The rationale for the order of draw following skin puncture is to minimize platelet clumping of hematology specimens and clotting in specimens collected in anticoagulant. Order of draw following skin puncture is: 1) hematology specimens collected first; 2) other anticoagulant microcollection containers; 3) serum specimens.
[Garza 10e, p385-386]

385. b If the correct order of draw is not followed, additive carryover can affect test results. For example, citrate carried over into a subsequent evacuated tube can potentially affect analyses for alkaline phosphatase, calcium, and phosphorous. In addition to following the correct order of draw to minimize additive carryover, phlebotomists should keep the patient's arm in a downward position to prevent reflux.
[McCall 7e, p208-210, 229, 291]

386. a If the correct order of draw is not followed, additive carryover can affect test results. For example, citrate carried over into a subsequent evacuated tube can potentially affect analyses for alkaline phosphatase, calcium, and phosphorous. In addition to following the correct order of draw to minimize additive carryover, phlebotomists should keep the patient's arm in a downward position to prevent reflux.
[McCall 7e, p208-210, 229, 291]

387. b If the correct order of draw is not followed, additive carryover can affect test results. For example, citrate carried over into a subsequent evacuated tube can potentially affect analyses for alkaline phosphatase, calcium, and phosphorous. In addition to following the correct order of draw to minimize additive carryover, phlebotomists should keep the patient's arm in a downward position to prevent reflux.
[McCall 7e, p208-210, 229, 291]

388. a If the correct order of draw is not followed, additive carryover can affect test results. For example, EDTA carried over into a subsequent evacuated tube can potentially affect analyses for alkaline phosphatase, calcium, creatine kinase, potassium, and sodium. In addition to following the correct order of draw to minimize additive carryover, phlebotomists should keep the patient's arm in a downward position to prevent reflux.
[McCall 7e, p208-210, 229, 291]

389. b If the correct order of draw is not followed, additive carryover can affect test results. For example, EDTA carried over into a subsequent evacuated tube can potentially affect analyses for alkaline phosphatase, calcium, creatine kinase, potassium, and sodium. In addition to following the correct order of draw to minimize additive carryover, phlebotomists should keep the patient's arm in a downward position to prevent reflux.
[McCall 7e, p208-210, 229, 291]

Specimen Collection — Explanations

390. c If the correct order of draw is not followed, additive carryover can affect test results. For example, EDTA carried over into a subsequent evacuated tube can potentially affect analyses for alkaline phosphatase, calcium, creatine kinase, potassium, and sodium. In addition to following the correct order of draw to minimize additive carryover, phlebotomists should keep the patient's arm in a downward position to prevent reflux.
[McCall 7e, p208-210, 229, 291]

391. c If the correct order of draw is not followed, additive carryover can affect test results. For example, EDTA carried over into a subsequent evacuated tube can potentially affect analyses for alkaline phosphatase, calcium, creatine kinase, potassium, and sodium. In addition to following the correct order of draw to minimize additive carryover, phlebotomists should keep the patient's arm in a downward position to prevent reflux.
[McCall 7e, p208-210, 229, 291]

392. d If the correct order of draw is not followed, additive carryover can affect test results. For example, EDTA carried over into a subsequent evacuated tube can potentially affect analyses for alkaline phosphatase, calcium, creatine kinase, potassium, and sodium. In addition to following the correct order of draw to minimize additive carryover, phlebotomists should keep the patient's arm in a downward position to prevent reflux.
[McCall 7e, p208-210, 229, 291]

393. a If the correct order of draw is not followed, additive carryover can affect test results. For example, heparin carried over into a subsequent evacuated tube can potentially affect analyses for acid phosphatase, calcium, and partial thromboplastin time. In addition to following the correct order of draw to minimize additive carryover, phlebotomists should keep the patient's arm in a downward position to prevent reflux.
[McCall 7e, p208-210, 229, 291]

394. a If the correct order of draw is not followed, additive carryover can affect test results. For example, heparin carried over into a subsequent evacuated tube can potentially affect analyses for acid phosphatase, calcium, and partial thromboplastin time. In addition to following the correct order of draw to minimize additive carryover, phlebotomists should keep the patient's arm in a downward position to prevent reflux.
[McCall 7e, p208-210, 229, 291]

395. d If the correct order of draw is not followed, additive carryover can affect test results. For example, heparin carried over into a subsequent evacuated tube can potentially affect analyses for acid phosphatase, calcium, and partial thromboplastin time In addition to following the correct order of draw to minimize additive carryover, phlebotomists should keep the patient's arm in a downward position to prevent reflux.
[McCall 7e, p208-210, 229, 291]

Explanations   Specimen Collection

396. b The additive most frequently implicated in issues associated with additive carryover is EDTA.
[McCall 7e, p209]

397. d Royal blue stopper evacuated tubes may be collected separately to minimize contamination due to carryover. Royal blue Hemogard evacuated tubes are specially formulated to contain low levels of trace elements, including zinc. Specific levels of trace elements in royal blue Hemogard evacuated tubes are included in product information. Manufacturer's recommendations must always be followed.
[Garza 10e, p267]

398. d According to CLSI Standard GP41, filling evacuated tubes from a syringe using a transfer device follows the same order of draw used for blood specimen collection using an evacuated tube system.
[CLSI Standard GP41, p27]

399. d A patient who is diaphoretic is perspiring profusely. If a patient is pale, he is manifesting pallor. A patient who is perspiring and pale is manifesting symptoms that may result in syncope, or fainting. The phlebotomist should lower the patient's head and instruct the patient to breathe deeply.
[Garza 10e, p298-299]

400. c Once a patient who has experienced syncope has regained consciousness, he should remain at the draw station for at least 15 minutes before being released and should be instructed to wait for at least 30 minutes before driving a vehicle.
[Garza 10e, p298]

401. b If a patient vomits during venipuncture, the procedure should be discontinued immediately.
[McCall 7e, p287]

402. c Sometimes patients faint at the thought or sight of having their blood drawn. This response may be compounded with certain other conditions such as dehydration, hypoglycemia, psychiatric issues, and certain medications.
[Garza 10e, p298-299]

403. b Hemolysis occurs when red blood cell membranes are ruptured and the contents released into the plasma or serum turning the plasma or serum from a light yellow color to pink or red. Some clinical conditions may cause hemolysis, but it is frequently due to collection error. If a specimen is hemolyzed, some analyses will be adversely affected, requiring the specimen to be redrawn.
[Garza 10e, p301-302]

Specimen Collection — Explanations

404. c The phlebotomist should immediately consider the patient's left antecubital area (antecubital fossa) for venipuncture. An arm with an intravenous (IV) line should not be considered as a site for venipuncture because drawing blood from an arm with an IV can potentially contaminate or dilute the blood specimen, causing erroneous results. If a patient has an IV running in one arm, the phlebotomist should consider the other arm as a site for venipuncture. If a suitable vein is not available in the left antecubital area (antecubital fossa), the second site the phlebotomist may consider is the left hand. CLSI Standard GP41 acknowledges that the larger, fuller median, median cubital, cephalic, and accessory cephalic veins of the antecubital area are used most frequently, but dorsal hand veins are also acceptable. Veins on the underside of the wrist must never be used.
[CLSI Standard GP41, p15, 17, 20, 44; Garza 10e, p301, 330-333]

405. c The phlebotomist should first consider the patient's left antecubital area (antecubital fossa) for venipuncture. An arm with an intravenous (IV) line should not be considered as a site for venipuncture because drawing blood from an arm with an IV can potentially contaminate or dilute the blood specimen, causing erroneous results. If a patient has an IV running in one arm, the phlebotomist should consider the other arm as a site for venipuncture. If a suitable vein is not available in the left antecubital area, the second site the phlebotomist may consider is the left hand. CLSI Standard GP41 acknowledges that the larger, fuller median, median cubital, cephalic, and accessory cephalic veins of the antecubital area are used most frequently, but dorsal hand veins are also acceptable. Veins on the underside of the wrist must never be used.
[CLSI Standard GP41, p15, 17, 20, 44; Garza 10e, p301, 330-333]

406. c The phlebotomist should first consider the patient's left antecubital area (antecubital fossa) for venipuncture and if a suitable vein is not available, then the second site to examine is the patient's left hand. An arm with an intravenous (IV) line should not be considered as a site for venipuncture because drawing blood from an arm with an IV can potentially contaminate or dilute the blood specimen, causing erroneous results. CLSI Standard GP41 acknowledges that the larger, fuller median, median cubital, cephalic, and accessory cephalic veins of the antecubital area are used most frequently, but dorsal hand veins are also acceptable. Veins on the underside of the wrist must never be used.
[CLSI Standard GP41, p15, 17, 20, 44; Garza 10e, p301, 330-334]

407. b If the specimen ordered cannot be collected by skin puncture, then the last site the phlebotomist should consider is the patient's right hand below the IV in strict adherence to institutional policy and in cooperation with the patient's nurse and physician. CLSI Standard GP41 acknowledges that the larger, fuller median, median cubital, cephalic, and accessory cephalic veins of the antecubital area (antecubital fossa) are used most frequently, but dorsal hand veins are also acceptable. Veins on the underside of the wrist must never be used.
[CLSI Standard GP41, p15, 17, 20, 44; Garza 10e, p301, 330-334]

Explanations
Specimen Collection

408. c The phlebotomist should examine the right antecubital area (antecubital fossa) for a suitable vein. A fistula results when an artery and a vein have been surgically and permanently fused in preparation for ongoing kidney dialysis. An arm with a fistula should never be considered as a potential venipuncture site. Moreover, tourniquets should never be applied to an arm containing a fistula. In these circumstances, phlebotomists should strictly adhere to institutional policy.
[CLSI Standard GP41, p15, 17, 20, 44; Garza 10e, p301, 330-334, 499]

409. c The procedure should be discontinued immediately. Systemic arterial blood is typically bright orange red in color. The color of the blood in the tube indicates that the phlebotomist is drawing blood from an artery instead of the basilic vein, which may lead to a number of complications, including excessive bleeding and hematoma formation. After stopping the procedure, the phlebotomist should apply pressure to the puncture site for at least 5 minutes and advise the patient's designated healthcare provider (often a nurse) of the incident.
[Garza 10e, p224-225, 230, 335, 504, 623]

410. d Since both arms are not available for venipuncture, the phlebotomist may follow the institution's policy for obtaining the physician's permission to perform the venipuncture on the patient's ankle or foot veins, including the great saphenous vein. The phlebotomist must be mindful that venipuncture in a patient's ankle or foot includes an increased risk of thrombophlebitis and thrombosis.
[Garza 10e, p224, 336]

411. d If the specimen ordered cannot be collected by skin puncture, then the phlebotomist should consider one of the patient's hands below the IV in strict adherence to institutional policy and in cooperation with the patient's nurse and physician. CLSI Standard GP41 acknowledges that the larger, fuller median, median cubital, cephalic, and accessory cephalic veins of the antecubital area (antecubital fossa) are used most frequently, but dorsal hand veins are also acceptable. Veins on the underside of the wrist (palmar surface) must never be used.
[CLSI Standard GP41, p15, 17, 20, 44; Garza 10e, p301, 330-334]

412. c The symptoms presented are consistent with nerve involvement during the venipuncture procedure. Symptoms of accidentally nicking a nerve include intense pain, which is often described as a shooting electrical sensation that may be associated with tingling or numbness. The procedure should be stopped immediately and the patient's designated healthcare provider (often a nurse) notified. Applying an ice pack to the site may reduce the inflammation and associated symptoms.
[CLSI Standard GP41, p36; Garza 10e, p335]

Specimen Collection — Explanations

413. **a**   The evacuated tube should be held so the blood enters the tube filling it from the bottom up. The blood should not be allowed to contact the needle or be moved in the holder during specimen collection because this may cause additive carryover and/or reflux. Reflux is prevented if the tube is held horizontally or slightly downward to facilitate filling the tube from the bottom up.
[McCall 7e, p229, 291; Garza 10e, p298, 344, 356]

414. **b**   After needle withdrawal, pressure should be applied to the puncture site for at least 3-5 minutes.
[McCall 7e, p285-286, 317]

415. **d**   If the venipuncture site continues to bleed after 3 minutes, the patient should be instructed to continue to apply pressure and the phlebotomist should notify the patient's designated healthcare provider (often a nurse) of the prolonged bleeding.
[McCall 7e, p285-286, 317]

416. **c**   Once the bleeding has stopped from a venipuncture site, the site should be bandaged and the patient instructed to leave the bandage on for at least 15 minutes.
[CLSI Standard GP41, p30; Garza 10e, p358-359]

417. **b**   Using a large volume evacuated tube with a small gauge needle, like a winged infusion needle, may cause hemolysis of the specimen collected.
[Garza 10e, p301-302, 349]

418. **a**   A patient may suffer a hematoma if the needle transfixes a vein during venipuncture.
[CLSI Standard GP41, p37; Garza 10e, p297-299, 361]

419. **a**   During pregnancy, the increase of body fluids may cause a patient's red blood cell count (RBC) to decrease (dilutional effect).
[McCall 7e, p277]

420. **d**   Hemoconcentration of a specimen may be caused by a variety of factors including sclerosed veins, prolonged tourniquet application, probing with the needle, and vigorous hand pumping by the patient during venipuncture.
[Garza 10e, p300, 340, 631]

421. **d**   Hemoconcentration of a specimen may be caused by a variety of factors including sclerosed veins, prolonged tourniquet application, probing with the needle, and vigorous hand pumping by the patient during venipuncture.
[Garza 10e, p300, 340, 631]

422. **d**   If a phlebotomist transfixes a vein, the result may be a short draw. There may be a spurt of blood or none at all in the evacuated tube.
[Garza 10e, p263, 297-299, 361]

Explanations
Specimen Collection

423. a The specimen should be recollected by a colleague. Attempts to successfully complete a venipuncture should be limited to two and then a colleague should attempt to collect the specimen. Additive tubes that are incompletely filled should never be combined because the blood:anticoagulant ratio will be incorrect and the results will be inaccurate.
[Garza 10e, p353-354]

424. d Venipuncture should not be performed on the same side as a mastectomy, so the phlebotomist should consider the right arm as a venipuncture site. The patient is more susceptible to infection in the arm on the same side as the mastectomy. As part of a mastectomy surgical procedure, lymph nodes adjacent to the breast may be removed in addition to the breast tissue. If the lymph nodes are removed, lymph fluid may abnormally accumulate in the proximal arm, a condition called lymphedema, which may impact test results.
[CLSI Standard GP41, p17; Garza 10e, p249, 293]

425. c As part of a mastectomy surgical procedure, lymph nodes adjacent to the breast may be removed in addition to the breast tissue. If the lymph nodes are removed, lymph fluid may abnormally accumulate in the proximal arm, a condition called lymphostasis.
[CLSI Standard GP41, p17; Garza 10e, p249, 632]

426. a If the phlebotomist notices a purple swelling around the puncture site after the needle is inserted and the evacuated tube engaged, the phlebotomist should discontinue the procedure immediately.
[Garza 10e, p297-300, 358-359]

427. a Erroneous test results may occur if analysis is performed on a specimen collected through a hematoma. If a hematoma is present, the phlebotomist should select another site without a hematoma or draw distal to the hematoma.
[CLSI Standard GP41, p17; Garza 10e, p361]

428. c The phlebotomist should select another site if a site examined for venipuncture is edematous. Edematous areas should be avoided for venipuncture because site selection will be very challenging and the specimen may be contaminated with excess tissue fluid. The patient's physician should be consulted before collecting the blood specimen.
[Garza 10e, p293]

429. a Edematous areas should be avoided for venipuncture because site selection will be very challenging and the specimen may be contaminated with excess tissue fluid. The patient's physician should be consulted before collecting the blood specimen.
[Garza 10e, p293]

430. b A specimen may be hemolyzed if it was collected through a hematoma.
[CLSI Standard GP41, p17; Garza 10e, p361]

Specimen Collection — Explanations

431. b Certain physiologic conditions may result in hemolysis of a patient's blood sample, including transfusion reaction, sickle cell anemia, and heart valve transplantation.
[Garza 10e, p301]

432. c If a phlebotomist palpates a vein and determines that it is sclerosed, the phlebotomist should select another site for venipuncture. Drawing from a sclerosed vein will be extremely challenging.
[Garza 10e, p290-291]

433. a Sclerosed veins may be caused by frequent venipuncture procedures.
[Garza 10e, p290-291]

434. c One cause of hemolysis is frothing between the hub of a needle and a syringe during venipuncture.
[Garza 10e, p361]

435. b The specimen was not mixed adequately with the anticoagulant (EDTA) immediately following collection, resulting in specimen clotting. Additive tubes require mixing immediately following specimen collection by gently inverting the tube the number of times recommended by the manufacturer.
[McCall 7e, p314]

436. c If a phlebotomist has determined that a venipuncture attempt was unsuccessful, he should untie the tourniquet, place a clean gauze pad over the site, and withdraw the needle. The phlebotomist should evaluate the situation and try again using a different site.
[Garza 10e, p345, 353-354]

437. b If a phlebotomist engages an evacuated tube and no blood appears, he must first assess the situation to determine the location of the vein relative to the needle. Under no circumstances should the phlebotomist reposition a needle without first identifying the exact location of the vein.
[CLSI Standard GP41, p32; Garza 10e, 353-354]

438. c Petechiae are tiny, pinpoint bruises located on a patient's skin. The presence of petechiae suggests a coagulation abnormality, including capillary wall defects and platelet abnormalities.
[Garza 10e, p634]

439. d The blood should not be allowed to contact the needle or be moved in the holder during specimen collection because this may cause reflux, or the flow of blood from the collection tube back into the patient's veins. Reflux is prevented if the tube is held horizontally or slightly downward to facilitate filling the tube from the bottom up.
[Garza 10e, p298, 344, 356]

Explanations
Specimen Collection

440. b If an evacuated tube with additive is vigorously shaken, the specimen may become hemolyzed. Evacuated tubes containing additives should be mixed with the patient's blood by gentle inversion immediately upon removal from the evacuated tube holder.
[Garza 10e, p302]

441. b Erroneous test results due to hemolysis may occur if analysis is performed on a specimen collected through a hematoma. If a hematoma is present, the phlebotomist should select another site without a hematoma or draw distal to the hematoma.
[CLSI Standard GP41, p17, 37; Garza 10e, p333, 361]

442. a If a specimen collected for arterial blood gas analysis contains air bubbles, it will be rejected for testing.
[McCall 7e, p449-450]

443. d Clinically significant changes will occur in a specimen collected for ABG analysis if the specimen is left at room temperature (22°C) for more than 30 minutes prior to analysis.
[McCall 7e, p450]

444. c If the first drop of blood generated after skin puncture is not wiped away prior to specimen collection, residual alcohol on the site contaminating the first drop of blood will contaminate the specimen and cause hemolysis.
[Garza 10e, p302, 382, 441]

445. c A potential complication of accidentally puncturing the calcaneus bone during a heel puncture, characterized by inflammation of the bone and bone marrow, is called osteomyelitis.
[Garza 10e, p436]

446. b A potential complication of accidentally puncturing the calcaneus bone during skin puncture, characterized by inflammation of the bone and cartilage, is called osteochondritis.
[Garza 10e, p432, 436]

447. a A significant risk of injuring a bone during finger puncture is very likely in patients who are less than 1 year old. Infections, including gangrene, have been reported following finger puncture on neonates.
[Garza 10e, p432]

448. b There are several physiological variables that will introduce differences in reference ranges, including age, altitude, dehydration, and diet. Red blood cell counts are typically higher in newborn infants than in adults.
[Garza 10e, p273, 305]

Specimen Collection — Explanations

449. a There are several physiological variables that will introduce differences in reference ranges, including age, altitude, dehydration, diet, and stress. Red blood cell count values are typically higher in patient populations residing at higher elevations.
[McCall 7e, p273]

450. d There are several physiological variables that will introduce differences in reference ranges, including age, altitude, dehydration, diet, and stress. If a patient experiences high anxiety associated with a phlebotomy procedure, certain analytes will be temporarily affected. Studies have documented marked increases in white cell counts in infants who are violently crying in response to a heelstick procedure. One report documents increases over baseline WBC of 140% as a result of the baby's emotional stress.
[Garza 10e, p288-292]

451. b If residual alcohol left is on the skin puncture site prior to specimen collection, it may contaminate the specimen and cause hemolysis.
[Garza 10e, p302, 382, 441]

452. a Excessive squeezing, sometimes called "milking," can cause hemolysis of the blood specimen.
[Garza 10e, p435]

453. d Povidone-iodine should never be used to cleanse skin puncture sites prior to puncture. Povidone-iodine can significantly interfere with a number of test results including bilirubin, phosphorous, potassium, and uric acid.
[McCall 7e, p313]

454. c The purpose of tourniquet administration is to diminish venous blood flow, increase venous filling, allowing for easier venipuncture site selection through palpation.
[CLSI Standard GP41, p17-18; Garza 10e, p275, 336-337]

455. c A sphygmomanometer is a blood pressure cuff and may be used by those who have been trained instead of a tourniquet. When used instead of a tourniquet, the cuff should be inflated to a gauge reading below the patient's diastolic pressure.
[CLSI Standard GP41, p18]

456. c A sphygmomanometer is a blood pressure cuff and may be used by those who have been trained instead of a tourniquet. When used instead of a tourniquet, the cuff should be inflated to a gauge reading below the patient's diastolic pressure.
[CLSI Standard GP41, p18]

457. b The purpose of tourniquet administration is to diminish venous blood flow, increase venous filling, allowing for easier venipuncture site selection through palpation.
[CLSI Standard GP41, p17; Garza 10e, p275, 336-337]

Explanations
Specimen Collection

458. d A number of studies have suggested that tourniquets have the potential to transfer bacteria. Reusable tourniquets must be cleaned frequently using a 70% isopropyl alcohol swab or a 1:10 dilution of chlorine bleach and discarded if visibly soiled with blood or body fluids. To address infection control and latex sensitivity concerns, CLSI Standard GP41 recommends facilities use disposable, single use, latex free tourniquets.
[CLSI Standard GP41, p18; Garza 10e, p275-276]

459. c Recent data suggest that the source of bacteria transferred by reusable tourniquets is the phlebotomist's hands, suggesting better hand hygiene is required.
[McCall 7e, p190]

460. c Patients must always be asked prior to venipuncture if they have a latex allergy. Non-latex tourniquets such as nitrile or vinyl must be used routinely to prevent latex sensitivity. Additionally, if a patient reports a latex allergy, latex-free blood collection equipment must be used to collect the blood specimen.
[CLSI Standard GP41, p12-13 & 17-18]

461. d Patients must always be asked prior to venipuncture if they have a latex allergy. Non-latex tourniquets such as nitrile or vinyl must be used routinely to prevent latex sensitivity. Additionally, if a patient reports a latex allergy, latex-free blood collection equipment must be used to collect the blood specimen.
[CLSI Standard GP41, p12-13 & 17-18]

462. d Following venipuncture, the needle and evacuated tube holder must be immediately discarded in a sharps container.
[Garza 10e, p345, 359]

463. d Packaging from uncontaminated gauze and alcohol prep pads should be discarded in a wastebasket.
[Garza 10e, p359]

464. b Gauze used to apply pressure following a venipuncture procedure should be discarded in a biohazard bag.
[Garza 10e, p359]

465. a Larger gauge needles (16-18) are used for collecting units of blood (450 mL) from blood donors.
[Garza 10e, p270]

466. a The evacuated blood collection system is composed of a needle, holder, and tube containing a premeasured amount of vacuum.
[Garza 10e, p258-259]

467. b 1 & 1½ needle lengths are most commonly used for adult venipuncture.
[Garza 10e, p270]

Specimen Collection — Explanations

468. b Evacuated tubes are typically manufactured in volumes ranging from 1.0 - 10 mL.
[Garza 10e, p261]

469. b Multisample needles are double sided. The longer side is used to access a patient's vein. The shorter side is covered with a rubber sheath and is inserted into the evacuated tube. The rubber sheath retracts as the evacuated tube is engaged and expands once the tube is removed, covering the needle and preventing blood from flowing into the evacuated tube holder.
[Garza 10e, p272]

470. c The standard for measuring the diameter of the lumen of a needle is the needle gauge. The higher the gauge number, the smaller the needle; conversely, the lower the gauge, the larger the needle.
[Garza 10e, p270]

471. d The internal space of a needle is the lumen.
[McCall 7e, p191]

472. a The 18 gauge needle represents the largest needle lumen. The lower the gauge, the larger the needle and conversely, the higher the gauge, the smaller the needle.
[Garza 10e, p270]

473. d The 23 gauge needle represents the smallest needle lumen. The higher the gauge number, the smaller the needle; conversely, the lower the gauge, the larger the needle.
[Garza 10e, p270]

474. c The needle gauges most commonly used for routine venipuncture are 21 and 22.
[Garza 10e, p270]

475. c Noncontaminated needle caps should be discarded in a wastebasket.
[Garza 10e, p359]

476. c Needle safety features are engineering devices that must create a barrier between the needle and the phlebotomist's hands.
[Garza 10e, p270-272]

477. c An example of a needle shield activated by pressing the shield on a hard surface is the Venipuncture Needle-Pro®.
[McCall 7e, p192]

478. c An example of a needle shield activated by the phlebotomist using his thumb to move the shield over the needle is the Vacuette™ Quickshield Complete Plus Safety Tube Holder.
[Garza 10e, p271]

Explanations

Specimen Collection

479. d An example of a needle shield activated by a retraction mechanism is the VanishPoint®.
[Garza 10e, p270-271]

480. d Red is the most commonly used color for puncture resistant, leakproof containers suitable for discarding used sharps. Sharps containers are manufactured in a variety of colors but all are labeled with the biohazard symbol.
[McCall 7e, p188]

481. a The phlebotomist should locate a sharps container that is not full and discard the contaminated needle there. The phlebotomist should never attempt to push materials in a sharps container down or move them around to accommodate a needle. If a sharps container is filled, the patient's nurse should be notified so she can contact housekeeping to replace the full container with an empty one.
[McCall 7e, p188]

482. b The phlebotomist should discard the needle in a sharps container.
[McCall 7e, p188]

483. c The evacuated tube system is used for routine venipuncture and includes a multisample needle, evacuated tube holder, and evacuated tube.
[Garza 10e, p258]

484. b A heel warmer is commonly used to prepare a site for skin puncture. Warming the site prior to skin puncture increases blood flow to the site, making blood collection following puncture easier and reducing the need to squeeze the site to generate the blood specimen. Warming the site prior to skin puncture arterializes the specimen and can increase blood flow to the site by as much as 7 times.
[McCall 7e, p307]

485. d Yellow stopper evacuated tubes containing the anticoagulant sodium polyanethol sulfonate may be used to collect specimens for blood culture analysis.
[Garza 10e, p263, 481, 654-655]

486. d Yellow stopper evacuated tubes containing the anticoagulant sodium polyanethol sulfonate (SPS) may be used to collect specimens for blood culture analysis. SPS prevents coagulation by binding calcium. It also binds, or inactivates, complement, a protein that destroys bacteria.
[Garza 10e, p262-264, 481, 654-655]

487. a The Bactec system is a blood culture collection system that includes two vials, one for anaerobic bacteria and one for aerobic bacteria. The vials are inoculated using either a syringe or a winged infusion needle. If a syringe is used, the anaerobic bottle should be inoculated first. If a winged infusion needle is used, the aerobic bottle should be inoculated first.
[Garza 10e, p482-483, 623]

Specimen Collection — Explanations

488. a The Hemogard closure of an evacuated tube manufactured by Becton-Dickinson containing clot activator and serum separator gel is gold.
[Garza 10e, p262, 264, 654]

489. c The Hemogard closure of an evacuated tube manufactured by Becton-Dickinson containing thrombin is orange.
[Garza 10e, p262, 265, 654]

490. b The Hemogard closure of an evacuated tube manufactured by Becton-Dickinson containing heparin and plasma separator gel is light green.
[Garza 10e, p262, 265, 654]

491. a Plastic evacuated tubes with red stoppers contain silica particles, which serve as clot activators.
[Garza 10e, p262, 265, 654]

492. d The ratio of blood to anticoagulant in sodium citrate tubes is a critical 9:1 ratio. Underfilling sodium citrate evacuated tubes can cause erroneously prolonged clotting times.
[McCall 7e, p205]

493. c Evacuated tubes with green conventional stoppers contain heparin, in one of the following three forms: ammonium, lithium, or sodium heparin.
[Garza 10e, p262, 265, 654]

494. c Evacuated tubes with gray conventional stoppers contain sodium fluoride, which acts as an antiglycolytic agent.
[Garza 10e, p262, 267, 654]

495. d Conventional evacuated tubes with yellow stoppers contain the anticoagulant sodium polyanethol sulfonate (SPS) and may be used to collect specimens for blood culture analysis. SPS prevents coagulation by binding calcium. It also binds, or inactivates, complement, a protein that destroys bacteria.
[Garza 10e, p262-263, 654]

496. c Sodium fluoride is usually found in grey top evacuated tubes and serves as a glycolytic inhibitor.
[Garza 10e, p262, 267, 654-655]

497. d Heparin functions as an anticoagulant by inhibiting thrombin. It is usually found in green top evacuated tubes, in one of the following three forms: ammonium, lithium, or sodium heparin.
[Garza 10e, p262, 265-266, 654-655]

498. c Royal blue Hemogard evacuated tubes are specially formulated to contain low levels of trace elements. Specific levels of trace elements in royal blue Hemogard evacuated tubes are specified with individual package inserts and are manufactured to minimize contamination of the specimen.
[CLSI Standard GP41, p26-27; Garza 10e, p262, 267, 654-655]

Explanations
Specimen Collection

499. d Tan Hemogard evacuated tubes are specially formulated to contain low levels of lead. Levels of lead in tan Hemogard evacuated tubes are specified with individual package inserts and are manufactured to minimize contamination of the specimen.
[CLSI Standard GP41, p26-27; Garza 10e, p262, 267, 654-655]

500. c Ethylenediamine tetraacetic acid (EDTA) functions as an anticoagulant by binding or chelating calcium. It is the additive of choice for hematology testing because it preserves cellular morphology and inhibits platelet aggregation. EDTA is usually found in lavender top evacuated tubes.
[Garza 10e, p262, 266-267, 654-655]

501. a The only evacuated tube color with two different additives is yellow. Acid citrate dextrose (ACD) is found in an evacuated tube with a yellow stopper. Acid citrate dextrose is used to collect specimens for immunohematology testing and human leukocyte antigen (HLA) typing used in paternity testing and to determine transplant compatibility. The second additive that may be found in an evacuated tube with a yellow stopper is sodium polyanethol sulfonate (SPS) used to collect blood specimens for blood culture analysis.
[Garza 10e, p262, 263, 654-655]

502. d Sodium citrate functions as an anticoagulant by binding or chelating calcium. It is the additive of choice for most routine coagulation testing because it preserves labile coagulation factors. Sodium citrate is usually found in light blue top evacuated tubes. Sodium citrate evacuated tubes must be completely filled to ensure accurate results.
[Garza 10e, p262, 264, 654-655]

503. c Evacuated tubes with gray conventional stoppers contain sodium fluoride, which acts as an antiglycolytic agent, preserving glucose levels until the analysis can be performed.
[Garza 10e, p262, 267, 654-655]

504. d Evacuated tubes with orange conventional stoppers or grey and yellow Hemogard tubes contain thrombin, which acts as a clotting agent. Evacuated tubes containing thrombin are characteristically used in emergency situations because the thrombin will cause the specimen to clot very quickly, usually within 5 minutes, significantly reducing the turnaround time.
[Garza 10e, p262, 654-655]

505. c The red top tube will yield a specimen consisting of red cells and serum. The red top tube contains a clot activator, which promotes clotting and the fluid portion of the specimen is called serum. There is no barrier gel in a red top tube so the cells may be accessed also, if needed.
[Garza 10e, p262, 265, 654-655]

Specimen Collection — Explanations

506. d According to evacuated tube manufacturer Becton-Dickinson, the phlebotomist must invert the tube completely, moving his/her wrist back and forth in a 180° motion.
[McCall 7e, p203-204]

507. a If an EDTA evacuated tube is underfilled, the blood:anticoagulant ratio will be incorrect causing an excess of EDTA in the specimen. Excess EDTA in the specimen may result in red cell shrinkage and a decrease in red cell size, a parameter measured on a routine complete blood count (CBC).
[Garza 10e, p262, 266-267, 654-655]

508. a Ethylenediamine tetraacetic acid (EDTA) functions as an anticoagulant by binding or chelating calcium. It is the additive of choice for hematology testing because it preserves cellular morphology and inhibits platelet aggregation. EDTA is found in lavender top evacuated tubes.
[Garza 10e, p262, 266-267, 654-655]

509. c Sodium citrate functions as an anticoagulant by binding or chelating calcium. It is the additive of choice for most routine coagulation testing because it preserves labile coagulation factors. Sodium citrate is usually found in light blue top evacuated tubes. Sodium citrate evacuated tubes must be completely filled to ensure accurate results.
[Garza 10e, p262, 264, 654-655]

510. c Heparinized evacuated tubes should not be used to collect specimens for blood smear analysis after being stained with Wright stain. Heparin causes the Wright stain to have a blue background, unsuitable for differential analysis and evaluation of red cell morphology.
[Garza 10e, p262, 266, 654-655]

511. a A winged infusion needle is commonly referred to as a butterfly needle because the winged infusion needle resembles the shape of a butterfly.
[McCall 7e, p202]

512. d The needle posing the greatest risk to phlebotomists is the winged infusion needle because failure to activate the safety feature according to manufacturer's recommendations may result in a higher incidence of needlestick injuries.
[CLSI Standards GP41, p54-55; Garza 10e, p110-112, 273, 317, 350]

513. a The most common lengths of winged infusion needles are 1/2 or 3/4 inch.
[McCall 7e, p201]

514. c According to CLSI Standard GP41, needles should never be disposed of by bending, cutting, or resheathing. Safety features for proper disposal of winged infusion needles include blunting, needle retracting, and locking needle shields.
[CLSI Standard GP41, p28]

Explanations
Specimen Collection

515. c A syringe is most commonly employed to collect a blood specimen when a patient has very thin, fragile veins because the phlebotomist can control the amount of pressure exerted on the patient's vein by adjusting the speed at which the plunger is withdrawn.
[Garza 10e, p268-270, 351]

516. a The use of syringes should be limited because they pose an increased risk of accidental needlestick injury to the phlebotomist.
[CLSI Standard GP41, p25; Garza 10e, p268-270, 353]

517. d Syringes for venous blood collection must always be used with a safety transfer device. The safety transfer device is used to transfer the specimen from the syringe into the appropriate evacuated tubes.
[CLSI Standard GP41, p27; Garza 10e, p268-270, 353]

518. a Equipment needed for a skin puncture includes a heel warmer, alcohol, and sterile gauze.
[Garza 10e, p381]

519. b Equipment needed for a skin puncture includes a safety lancet, microcollection container, and sterile gauze.
[Garza 10e, p278, 376, 381]

520. d The temperature of commercial heel warmers should not exceed 42°C. Temperatures exceeding 42°C can burn an infant's sensitive skin.
[Garza 10e, p434]

521. a To prevent accidental injury to an infant's bone, the depth of a puncture on an infant's heel should never exceed 2.0 mm. Additionally, skin punctures for heelstick procedures must be performed on the most medial or lateral aspects of the plantar surface of the infant's heel.
[Garza 10e, p278-279, 432-434]

522. b A sharp device used to puncture the skin prior to capillary blood collection is called a safety lancet.
[Garza 10e, p278, 632]

523. b Permanently retractable blades are mandated on safety lancets as an engineering control prescribed by OSHA to reduce accidental sharps injury.
[Garza 10e, p278]

524. d Surgical blades should never be used instead of a safety lancet to perform a skin puncture.
[Garza 10e, p278]

525. d Patients are classified as obese if their body mass index exceeds 30 kg/m^2.
[Garza 10e, p290]

526. b Occluded veins are blocked and prevent blood flow.
[Garza 10e, p290-291]

Specimen Collection — Explanations

527. d Sclerosed, or hardened veins are often the result of frequent, multiple venipuncture procedures and the resulting inflammatory response.
[Garza 10e, p290-291]

528. b Certain blood component levels may fluctuate throughout the day (diurnal) or over a 24-hour cycle (circadian).
[Garza 10e, p292-293]

529. c Petechiae are small, pinpoint bruises in the skin indicative of a coagulation abnormality. If a phlebotomist notes petechiae on a patient's skin, she should anticipate that the patient will bleed longer than usual following venipuncture.
[Garza 10e, p634]

530. c Hemolysis occurs when red blood cell membranes are ruptured and the contents released into the plasma or serum turning the plasma or serum from yellow to pink or red. Some clinical conditions may cause hemolysis, but it is frequently due to collection error. If a specimen is hemolyzed, some analytes will be adversely affected.
[Garza 10e, p301-302]

531. c Syncope means fainting and includes symptoms such as diaphoresis and pallor. In the event a patient experiences syncope, the phlebotomist should lower the patient's head and instruct her to breathe deeply.
[Garza 10e, p298-299, 320-321, 362]

532. c The angle formed between the patient's arm and the needle is called the angle of insertion.
[CLSI Standard 39, p24]

533. a Swelling caused by an abnormal accumulation of fluid is called edema.
[Garza 10e, p293, 629]

534. b A substance that prevents the breakdown of glucose by red blood cells is a glycolytic inhibitor. [CLSI Standard 39, p2; Garza 10e, p267]

535. c The international normalized ratio (INR) represents a comparison of a patient's prothrombin time result to a reference range result. It is used most frequently to monitor a patient's warfarin (Coumadin®) therapy.
[Garza 10e, p240, 467-468, 632]

536. b Geriatrics is the medical specialty that focuses on the care and treatment of the elderly.
[Garza 10e, p450, 630]

537. c Vein patency refers to the state of being freely open; is the opposite of occluded.
[McCall 7e, p492]

Explanations
Specimen Collection

538. a A method of medication administration which involves piercing the skin or mucous membranes is called parenteral.
[Garza 10e, p633]

539. a The antecubital area (antecubital fossa) is the shallow depression located in front of—or anterior to—the elbow when the patient is in anatomic position.
[Garza 10e, p172-173, 330, 626]

540. c Reflux, or the backwash of contents from an evacuated tube into a patient's vein may be prevented if a patient's arm is positioned downward during venipuncture.
[McCall 7e, p291]

541. a By identifying the meaning of the word root and suffix, the meaning of the word can be constructed. The root word *hemat* means "blood." The suffix *-oma* means "tumor." Literally translated, *hematoma* means "blood tumor." Hematoma, a common complication of venipuncture, results when blood leaves the blood vessels and seeps into the surrounding tissues, evidenced by a purple swelling around the puncture site.
[CLSI Standard GP41, p37; Garza 10e, p247, 297, 299-300, 361]

542. a A substance being tested or analyzed is an analyte.
[Garza 10e, p626]

543. c By identifying the meaning of the word root and suffix, the meaning of the word can be constructed. The root word *glyc* means "glucose" or "sugar." The suffix *-lysis* means "breakdown." The vowel "o" serves is the combining vowel joining the 2 word components. Therefore, *glycolysis* means "breakdown of sugar."
[McCall 7e, p105]

544. b Daily changes that occur during daytime hours in the body and reflecting significant differences in certain test results, most notably hormones, are called diurnal rhythms.
[Garza 10e, p292-293]

545. b Hemoconcentration is the condition when the plasma portion of the blood filters into the tissues resulting in an erroneous decrease in the fluid portion of a blood specimen and an increase in the concentration of cells and large molecules. Prolonged tourniquet application can cause hemoconcentration.
[Garza 10e, p300, 340]

546. d Blood cultures are used to confirm the presence of microorganisms and/or toxins in the patient's bloodstream, a very serious condition often manifested in patients as fevers of unknown origin (FUO).
[Garza 10e, p474]

Specimen Collection — Explanations

547. d The presence of bacteria and their toxins in the bloodstream is called septicemia, a leading cause of death in the United States.
[Garza 10e, p474]

548. b By identifying the meaning of the word root and suffix, the meaning of the word can be constructed. The prefix *an-* means "without." The root word *aer* means "air." The suffix *-ic* means "pertaining to." The vowel "o" serves as the combining vowel joining the word components. Therefore, *anaerobic* means "pertaining to without air." The term that means "without air" is anaerobic.
[Garza 10e, p478-479, 482-483]

549. a By identifying the meaning of the word root and suffix, the meaning of the word can be constructed. The root word *aer* means "air." The suffix *-ic* means "pertaining to." The vowel "o" serves is the combining vowel joining the word components. Therefore, *aerobic* means "pertaining to air." Aerobic is the term that refers to microbes requiring oxygen in order to survive.
[Garza 10e, p478-479, 482-483, 626]

550. b The agency responsible for developing standards of practice in clinical laboratory testing is the Clinical Laboratory Standards Institute. The standard of care for phlebotomy is established by the standards created and published by this agency.
[CLSI Standard GP41, p2]

551. c Extreme, deep, sideways redirection of the needle is probing. Probing is extremely painful for the patient and increases the risk of injury to arteries, nerves, and other structures surrounding the vein. Phlebotomists should never probe in an effort to locate a vein.
[CLSI Standard GP41, p32-33; Garza 10e, p353]

552. a If a skin puncture site is warmed prior to blood collection, the specimen is said to be arterialized. This is a critical step in quality collection of capillary blood gases. Warming the site prior to skin puncture increases the arterial blood flow to the capillary beds.
[McCall 7e, p307]

553. a To achieve standardization consistent with the International Standards Organization (ISO), the Clinical Laboratory Standards Institute describes the laboratory work flow within the context of specimen examination processes, instead of phases. The laboratory workflow takes place in three processes: 1) preexamination/preanalytical process; 2) examination process; 3) postexamination/postanalytical process.
[Garza 10e, p9]

Explanations
Specimen Collection

554. d The preexamination/preanalytical process includes practices completed before laboratory analysis beginning with the requisition from the patient's physician and ending with specimen delivery to the laboratory for accessioning and processing. The preexamination/preanalytical process is the essential domain of every phlebotomist and absolutely vital to quality test results.
[Garza 10e, p9]

555. d The preexamination/preanalytical process includes practices completed before laboratory analysis beginning with the requisition from the patient's physician and ending with specimen delivery to the laboratory for accessioning and processing. The preexamination/preanalytical process is the essential domain of every phlebotomist and absolutely vital to quality test results.
[Garza 10e, p9]

556. d Sometimes referred to as "normal limits," reference ranges are a range of values compiled from data based on results obtained from healthy individuals including high and low limits. The physician evaluates the patient's results within the context of reference ranges to determine if the patient's results are within the values expected.
[Garza 10e, p239-242, 588-591, 635]

557. d Patients are in basal state early in the morning, when a patient is resting, fasting for approximately 12 hours and in a supine position. Reference ranges are established while persons are in basal state so basal state specimens are ideal for testing.
[McCall 7e, p275]

558. a Accession numbers, unique to each specimen and corresponding paperwork, are used to unmistakably correlate the specimen and all procedures conducted on the specimen with the patient.
[McCall 7e, p218, 375]

559. b The term describing adverse effects of medical treatment is iatrogenic. Iatrogenic blood loss refers to the amount of blood a patient loses as the result of blood specimen collection for laboratory testing. Most patients tolerate blood loss due to specimen collection very well. However, some patients are at high risk for complication due to blood collection, including neonates, critically ill patients, and patients with poor prognosis. Patients at high risk for adverse effects of blood collection must be closely monitored for blood loss through specimen collection.
[Garza 10e, p285, 360, 373, 431-432, 596-597, 616, 631]

Specimen Collection — **Explanations**

560. b Extensive loss of blood resulting in death is exsanguination. A patient's life may be threatened if more than 10% of his/her blood volume is lost in a short period of time. Blood collection from neonates and especially premature neonates are at high risk of iatrogenic blood loss that could potentially lead to exsanguination. Withdrawing 10 mL of blood from a premature or newborn infant equates to 5-10% of the infant's total blood volume. Close monitoring of blood volume collected for laboratory analysis is critically important for all patients at risk of iatrogenic blood loss, but especially for infants.
[Garza 10e, p360, 431-432, 597, 631]

561. a Any ingredient added to an evacuated tube to perform a specific function, such as prevention or promotion of coagulation is called an additive.
[CLSI Standard GP39-A6, p1]

Specimen Handling, Transport & Processing

The following items have been identified as appropriate for those preparing for the PBT examination.

1. Laboratory processes include:
   a. preexamination/preanalytical, examination, and postexamination/postanalytical
   b. quality control, quality assurance, quality standards
   c. turnaround time, preexamination/preanalytical processes, phlebotomist expertise
   d. blood culture contamination rates, turnaround time, examination processes

2. The laboratory process with the highest degree of errors is:
   a. preexamination/preanalytical
   b. postexamination/postanalytical
   c. quality assurance
   d. quality control

3. What percentage of errors in laboratory testing during the preexamination/preanalytical process?
   a. 1-3%
   b. 13-15%
   c. 25-40%
   d. 46-68%

4. Preexamination/preanalytical tasks include:
   a. entering laboratory result data
   b. performing quality control in instrumentation
   c. specimen collection
   d. troubleshooting equipment

5. What percentage of errors in laboratory testing occur during the examination process?
   a. 1-3%
   b. 13-15%
   c. 25-40%
   d. 46-68%

Specimen Handling, Transport & Processing — Questions

6. A phlebotomist forgets to deliver a specimen for electrolyte analysis. He leaves it on his cart and goes to lunch. What category of error does this represent?
   - a examination
   - b postexamination/postanalytical
   - c preexamination/preanalytical
   - d quality control

7. A phlebotomist does not adhere to the correct order of draw when collecting multiple specimens following venipuncture. What type of error will this introduce into the specimen?
   - a examination
   - b postexamination/postanalytical
   - c preexamination/preanalytical
   - d quality control

8. A nurse does not instruct an outpatient to fast prior to collection of a first-morning glucose specimen. What type of error will this introduce into the specimen?
   - a examination
   - b postexamination/postanalytical
   - c preexamination/preanalytical
   - d quality control

9. Which of the following analyses requires the patient to fast prior to collection?
   - a cholesterol
   - b hemoglobin A1C
   - c renin
   - d serum gastrin

10. Which of the following analyses requires the patient to fast prior to collection?
    - a theophylline
    - b thrombin time
    - c tobramycin
    - d triglycerides

11. If the serum of a specimen collected for electrolytes is hemolyzed, the specimen will be:
    - a used to perform the type and crossmatch
    - b used to perform a type and screen only
    - c referred to a reference lab
    - d rejected

12. A specimen was collected for therapeutic drug monitoring (TDM) in a red top evacuated tube. The appropriate course of action is to:
    - a accept the specimen
    - b reject the specimen
    - c warm the specimen
    - d send the specimen to a reference lab

Questions
Specimen Handling, Transport & Processing

13. Which of the following specimens would be accepted for lactate dehydrogenase analysis in the clinical laboratory?
    a   plasma in a sodium citrate evacuated tube
    b   serum in a gold Hemogard gel barrier evacuated tube
    c   whole blood in an EDTA tube (pink)
    d   whole blood in a potassium oxalate/sodium fluoride tube

14. Which of the following specimens would be accepted for ABO group and Rh typing in the clinical laboratory?
    a   plasma in a heparinized evacuated tube
    b   plasma in a sodium citrate evacuated tube
    c   whole blood in an EDTA tube (pink)
    d   whole blood in a potassium oxalate/sodium fluoride tube

15. Which of the following specimens would be accepted for a partial thromboplastin time testing in the clinical laboratory?
    a   plasma in a heparinized evacuated tube
    b   plasma in a sodium citrate evacuated tube
    c   whole blood in an EDTA tube (lavender)
    d   whole blood in an EDTA tube (pink)

16. Which of the following specimens would be accepted for prothrombin time (PT) testing in the clinical laboratory?
    a   plasma in a heparinized evacuated tube
    b   plasma in a sodium citrate evacuated tube
    c   whole blood in an EDTA tube (lavender)
    d   whole blood in an EDTA tube (pink)

17. Which of the following specimens would be accepted for complete blood count (CBC) testing in the clinical laboratory?
    a   plasma in a heparinized evacuated tube
    b   plasma in a sodium citrate evacuated tube
    c   whole blood in an EDTA tube (lavender)
    d   whole blood in a potassium oxalate/sodium fluoride tube

18. Which of the following specimens would be accepted for reticulocyte count testing in the clinical laboratory?
    a   plasma in a heparinized evacuated tube
    b   plasma in a sodium citrate evacuated tube
    c   whole blood in an EDTA tube (lavender)
    d   whole blood in a potassium oxalate/sodium fluoride tube

19. Which of the following specimens would be accepted for erythrocyte sedimentation rate testing in the clinical laboratory?
    a   plasma in a heparinized evacuated tube
    b   plasma in a sodium citrate evacuated tube
    c   whole blood in an EDTA tube (lavender)
    d   whole blood in a potassium oxalate/sodium fluoride tube

Specimen Handling, Transport & Processing — Questions

20. Which of the following specimens would be accepted for hemoglobin electrophoresis in the clinical laboratory?
    a plasma in an EDTA tube (pink)
    b plasma in a heparinized evacuated tube
    c plasma in a sodium citrate evacuated tube
    d whole blood in an EDTA tube (lavender)

21. Which of the following specimens would be accepted for platelet count in the clinical laboratory?
    a plasma in an EDTA tube (pink)
    b plasma in a heparinized evacuated tube
    c plasma in a sodium citrate evacuated tube
    d whole blood in an EDTA tube (lavender)

22. Which of the following specimens would be accepted for electrolyte analysis in the clinical laboratory?
    a plasma in a heparinized evacuated tube
    b plasma in a sodium citrate evacuated tube
    c whole blood in an EDTA tube (pink)
    d whole blood in an EDTA tube (lavender)

23. Which of the following specimens would be accepted for glucose analysis in the clinical laboratory?
    a plasma in a potassium oxalate and sodium fluoride evacuated tube
    b plasma in a sodium citrate evacuated tube
    c whole blood in a gel barrier tube
    d whole blood in an EDTA tube (lavender)

24. Which of the following specimens would be accepted for a basic metabolic panel (BMP) analysis in the clinical laboratory?
    a plasma in a lithium heparin evacuated tube
    b plasma in a sodium heparin evacuated tube
    c whole blood in a sodium citrate evacuated tube
    d whole blood in an EDTA tube (lavender)

25. Which of the following specimens would be accepted for a glycosylated hemoglobin (hemoglobin A1c) analysis in the clinical laboratory?
    a plasma in a potassium oxalate and sodium fluoride evacuated tube
    b plasma in a sodium citrate evacuated tube
    c serum in a gel barrier tube
    d whole blood in an EDTA tube (lavender)

26. Which of the following specimens would be accepted for a creatinine analysis in the clinical laboratory?
    a plasma in a potassium oxalate and sodium fluoride evacuated tube
    b plasma in a sodium citrate evacuated tube
    c serum in a gel barrier tube
    d whole blood in an EDTA tube (lavender)

Questions
Specimen Handling, Transport & Processing

27. Which of the following specimens would be accepted for a carcinoembryonic antigen (CEA) analysis in the clinical laboratory?
    a   plasma in a potassium oxalate and sodium fluoride evacuated tube
    b   plasma in a sodium citrate evacuated tube
    c   serum in a gel barrier tube
    d   whole blood in an EDTA tube (lavender)

28. Which of the following specimens would be accepted for an eosinophil count in the clinical laboratory?
    a   plasma in a evacuated tube
    b   plasma in a sodium citrate evacuated tube
    c   serum in a gel barrier tube
    d   whole blood in an EDTA tube (lavender)

29. Which of the following specimens would be accepted for a fibrinogen level analysis in the clinical laboratory?
    a   plasma in a heparinized evacuated tube
    b   plasma in a sodium citrate evacuated tube
    c   serum in a gel barrier tube
    d   whole blood in an EDTA tube (lavender)

30. Which of the following specimens would be accepted for a human chorionic gonadotropin (HCG) analysis in the clinical laboratory?
    a   plasma in a potassium oxalate and sodium fluoride evacuated tube
    b   plasma in a sodium citrate evacuated tube
    c   serum in a gel barrier tube
    d   whole blood in an EDTA tube (lavender)

31. Which of the following specimens would be accepted for a fluorescent treponemal antibody absorption analysis in the clinical laboratory?
    a   blood smear stained with Wright stain
    b   plasma in a sodium citrate evacuated tube
    c   serum in an evacuated tube without additive
    d   whole blood in an EDTA tube (pink)

32. Which of the following specimens would be accepted for a creatine kinase MB analysis in the clinical laboratory?
    a   plasma in a potassium oxalate and sodium fluoride evacuated tube
    b   plasma in a sodium citrate evacuated tube
    c   serum in a gel barrier tube
    d   whole blood in an EDTA tube (lavender)

33. Which of the following specimens would be accepted for an antithrombin III analysis in the clinical laboratory?
    a   blood smear stained with Wright stain
    b   plasma collected in an EDTA tube (lavender)
    c   plasma in an EDTA tube (pink)
    d   plasma in a sodium citrate evacuated tube

Specimen Handling, Transport & Processing — Questions

34. Which of the following specimens would be accepted for a blood urea nitrogen (BUN) analysis in the clinical laboratory?
    a   plasma in a potassium oxalate and sodium fluoride evacuated tube
    b   plasma in a sodium citrate evacuated tube
    c   serum in a gel barrier tube
    d   whole blood in an EDTA tube (lavender)

35. Which of the following specimens would be accepted for a differential white cell count in the clinical laboratory?
    a   blood smear stained with Wright stain
    b   plasma in a sodium fluoride tube
    c   plasma in a sodium heparin tube
    d   whole blood in a sodium citrate evacuated tube

36. Which of the following specimens would be accepted for an alanine aminotransferase (ALT) analysis in the clinical laboratory?
    a   plasma in a potassium oxalate and sodium fluoride evacuated tube
    b   plasma in a sodium citrate evacuated tube
    c   serum in a gel barrier tube
    d   whole blood in an EDTA tube (lavender)

37. Which of the following specimens would be accepted for an hematocrit level in the clinical laboratory?
    a   blood smear stained with Wright stain
    b   plasma in an EDTA tube (pink)
    c   plasma in a sodium citrate evacuated tube
    d   whole blood in an EDTA tube (lavender)

38. Which of the following specimens would be accepted for an alkaline phosphatase analysis in the clinical laboratory?
    a   plasma in an EDTA evacuated tube
    b   plasma in a sodium citrate evacuated tube
    c   serum in an evacuated tube without additive
    d   whole blood in a gel separator tube

39. Which of the following specimens would be accepted for an Anti-Rh antibody screen in the clinical laboratory?
    a   blood smear stained with Wright stain
    b   plasma in a sodium citrate evacuated tube
    c   serum in an evacuated tube without additive
    d   whole blood in a gel barrier tube (pink)

40. Which of the following specimens would be accepted for an amylase analysis in the clinical laboratory?
    a   plasma in an EDTA evacuated tube
    b   plasma in a sodium citrate evacuated tube
    c   serum in a gel barrier tube
    d   whole blood in a gel separator tube

Questions
Specimen Handling, Transport & Processing

41. Which of the following specimens would be accepted for an acid phosphatase analysis in the clinical laboratory?
    a   plasma in a potassium oxalate and sodium fluoride evacuated tube
    b   plasma in a sodium citrate evacuated tube
    c   serum in a gel barrier tube
    d   whole blood in an EDTA tube (lavender)

42. Which of the following specimens would be accepted for red cell index analysis in the clinical laboratory?
    a   blood smear stained with Wright stain
    b   plasma in an EDTA tube (pink)
    c   plasma in a sodium citrate tube
    d   whole blood in an EDTA tube (lavender)

43. Which of the following specimens would be accepted for an aspartate aminotransferase (AST) analysis in the clinical laboratory?
    a   plasma in a potassium oxalate and sodium fluoride evacuated tube
    b   plasma in a sodium citrate evacuated tube
    c   serum in a gel barrier tube
    d   whole blood in an EDTA tube (lavender)

44. Which of the following specimens would be accepted for a mononucleosis screen analysis in the clinical laboratory?
    a   blood smear stained with Wright stain
    b   plasma in an EDTA tube (lavender)
    c   serum in an EDTA tube (pink)
    d   whole blood in a sodium citrate evacuated tube

45. Which of the following specimens would be accepted for a bilirubin analysis in the clinical laboratory?
    a   plasma in an EDTA evacuated tube
    b   plasma in a sodium citrate evacuated tube
    c   serum in a gel barrier tube
    d   whole blood in a gel separator tube

46. Which of the following specimens would be accepted for a lipase analysis in the clinical laboratory?
    a   plasma in an EDTA evacuated tube
    b   plasma in a sodium citrate evacuated tube
    c   serum in an evacuated tube without additive
    d   whole blood in a gel separator tube

47. Which of the following specimens would be accepted for a high-density lipoprotein analysis in the clinical laboratory?
    a   plasma in a potassium oxalate and sodium fluoride evacuated tube
    b   plasma in a sodium citrate evacuated tube
    c   serum in a gel barrier tube
    d   whole blood in an EDTA tube (lavender)

Specimen Handling, Transport & Processing — Questions

48. Which of the following specimens would be accepted for a total white cell count in the clinical laboratory?
    a   blood smear stained with Wright stain
    b   plasma in an EDTA tube (lavender)
    c   serum in an EDTA tube (pink)
    d   whole blood in an EDTA tube (lavender)

49. Which of the following specimens would be accepted for a C-reactive protein analysis in the clinical laboratory?
    a   blood smear stained with Wright stain
    b   plasma in an EDTA tube (lavender)
    c   serum in an EDTA tube (lavender)
    d   serum in an evacuated tube without additive

50. Which of the following specimens would be accepted for a cholesterol analysis in the clinical laboratory?
    a   plasma in an EDTA evacuated tube
    b   plasma in a sodium citrate evacuated tube
    c   serum in an evacuated tube without additive
    d   whole blood in a gel separator tube

51. Which of the following specimens would be accepted for an antistreptolysin O analysis in the clinical laboratory?
    a   blood smear stained with Wright stain
    b   plasma in an EDTA tube (lavender)
    c   serum in an EDTA tube (lavender)
    d   serum in an evacuated tube without additive

52. Which of the following specimens would be accepted for a prostate-specific antigen analysis in the clinical laboratory?
    a   plasma in an EDTA evacuated tube
    b   plasma in a sodium citrate evacuated tube
    c   serum in a gel separator tube
    d   whole blood in an evacuated tube without additive

53. If a patient finishes drinking a glucose solution during a 3-hour glucose tolerance test (GTT) at 7:30 AM, what time should the first specimen be drawn?
    a   7:45 AM
    b   8:00 AM
    c   8:15 AM
    d   8:30 AM

Questions
Specimen Handling, Transport & Processing

54. If a patient finishes drinking a glucose solution during a 3-hour glucose tolerance test (GTT) at 7:30 AM, what time should the last specimen be drawn?
    a   8:00 AM
    b   8:30 AM
    c   9:30 AM
    d   10: 30 AM

55. If a physician orders a 3-hour glucose tolerance test on a patient, how many blood collection procedures must be performed as part of the GTT?
    a   2
    b   3
    c   4
    d   5

56. A patient finishes eating a breakfast of approximately 80 g of glucose and a specimen for plasma glucose was collected 120 minutes later. This test is called a:
    a   glucose tolerance test
    b   lactose tolerance test
    c   postprandial glucose level
    d   sweat chloride test

57. Which of the following test procedures is preceded by a glucose tolerance test (GTT)?
    a   glucagon tolerance test
    b   lactose tolerance test
    c   sweat chloride test
    d   D-xylose test

58. Phlebotomists must ensure that patients have access to which of the following during a lactose tolerance test?
    a   iPad
    b   lavatory
    c   television
    d   water cooler

59. Lactose tolerance may also be performed on what kind of sample?
    a   breath
    b   sputum
    c   stool
    d   urine

Specimen Handling, Transport & Processing — **Questions**

60. Which of the following tests is usually ordered as a series of samples collected at timed intervals?
    a   blood cultures
    b   cold agglutinin titers
    c   cryoglobulin levels
    d   fibrin degradation products

61. Manufacturers of blood culture specimen bottles recommend using either a winged infusion set or a syringe to prevent which of the following?
    a   hemoconcentration
    b   hemolysis
    c   lipemia
    d   reflux

62. Which blood culture bottle should be collected first when collecting a blood culture specimen using a winged infusion set?
    a   aerobic
    b   anaerobic
    c   antisepsis
    d   anticoagulant

63. Which of the following characteristics applies to a drug that is monitored by a therapeutic drug monitoring (TDM) system?
    a   administered IV only
    b   administered "STAT"
    c   narrow therapeutic/toxic ranges
    d   predictable dose-response relationships

64. Which of the following drugs is characteristically incorporated into a TDM program?
    a   acetaminophen
    b   aminoglycosides
    c   morphine
    d   salicylate

65. Which of the following is a common reason for rejection of specimens collected as part of a TDM program?
    a   failure to collect specimen at the appropriate time
    b   failure to mix blood with additive
    c   incorrect specimen tube
    d   insufficient specimen

66. Before a specimen for TDM can be collected, there must be verification of the patient's last:
    a   meal
    b   medication dose
    c   therapy session
    d   venipuncture

Questions
Specimen Handling, Transport & Processing

67. A phlebotomist is to collect a trough blood specimen at 7:00 AM as part of a TDM program. The phlebotomist has several specimens to collect at that time. How many minutes before the hour can she or he collect the specimen?
    a   15
    b   20
    c   25
    d   30

68. Which category of tests are typically ordered by a physician to assess environmental exposure, nutritional deficiencies, or the metal-on-metal wear of artificial joints?
    a   basic metabolic panel
    b   lipid profile
    c   therapeutic drug monitoring
    d   trace metal analysis

69. Which of the following analytes are considered trace metals?
    a   amylase, lipase, creatine kinase
    b   alanine aminotransferase, aspartate aminotransferase, alkaline phosphatase
    c   bilirubin, ferritin, urobilinogen
    d   cobalt, chromium, copper

70. Specimens for which of the following elements may be contaminated by substances commonly found in evacuated tube components, ie, stoppers, glass or plastic?
    a   lead
    b   lithium
    c   potassium
    d   sodium

71. Listed below are colors of Hemogard stoppers for evacuated tubes. Which Hemogard stoppered evacuated tube is most suitable for lead level determinations?
    a   gold
    b   gray
    c   red
    d   tan

72. Listed below are colors of Hemogard stoppers for evacuated tubes. Which Hemogard evacuated tube is most suitable for zinc level determinations?
    a   brown
    b   gold
    c   light blue
    d   royal blue

73. Which of the following specimens require timed collections based on circadian rhythms?
    a   carotene
    b   complete blood count
    c   cortisol
    d   creatinine

74. A phlebotomist attempted to collect a cortisol level from a patient at 8:00 AM. She was unsuccessful twice. The appropriate course of action is to:
    a   leave the tubes and requisitions at the nurse's station so the nurses can collect the specimen
    b   leave the tubes and requisitions at the nurse's station so the physician can collect the specimen
    c   immediately page another phlebotomist to collect the specimen
    d   bring the requisition down to the lab marked "unsuccessful"

75. Which of the following specimens must be collected after a patient has been in a supine position for at least 30 minutes prior to specimen collection?
    a   aldosterone
    b   aldolase
    c   cortisol
    d   creatinine

76. Which of the following specimens must be collected in a plastic evacuated tube?
    a   aldosterone
    b   aldolase
    c   cortisol
    d   creatinine

77. Neonatal specimens for phenylketonuria (PKU) analysis should be collected using:
    a   filter paper
    b   glass slides
    c   microtainer tubes
    d   unopette system

78. Following collection, newborn screening specimens should be dried at which of the following temperatures?
    a   4°C
    b   22°C
    c   37°C
    d   56°C

Questions
Specimen Handling, Transport & Processing

79. Following collection, newborn screening specimens should be dried horizontally for at least how long?
    a   1 hour
    b   2 hours
    c   3 hours
    d   6 hours

80. Within how many hours must filter paper specimens be mailed to the laboratory following collection?
    a   6
    b   12
    c   24
    d   48

81. A phlebotomist performs a skin puncture on a baby to collect a specimen for neonatal screening tests. How should the specimen be allocated to the filter paper?
    a   flip the filter paper back and forth and use both sides to completely fill the circles indicated
    b   use a capillary tube to collect the specimen and tap the capillary tube onto the filter paper to aliquot the specimen
    c   use only one side of the paper and a continuous flow of blood from the skin puncture site onto each circle until each is completely saturated
    d   repeatedly tap the baby's heel onto the filter paper until the circles are completely saturated

82. Specimens for neonatal screening must be collected before the baby is:
    a   24 hours old
    b   48 hours old
    c   72 hours old
    d   96 hours old

83. Which of the following clinical circumstances will cause a neonatal screen specimen to provide invalid results?
    a   blood transfusion
    b   intravenous fluids
    c   phototherapy
    d   RhoGam administration

84. Which of the following diseases is characteristically included in a newborn screening panel?
    a   cystic fibrosis
    b   hemolytic disease of the newborn
    c   hyperthyroidism
    d   thalassemia

85. Chain of custody procedures are most frequently used for which type of specimen?
    a   forensic
    b   newborn screening
    c   routine
    d   STAT

86. Which of the following forms may be used to document the handling and storage of a specimen from the time the specimen is given to a collector until the specimen is disposed?
    a   Federal Drug Testing Custody and Control Form (CCF)
    b   State Drug Testing Custody and Control Form (CCF)
    c   Incident Report Form
    d   Evidence Report Form

87. Which of the following agencies defines requirements for the collection, processing, and testing of urine drug screens?
    a   ASCP
    b   ASMT
    c   NCCLS
    d   NIDA

88. The minimum acceptable volume of urine specimen for drug screening for the Department of Transportation is:
    a   25 mL
    b   35 mL
    c   45 mL
    d   55 mL

89. The temperature of a urine specimen must be measured following collection of a specimen for drug screening within:
    a   1 minute
    b   2 minutes
    c   4 minutes
    d   8 minutes

90. The temperature of a urine specimen measured following collection of a specimen for drug screening must fall within the following range:
    a   32-38°C
    b   31-39°C
    c   32-40°C
    d   33-41°C

91. The process of recording [specimens] in the order received is called:
    a   accessioning
    b   triaging
    c   quality assurance
    d   quality control

Questions — Specimen Handling, Transport & Processing

92. The accessioning process documents correlation of the specimen to the:
    a patient
    b physician
    c physician and nurse
    d physician, nurse, and discharge date

93. The character used to unmistakably connect a specimen to a patient is an accession:
    a icon
    b letter
    c number
    d symbol

94. The accession number assigned to a specimen is generated by the:
    a HIPAA compliance officer
    b laboratory director
    c laboratory information system (LIS)
    d legal department

95. An EDTA specimen for complete blood count (CBC) was delivered to the laboratory. Once accessioned, the specimen should be placed:
    a on a test tube rocker
    b in a centrifuge
    c in a 37°C incubator
    d in a refrigerator

96. A specimen for STAT troponin level was drawn in a gel separation tube at 9:30 AM and delivered to the laboratory at 9:45 AM. The patient is not on anticoagulant therapy. How soon can the phlebotomist centrifuge the specimen for quality results?
    a 10:00 AM
    b 10:15 AM
    c immediately
    d the specimen should be redrawn

97. A specimen for STAT creatine-kinase MB was drawn in an evacuated tube containing thrombin at 9:30 AM and delivered to the laboratory at 9:45 AM The patient is not on anticoagulant therapy. How soon can the phlebotomist centrifuge the specimen for quality results?
    a 10:00 AM
    b 10:15 AM
    c immediately
    d the specimen should be redrawn

98. The practice of removing an evacuated stopper and using a wooden applicator stick to remove specimen from the top of the evacuated tube is called:
    a   reflux
    b   rhizotomy
    c   rimming
    d   rockery

99. Rimming is:
    a   an acceptable practice
    b   an acceptable practice in STAT situations only
    c   contraindicated due to the danger of aerosol formation
    d   contraindicated due to microclot formation

100. A specimen was not allowed to clot completely before centrifugation. As a result, the serum may be contaminated with:
    a   fibrin
    b   fibrinogen
    c   plasminogen
    d   thrombin

101. A specimen was collected in a gel barrier evacuated tube from a patient receiving heparin therapy. The clotting time for this patient's specimen is expected to be:
    a   lipemic
    b   prolonged
    c   shortened
    d   unaffected

102. When should specimen labels be affixed to specimen tubes?
    a   before collecting the specimen, while preparing supplies
    b   before collecting the specimen, at the patient's bedside
    c   after collecting the patient's specimen and after arriving in the laboratory
    d   after collecting the patient's specimen and before leaving or dismissing the patient

103. Which of the following pieces of information must always be included on a patient specimen label?
    a   patient address
    b   patient blood type
    c   phlebotomist initials
    d   physician name

Questions
Specimen Handling, Transport & Processing

104. Collection of blood specimens for which of the following tests may incorporate the use of a temporary identification number and a three-part identification band?
    a   blood cultures
    b   glucose tolerance testing
    c   fibrin split products
    d   type and crossmatch

105. Which of the following would appear in addition to routine labeling information on a specimen collected as part of a GTT?
    a   skin puncture site selected
    b   time interval of the specimen
    c   Typenex numbers
    d   venipuncture site selected

106. When labeling a blood culture specimen, what information should a phlebotomist record, in addition to routine labeling information?
    a   time of last venipuncture
    b   date of last venipuncture
    c   initials of the patient's designated healthcare provider (often a nurse)
    d   venipuncture site used

107. A patient's requisition form reads, "Jane Jones." A specimen submitted to the laboratory corresponding to the requisition is labeled "J. Jones." What is the appropriate course of action?
    a   ask the PBT to use full names on all future labels and analyze
    b   accept the specimen
    c   change the label
    d   reject the specimen

108. An EDTA specimen from a 50-year-old female patient was submitted for hemoglobin testing. The hemoglobin result generated was 5.8 g/dL. What is the appropriate course of action?
    a   report the results and notify the patient's physician at once
    b   panic because this is a critical (panic) value
    c   repeat the quality control procedures on the analyzer
    d   report the result following routine procedures

109. An EDTA specimen from a 30-year-old female patient was submitted for hemoglobin testing. The hemoglobin result generated was 6.8 g/dL. The patient's specimen was redrawn and the second result was a 12.1 g/dL. This discrepancy most likely occurred because the first specimen was:
    a   clotted
    b   hemolyzed
    c   transported at 37°C
    d   transported on ice

110. An EDTA specimen from a 30-year-old female patient was submitted for hemoglobin testing. The hemoglobin result generated was 6.8 g/dL. The patient's specimen was redrawn and the second result was a 12.1 g/dL. The error that caused this discrepancy is most likely:
    a   examination
    b   postexamination/postanalytical
    c   preexamination/preanalytical
    d   supervisory

111. What is the most common reason for specimen rejection in the chemistry department of the clinical laboratory?
    a   clotting
    b   hemoconcentration
    c   hemolysis
    d   lipemia

112. What is the most common reason for specimen rejection in the chemistry department of the clinical laboratory from the list below?
    a   hemoconcentration
    b   lipemia
    c   QC
    d   QNS

113. What is the most common reason for specimen rejection in the hematology department of the clinical laboratory?
    a   clotting
    b   hemoconcentration
    c   hemolysis
    d   lipemia

114. Which of the following analytes would be falsely increased in a hemolyzed specimen?
    a   ammonia
    b   antinuclear antibodies
    c   blood urea nitrogen
    d   uric acid

115. Which of the following analytes would be falsely increased in a hemolyzed specimen?
    a   carcinoembryonic antigen
    b   digoxin
    c   dilantin
    d   potassium

Questions — Specimen Handling, Transport & Processing

116. Which of the following analytes would be falsely increased in a hemolyzed specimen?
    a   amylase
    b   antinuclear antibodies
    c   blood urea nitrogen
    d   uric acid

117. Which of the following analytes would be falsely increased in a hemolyzed specimen?
    a   human chorionic gonadotropin
    b   human leukocyte antigen B-27
    c   lactate dehydrogenase
    d   lipoprotein

118. Which of the following analytes would be falsely increased in a hemolyzed specimen?
    a   hepatitis B surface antibody
    b   hepatitis B surface antigen
    c   iron
    d   tobramycin

119. A specimen was collected for alanine and aspartate aminotransferase (ALT & AST) analyses. A serum separator evacuated tube was used to collect the specimen and was filled to approximately 60% of scheduled volume. The patient has an extremely high hematocrit due to polycythemia. The medical laboratory scientist requested a redraw. What is the most likely reason a redraw was requested?
    a   concentrated specimen
    b   diluted specimen
    c   PVC
    d   QNS

120. An EDTA specimen for a complete blood count (CBC) was delivered to the hematology laboratory. The specimen was analyzed using an automated cell counting method. During analysis, the sample probe was occluded. What is the most likely explanation?
    a   the phlebotomist did not adequately mix the specimen following collection
    b   the specimen was not allowed to clot prior to centrifugation
    c   the technologist did not follow quality control protocols
    d   there was no error committed because this is a normal circumstance

Specimen Handling, Transport & Processing **Questions**

121. A specimen was collected in a green top evacuated tube for an electrolyte level. The results generated included a critical (panic) value for sodium. The first action the technologist should take is to:
    a   call the patient's physician immediately
    b   call the patient's designated healthcare provider (often a nurse) and instruct that the patient's IV be discontinued
    c   examine the green top evacuated tube used to collect the specimen
    d   rerun the specimen to confirm the result

122. A specimen for an erythrocyte sedimentation rate was submitted in a lavender microcollection container following skin puncture. Why was the specimen rejected for analysis?
    a   concentrated
    b   diluted
    c   QNS
    d   suitable for testing

123. A specimen for bilirubin analysis was collected in a gel separator tube and transported to the laboratory 60 minutes after collection. It was not shielded from the light. As a result, the bilirubin levels in the specimen will be falsely:
    a   decreased by as much as 50%
    b   decreased by as much as 75%
    c   increased by as much as 10%
    d   increased by as much as 25%

124. Listed below are colors of conventional stoppers for evacuated tubes. Which stopper color would be selected most often to collect specimens analyzed in the chemistry department?
    a   gray
    b   lavender
    c   light blue
    d   red and gray

125. Listed below are colors of conventional stoppers for evacuated tubes. Which stopper color would be selected most often to collect specimens analyzed by the hematology department?
    a   gray
    b   lavender
    c   light blue
    d   red SST

Questions

Specimen Handling, Transport & Processing

126. Which of the following departments in the clinical laboratory performs antistreptolysin-O (ASO) titers, cold agglutinin titers, and rapid plasma reagin analyses?
    a   clinical chemistry
    b   hematology
    c   immunology
    d   microbiology

127. Which of the following laboratory departments offers a profile of tests that typically includes electrolytes, glucose, ALT, AST, BUN, calcium, and creatinine?
    a   clinical chemistry
    b   hematology
    c   immunology
    d   microbiology

128. Which of the following departments in the clinical laboratory is most often responsible for analyzing specimens for prothrombin and partial thromboplastin time analysis?
    a   clinical chemistry
    b   coagulation
    c   immunology
    d   microbiology

129. Which department of the clinical laboratory is most likely to perform a culture and sensitivity?
    a   clinical chemistry
    b   hematology
    c   immunology
    d   microbiology

130. Which of the following colored conventional stoppers for evacuated tubes would most likely be delivered to microbiology for analysis?
    a   lavender
    b   light blue
    c   red & gray
    d   yellow SPS tube

131. Which of the following departments would most likely perform a type and crossmatch analysis?
    a   clinical chemistry
    b   hematology
    c   immunology
    d   immunohematology

Specimen Handling, Transport & Processing — Questions

132. Listed below are colors of conventional stoppers for evacuated tubes. Which stopper color would be selected most often to collect specimens analyzed in the immunohematology department?
    a   pink
    b   red SST
    c   light blue
    d   royal blue

133. Listed below are colors of conventional stoppers for evacuated tubes. Which stopper color would be selected most often to collect specimens analyzed in the coagulation department?
    a   green
    b   red
    c   light blue
    d   royal blue

134. Which of the following analyses is always transported and analyzed STAT?
    a   ABG
    b   BUN
    c   CBC
    d   RPR

135. Arterial blood gas specimens require special transport to prevent changes in:
    a   bilirubin levels
    b   carotene levels
    c   glucose levels
    d   pH levels

136. What advantage does a pneumatic tube delivery system offer?
    a   decreases specimen delivery time
    b   increases specimen delivery time
    c   reduces contamination risks to personnel
    d   reduces the number of hemolyzed blood specimens

137. An EDTA specimen was collected for a complete blood count (CBC) in a microcollection container. Within what time frame should the specimen be analyzed?
    a   1 hour
    b   2 hours
    c   4 hours
    d   8 hours

138. An EDTA specimen was collected for a complete blood count (CBC) in an evacuated tube. How long will the specimen be stable at 22°C?
    a   2 hours
    b   4 hours
    c   12 hours
    d   24 hours

Questions
Specimen Handling, Transport & Processing

139. An EDTA specimen was collected for an erythrocyte sedimentation rate (ESR) in an evacuated tube. How long will the specimen be stable at 22°C?
    a   2 hours
    b   4 hours
    c   12 hours
    d   24 hours

140. An EDTA specimen was collected for an erythrocyte sedimentation rate (ESR) in an evacuated tube. How long will the specimen be stable at 4°C?
    a   2 hours
    b   4 hours
    c   12 hours
    d   24 hours

141. A sodium fluoride specimen was collected for a glucose level. How long will the specimen be stable at 22°C?
    a   2 hours
    b   4 hours
    c   12 hours
    d   24 hours

142. A sodium citrate specimen was collected for a prothrombin time (PT). How long will the specimen be stable at 22°C?
    a   2 hours
    b   4 hours
    c   12 hours
    d   24 hours

143. A sodium citrate specimen was collected for a partial thromboplastin time (PTT). How long will the specimen be stable at 22°C?
    a   2 hours
    b   4 hours
    c   12 hours
    d   24 hours

144. At what temperature should specimens for cold agglutinin titers be transported?
    a   4°C
    b   22°C
    c   37°C
    d   56°C

145. Which of the following specimens must be transported at 37°C?
    a   carotene
    b   catecholamines
    c   cold agglutinin titers
    d   creatine phosphokinase

Specimen Handling, Transport & Processing — Questions

146. Which of the following specimens must be transported at 37°C?
     a carotene
     b catecholamines
     c creatine phosphokinase
     d cryoglobulin

147. Which of the following specimens must be transported at 37°C?
     a carotene
     b catecholamines
     c creatine phosphokinase
     d cryofibrinogen

148. What is the best method to transport specimens at 37°C?
     a ice bath
     b heat block
     c wrapped in a towel
     d wrapped in a washcloth dampened with warm water

149. Specimens that must be transported chilled should be transported:
     a on dry ice
     b in a plastic bag filled with ice cubes
     c in a crushed ice slurry
     d wrapped in a cold pack

150. Which of the following specimens requires chilled transport?
     a albumin
     b ammonia
     c amylase
     d antibody screen

151. Which of the following specimens requires chilled transport?
     a acid phosphatase
     b adrenocorticotropic hormone (ACTH)
     c aldosterone
     d α-fetoprotein (AFP)

152. Which of the following specimens requires chilled transport?
     a alanine aminotransferase (ALT)
     b amylase
     c magnesium
     d parathyroid hormone (PTH)

153. Which of the following specimens requires chilled transport?
     a alanine aminotransferase (ALT)
     b amylase
     c angiotensin-converting enzyme (ACE)
     d aspartate aminotransferase (AST)

Questions
Specimen Handling, Transport & Processing

154. Which of the following specimens requires chilled transport?
    a   acetone
    b   alanine aminotransferase (ALT)
    c   amylase
    d   aspartate aminotransferase (AST)

155. Which of the following specimens requires chilled transport?
    a   catecholamines
    b   carotene
    c   cold agglutinin
    d   cryoglobulins

156. Which of the following specimens requires chilled transport?
    a   lactic acid
    b   lactate dehydrogenase
    c   lipase
    d   lithium

157. Which of the following specimens requires chilled transport?
    a   hemoglobin
    b   hematocrit
    c   hemoglobin electrophoresis
    d   homocysteine

158. Which of the following specimens requires chilled transport?
    a   gastrin
    b   gentamicin
    c   glucose
    d   glucose-6-phosphate dehydrogenase

159. Which of the following specimens requires chilled transport?
    a   rapid plasma reagin
    b   renin
    c   reticulocyte count
    d   RhoGAM workup

160. A specimen for potassium was collected in a gel separation evacuated tube in a physician's office. The centrifuge was broken so the phlebotomist placed the specimen in the refrigerator for the courier. What effect will this have on the specimen?
    a   falsely decrease the potassium
    b   falsely elevate the potassium
    c   none because the gel barrier preserved the potassium level
    d   none because the specimen was processed appropriately

Specimen Handling, Transport & Processing — **Questions**

161. A specimen for prothrombin time was collected in a sodium citrate evacuated tube in a physician's office. The centrifuge was broken so the phlebotomist placed the specimen in the rack on the counter for the courier. What effect will this have on the specimen?
    a falsely decrease the prothrombin time
    b falsely increase the prothrombin time
    c none because the gel barrier preserved the prothrombin level
    d none because the specimen was processed appropriately

162. Which of the following materials is most commonly used to transport specimens shielded from light?
    a aluminum foil
    b paper cup
    c paper towel
    d plastic bag

163. Which of the following specimens requires transport shielded from light?
    a alkaline phosphatase
    b bilirubin
    c cold agglutinin
    d fibrinogen

164. Which of the following specimens requires transport shielded from light?
    a acid phosphatase
    b β-carotene
    c blood urea nitrogen
    d fibrin split products

165. Which of the following specimens requires transport shielded from light?
    a ammonia
    b electrolytes
    c gastrin
    d folate

166. Which of the following specimens requires transport shielded from light?
    a acid phosphatase
    b blood urea nitrogen
    c fibrin split products
    d vitamin B_{12}

167. Which of the following specimens requires transport shielded from light?
    a acetone
    b blood urea nitrogen
    c fibrin split products
    d vitamin B_6

Questions
Specimen Handling, Transport & Processing

168. Which of the following specimens requires transport shielded from light?
- a cold agglutinins
- b gastrin
- c homocysteine
- d vitamin C

169. Which of the following analytes will be falsely elevated if the specimen is stored uncentrifuged at 4°C?
- a plasminogen
- b phosphorous
- c red blood cell count
- d white blood cell count

170. According to CLSI, what is the maximum time that may elapse between collection of a blood specimen and separation of the cells from the sera for most specimens?
- a 30 minutes
- b 45 minutes
- c 1 hour
- d 2 hours

171. Which of the following test results will be falsely decreased if cells are not promptly separated from serum?
- a CBC
- b WBC
- c glucose
- d vancomycin

172. A specimen for glucose analysis is collected in an evacuated tube with a serum separator gel. The specimen was centrifuged 1.5 hours following collection. As a result, the serum glucose values were:
- a falsely decreased
- b falsely increased
- c impossible to analyze
- d unaffected

173. Which of the following test results will be falsely decreased if cells are not promptly separated from serum or plasma?
- a fibrin split products
- b hemoglobin electrophoresis
- c ionized calcium
- d lactate dehydrogenase

174. Which of the following test results will be falsely elevated if cells are not promptly separated from serum or plasma?
    a   fibrin split products
    b   hemoglobin electrophoresis
    c   ionized calcium
    d   lactate dehydrogenase

175. Which of the following test results will be falsely decreased if cells are not promptly separated from serum or plasma?
    a   folate
    b   hepatitis B surface antibody
    c   phosphorous
    d   potassium

176. Which of the following test results will be falsely elevated if cells are not promptly separated from serum or plasma?
    a   bicarbonate (CO_2)
    b   folate
    c   hepatitis B surface antibody
    d   potassium

177. Which of the following test results will be falsely decreased if cells are not promptly separated from serum or plasma?
    a   bicarbonate (CO_2)
    b   creatinine
    c   Human chorionic gonadotropin (HCG)
    d   IgA immunoglobulin

178. Which of the following test results will be falsely elevated if cells are not promptly separated from serum or plasma?
    a   aspartate aminotransferase (AST)
    b   bicarbonate (CO_2)
    c   glucose
    d   ionized calcium (Ca^{++})

179. Which of the following test results will be falsely elevated if cells are not promptly separated from serum or plasma?
    a   alanine aminotransferase (ALT)
    b   folate
    c   glucose
    d   ionized calcium (Ca^{++})

180. Which of the following test results will be most affected by metabolism of the red blood cells if cells are not promptly separated from serum or plasma?
    a   aldosterone
    b   MCHC
    c   MCV
    d   WBC

Questions — Specimen Handling, Transport & Processing

181. A specimen for creatinine analysis is collected in a red and gray stopper serum separator evacuated tube. The specimen was centrifuged one hour after collection, but not analyzed immediately. As a result, the serum creatinine values were:
    a falsely decreased
    b falsely elevated
    c impossible to analyze
    d unaffected

182. A specimen for potassium analysis is collected in a heparinized (dark green) Hemogard tube. The specimen was centrifuged promptly, but not separated in a timely fashion. As a result, the serum potassium values were:
    a falsely decreased
    b falsely elevated
    c impossible to analyze
    d unaffected

183. A specimen for lactate dehydrogenase (LD) analysis is collected in a red top evacuated tube. The specimen was centrifuged 60 minutes after collection, but not separated in a timely fashion. As a result, the serum LD values were:
    a falsely decreased
    b falsely elevated
    c impossible to analyze
    d unaffected

184. A specimen for potassium analysis is collected in a red SST evacuated tube. The specimen was centrifuged 45 minutes after collection, but not analyzed in a timely fashion. As a result, the serum potassium values were:
    a falsely decreased
    b falsely increased
    c impossible to analyze
    d unaffected

185. A specimen for glucose analysis is collected in a gray top evacuated tube containing sodium fluoride. The specimen was centrifuged promptly, but not separated in a timely fashion. As a result, the glucose values were:
    a decreased
    b elevated
    c impossible to analyze
    d unaffected

Specimen Handling, Transport & Processing — Questions

186. A specimen for potassium analysis is collected in a mint green Hemogard tube. The specimen was obtained as a result of a venipuncture involving several needle readjustments and the specimen was hemolyzed. The potassium results will be:
    a falsely decreased
    b falsely elevated
    c impossible to analyze
    d unaffected

187. A specimen is collected at a patient service center for electrolyte analysis in a mint green Hemogard tube. How long after collection must the phlebotomist wait to centrifuge the evacuated tube?
    a 0 minutes
    b 30 minutes
    c 60 minutes
    d 120 minutes

188. A specimen is collected at a patient service center for high-density lipoprotein (HDL) and low-density lipoprotein (LDL) in a gold Hemogard tube. How long must the phlebotomist wait to centrifuge the evacuated tube?
    a 0 minutes
    b 15 minutes
    c 30 minutes
    d 90 minutes

189. A specimen is collected in a hospital from an inpatient for reticulocyte count in a lavender Hemogard tube. When should the tube be centrifuged?
    a never
    b 30-60 minutes after collection
    c 2-3 hours after collection
    d within 3 hours of collection

190. A phlebotomist collects a blood specimen from a home bound patient. How should the specimen be transported in the car?
    a in a leakproof bag in an upright position
    b in a leakproof bag in a horizontal position
    c in a portable centrifuge
    d on ice

191. A home health phlebotomist collects blood specimens from several patients. What should the phlebotomist use to transport the specimens in the car?
    a biohazard bag surrounded by an ice slurry
    b biohazard bag surrounded by a heel warmer
    c enclosed container
    d test tube rack

Questions — Specimen Handling, Transport & Processing

192. A phlebotomist is going to transport a specimen for a complete blood count (CBC) using a pneumatic tube system. She places the specimen in a leakproof bag. How should the specimen be transported?
    a packed in an ice slurry
    b surrounded by shock absorbent material
    c wrapped in a heel warmer
    d wrapped in aluminum foil

193. When shipping specimens to referral laboratories, which of the following containers must be watertight?
    a gas impermeable container
    b primary container
    c secondary container
    d shipping container

194. What material must be inserted between a primary and secondary shipping container?
    a absorbent material
    b biohazard bag
    c dry ice
    d heel warmer

195. What regulatory agency serves as the primary source for regulations governing specimen and biological shipments in the United States?
    a Centers for Disease Control (CDC)
    b Department of Defense (DOD)
    c Department of Transportation (DOT)
    d World Health Organization (WHO)

196. If blood specimens have been placed in a centrifuge correctly, they will be placed:
    a at random in the centrifuge
    b on the left side of the centrifuge
    c on the right side of the centrifuge
    d tubes of similar size & volume opposite each other

197. When a phlebotomist places evacuated tubes of similar size & volume across from each other in a centrifuge she is achieving a:
    a balance
    b bariatric
    c baseline
    d buffy coat

198. A phlebotomist has placed several blood specimens into the centrifuge and started it. The centrifuge begins to loudly vibrate, the phlebotomist should:
    a call a code
    b call the security department
    c pull the fire alarm
    d turn off the centrifuge

Specimen Handling, Transport & Processing — Questions

199. How many times may a serum specimen be frozen in anticipation of analysis?
    a   once
    b   twice
    c   never
    d   only once and after analysis

200. In addition to gloves, what personal protective equipment is required during evacuated tube stopper removal?
    a   gown & N95 mask
    b   a full length face shield & N95 mask
    c   a splash shield
    d   no additional PPE is required

201. A phlebotomist is placing specimens in a centrifuge. She should place the specimens in the centrifuge:
    a   with the stoppers removed
    b   with the stoppers intact
    c   in ascending order of size, with the smallest tube in car 1
    d   in descending order of size, with the largest tube in car 1

202. A specimen was collected into a heparinized evacuated tube containing an inert polymer gel. The specimen was removed from the centrifuge and the phlebotomist noticed the gel was on an angle across the interior of the evacuated tube. This indicates that the centrifuge was:
    a   balanced
    b   not properly balanced
    c   set at an incorrect speed
    d   set at an incorrect time

203. The condition when the patient is at rest, in a supine position, 12 hours after the last ingestion of food, exercise, or activity is:
    a   basal state
    b   diurnal rhythms
    c   normal
    d   reference value

204. Normal variations of blood constituents throughout the day are called:
    a   basal state
    b   diurnal rhythms
    c   normal
    d   reference value

205. Normal values for laboratory test results are called:
    a   basal state
    b   diurnal rhythms
    c   normal
    d   reference ranges

Questions
Specimen Handling, Transport & Processing

206. A clinical situation in which the water from the plasma portion of the blood filters into the tissues, causing nonfilterable values in the blood to falsely increase, is called:
   a   hemoconcentration
   b   hemolysis
   c   hematology
   d   hematoma

207. Cloudy serum or plasma caused by an increased lipid content is called:
   a   diurnal rhythms
   b   hemoconcentration
   c   hemolysis
   d   lipemic

208. Large laboratories that perform tests on specimens from many different facilities are called:
   a   point-of-care facilities
   b   reference laboratories
   c   satellite laboratories
   d   STAT laboratories

209. A therapeutic drug monitoring (TDM) specimen that is collected within 15 minutes of the next scheduled dose is for what type of medication level?
   a   peak
   b   random
   c   toxic
   d   trough

210. The term that means "immediately" is:
   a   ASAP
   b   FYI
   c   Med Emerg
   d   STAT

211. The department in the clinical laboratory that identifies disease of blood-forming tissues is:
   a   clinical chemistry
   b   hematology
   c   immunology
   d   microbiology

212. The department in the clinical laboratory, often housed in the hematology department, that monitors medication given as anticoagulant therapy is:
   a   clinical chemistry
   b   coagulation
   c   microbiology
   d   urinalysis

Specimen Handling, Transport & Processing — Questions

213. The department in the clinical laboratory that cultures and identifies bacterial pathogens is:
    a   clinical chemistry
    b   hematology
    c   microbiology
    d   urinalysis

214. The department in the clinical laboratory that analyses antibody-antigen reactions prior to the transfusion of blood or blood products is:
    a   clinical chemistry
    b   immunohematology
    c   immunology
    d   radioimmunoassay

215. The department in the clinical laboratory that assesses the body's response to certain infectious diseases through the analysis of antigen-antibody reactions is:
    a   clinical chemistry
    b   hematology
    c   immunohematology
    d   immunology

216. The department in the clinical laboratory that screens for the early detection of cancer cells is:
    a   clinical microscopy
    b   cytology
    c   hematology
    d   histology

217. The department in the clinical laboratory that prepares and processes tissue samples removed during surgical procedures is:
    a   clinical microscopy
    b   cytology
    c   hematology
    d   histology

218. Which of the following terms refers to removing part of a patient's specimen for analysis?
    a   accession
    b   aliquot
    c   centrifuge
    d   filter

219. The presence of microorganisms and/or toxins in a patient's blood is called:
    a   bacteremia
    b   septicemia
    c   false positive
    d   false negative

Questions
Specimen Handling, Transport & Processing

220. Which of the following patient conditions would likely result in a blood culture requisition issued by a physician:
    a   FBG
    b   FSP
    c   FTA
    d   FUO

221. In therapeutic drug monitoring, the time required to metabolize half the amount of the drug administered is called the:
    a   half-life
    b   quarter life
    c   peak level
    d   trough level

222. A substance that must be chilled immediately after collection to slow down metabolic processes at higher temperatures is called:
    a   thermokinematics
    b   thermolabile
    c   thermolysis
    d   thermesthesia

223. A substance that must be transported shielded from the light immediately after collection to prevent decomposition due to light exposure is called:
    a   photochromography
    b   photoproton
    c   photosensitive
    d   photostable

224. A patient's result on a laboratory test is so far outside the reference range it is life threatening, requiring immediate medical intervention. This value is called:
    a   equivocal
    b   normal
    c   critical (panic) value
    d   standard deviation

225. The time it takes to generate a laboratory result from the time it is ordered by a physician is called:
    a   report time
    b   quality assurance
    c   T3 resin uptake
    d   turnaround time

226. A specimen transportation system evaluated for breakage rates, carrier size, distance, shock absorbency and speed is the:
    a   collection tray
    b   phlebotomist
    c   pneumatic tube system
    d   point-of-care testing

Specimen Handling, Transport & Processing

227. Improper removal of an evacuated tube stopper can lead to the formation of
    a   aerosols
    b   additives
    c   adulteration
    d   aliquots

228. What term describes the specimen pictured?
    a   hemolyzed
    b   icteric
    c   lipemic
    d   normal

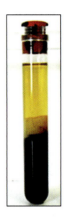

229. What term describes the specimen pictured?
    a   hemolyzed
    b   icteric
    c   lipemic
    d   normal

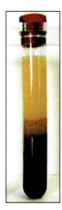

Questions
Specimen Handling, Transport & Processing

230. What term describes the specimen pictured?
    a   hemolyzed
    b   icteric
    c   lipemic
    d   normal

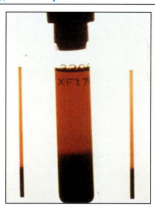

Specimen Handling, Transport & Processing — Explanations

The following items have been identified as appropriate for those preparing for the PBT examination.

1. **a** There are three processes to laboratory testing: preexamination/preanalytical process, examination process, and postexamination/postanalytical process.
   [Garza 10e, p9, 397]

2. **a** The preexamination/preanalytical process of laboratory testing has the highest error rate. The phlebotomist's domain falls in the preexamination/preanalytical process of laboratory testing.
   [McCall 7e, p393-384]

3. **d** The estimated percentage of laboratory error that occurs during the preexamination/preanalytical process is 46-68%.
   [McCall 7e, p393-384]

4. **c** The preexamination/preanalytical process includes tasks associated with requisitioning, patient preparation and specimen collection, processing, handling, and storage. The phlebotomist's domain falls in the preexamination/preanalytical process of laboratory testing.
   [Garza 10e, p9]

5. **b** The examination process includes the tasks associated with analyzing the specimen, including quality control procedures. This process has the lowest percentage of error associated with it, estimated at ~13% of all laboratory errors.
   [McCall 7e, p393-384]

6. **c** Delay in specimen delivery is a preexamination/preanalytical error. The phlebotomist's domain falls in the preexamination/preanalytical process of laboratory testing.
   [Garza 10e, p9]

7. **c** Errors in specimen collection, including incorrect order of draw, are preexamination/preanalytical errors, which fall in the domain of the phlebotomist.
   [Garza 10e, p9]

8. **c** Errors in specimen collection, including incorrect patient preparation are preexamination/preanalytical errors.
   [Garza 10e, p9]

9. **a** One analysis that requires a patient to fast prior to specimen collection is cholesterol. Correct patient preparation prior to specimen collection is a task associated with the preexamination/preanalytical process of laboratory workflow.
   [Garza 10e, p9, 364]

Explanations Specimen Handling, Transport & Processing

10. **d** A triglyceride analysis requires a patient to fast for 12-14 hours prior to specimen collection. Correct patient preparation prior to specimen collection is a task associated with the preexamination/preanalytical process of laboratory workflow.
[Garza 10e, p9, 364]

11. **d** Hemolysis may be caused by specimen collection errors. One element measured in an electrolyte panel is potassium, which is falsely elevated in hemolyzed specimens. The appropriate course of action is to reject the specimen and request a redraw.
[Garza 10e, p362-363, 420, 620]

12. **a** The red top (plain) evacuated tube is appropriate to use for collection of a therapeutic drug monitoring (TDM) specimen. Gel barrier evacuated tubes may adversely affect the results of a TDM analyses. Strict adherence to laboratory policies and procedures are required if a gel separator tube is used to collect a specimen for TDM analysis.
[Garza 10e, p494-495]

Please consult the explanation below for questions 13-52 regarding the sequence of filling evacuated tubes following venipuncture.

Questions 13-52 address the correct selection of evacuated tubes for venipuncture specimen collection. Correct selection of specimen collection tubes prior to specimen collection is a task associated with the preexamination/preanalytical process of laboratory workflow, which falls in the domain of the phlebotomist.

13. **b** Lactate dehydrogenase analysis is performed on plasma or serum samples so the appropriate collection container is the gold Hemogard gel barrier evacuated tube.
[Garza 10e, p9, 590; McCall 7e, 458-460, 476-479]

14. **c** ABO & Rh typing may be performed on whole blood samples so the appropriate collection container is the pink EDTA evacuated tube.
[Garza 10e, p9, 588; McCall 7e, 458-460, 476-479]

15. **b** Partial thromboplastin time is performed on citrated plasma samples so the appropriate collection container is the blue sodium citrate evacuated tube.
[Garza 10e, p9, 588; McCall 7e, 458-460, 476-479]

16. **b** Prothrombin time is performed on citrated plasma samples so the appropriate collection container is the blue sodium citrate evacuated tube.
[Garza 10e, p9, 591; McCall 7e, 458-460, 476-479]

17. **c** Complete blood count (CBC) is performed on whole blood specimens collected in EDTA so the appropriate collection container is the lavender EDTA evacuated tube.
[Garza 10e, p9, 590; McCall 7e, 458-460, 476-479]

Specimen Handling, Transport & Processing — Explanations

18. **c** Reticulocyte counts are performed on whole blood specimens collected in EDTA so the appropriate collection container is the lavender EDTA evacuated tube.
[Garza 10e, p9, 591; McCall 7e, 458-460]

Questions 13-52 address the correct selection of evacuated tubes for venipuncture specimen collection. Correct selection of specimen collection tubes prior to specimen collection is a task associated with the preexamination/preanalytical process of laboratory workflow, which falls in the domain of the phlebotomist.

19. **c** Erythrocyte sedimentation rate analyses are often performed on whole blood specimens collected in EDTA so the appropriate collection container is the lavender EDTA evacuated tube.
[Garza 10e, p9, 590; McCall 7e, 458-460]

20. **d** Hemoglobin electrophoresis is performed on whole blood specimens collected in EDTA so the appropriate collection container is the lavender EDTA evacuated tube.
[McCall 7e, 458-460]

21. **d** Platelet counts are performed on whole blood specimens collected in EDTA so the appropriate collection container is the lavender EDTA evacuated tube.
[Garza 10e, p9, 590; McCall 7e, 458-460]

22. **a** Electrolyte analysis is often performed on plasma specimens collected in an evacuated tube containing heparin.
[McCall 7e, 458-460]

23. **a** Glucose analysis is typically performed on plasma specimens collected in sodium fluoride.
[McCall 7e, 458-460]

24. **a** Basic metabolic panels (BMP) include electrolyte (Na, K, Cl, CO_2) analysis. Heparinized specimens for BMP analysis including electrolytes must be collected in lithium heparin tubes to prevent contamination with sodium.
[McCall 7e, 453-460, 476-479]

25. **d** Glycosylated hemoglobin analysis is performed on whole blood specimens collected into EDTA.
[McCall 7e, 453-460, 476-479]

26. **c** Creatinine analysis is performed on serum samples so the appropriate collection container is the gel barrier evacuated tube.
[McCall 7e, 453-460, 476-479]

27. **c** Carcinoembryonic antigen may be performed on serum samples so the appropriate collection container is the gel barrier evacuated tube.
[McCall 7e, 453-460, 476-479]

Explanations — Specimen Handling, Transport & Processing

28. **d** Eosinophil counts are performed on whole blood specimens collected in EDTA.
[McCall 7e, 453-460, 476-479]

29. **b** Fibrinogen levels are performed on plasma specimens collected in sodium citrate.
[McCall 7e, 453-460, 476-479]

30. **c** Human chorionic gonadotropin levels are performed on serum specimens collected in gel barrier evacuated tubes.
[McCall 7e, 453-460, 476-479]

31. **c** Fluorescent treponemal antibody absorption analysis is performed on serum specimens collected in red top evacuated tubes.
[McCall 7e, 453-460, 476-479]

32. **c** Creatine kinase MB is performed on serum specimens collected in gel barrier evacuated tubes.
[McCall 7e, 453-460, 476-479]

33. **d** Antithrombin III analysis is performed on plasma specimens collected in sodium citrate evacuated tubes.
[McCall 7e, 453-460, 476-479]

34. **c** Blood urea nitrogen (BUN) analysis is performed on serum specimens collected in gel barrier evacuated tubes.
[McCall 7e, 453-460, 476-479]

35. **a** Differential white blood cell counts are performed on blood smears collected in EDTA and stained with Wright stain.
[McCall 7e, 453-460, 476-479]

36. **c** Alanine aminotransferase analysis may be performed on serum specimens collected in gel barrier evacuated tubes.
[McCall 7e, 453-460, 476-479]

37. **d** Hematocrit analysis is performed on whole blood specimens collected in EDTA.
[McCall 7e, 453-460, 476-479]

38. **c** Alkaline phosphatase analysis may be performed on serum specimens collected in gel barrier evacuated tubes. Whole blood samples are not collected in gel barrier tubes.
[McCall 7e, 453-460, 476-479]

39. **c** Anti-RH antibody screen may be performed on serum specimens collected in evacuated tubes without additive.
[McCall 7e, 453-460, 476-479]

40. **c** Amylase analysis may be performed on serum specimens collected in gel barrier evacuated tubes.
[McCall 7e, 453-460, 476-479]

Specimen Handling, Transport & Processing — Explanations

41. **c** Acid phosphatase analysis is performed on serum specimens collected in gel barrier evacuated tubes.
[McCall 7e, 453-460, 476-479]

42. **d** Red cell index analysis is performed on whole blood specimens collected in EDTA.
[McCall 7e, 453-460, 476-479]

Questions 13-52 address the correct selection of evacuated tubes for venipuncture specimen collection. Correct selection of specimen collection tubes prior to specimen collection is a task associated with the preexamination/preanalytical process of laboratory workflow, which falls in the domain of the phlebotomist.

43. **c** Aspartate aminotransferase analysis may be performed on serum specimens collected in gel barrier evacuated tubes.
[McCall 7e, 453-460, 476-479]

44. **b** Mononucleosis screen analysis may be performed on plasma EDTA specimens collected in lavender top evacuated tubes.
[McCall 7e, 453-460, 476-479]

45. **c** Bilirubin analysis is performed on serum specimens collected in gel barrier evacuated tubes. Additionally, bilirubin samples must be transported shielded from light.
[McCall 7e, 453-460, 476-479]

46. **c** Lipase analysis may be performed on serum specimens collected in red top evacuated tubes.
[McCall 7e, 453-460, 476-479]

47. **c** High-density lipoprotein analysis is performed on serum specimens collected in gel barrier evacuated tubes.
[McCall 7e, 453-460, 476-479]

48. **d** Total white cell counts are performed on whole blood specimens collected in EDTA.
[McCall 7e, 453-460, 476-479]

49. **d** C-reactive protein analysis may be performed on serum specimens collected in red top evacuated tubes.
[McCall 7e, 453-460, 476-479]

50. **c** Cholesterol analysis may be performed on serum specimens collected in red top evacuated tubes.
[McCall 7e, 453-460, 476-479]

51. **d** Antistreptolysin-O analysis is performed on serum specimens collected in red top evacuated tubes.
[McCall 7e, 453-460, 476-479]

Explanations Specimen Handling, Transport & Processing

52. **c** Prostate-specific antigen analysis may be performed on serum specimens collected in gel barrier evacuated tubes.
[McCall 7e, 453-460, 476-479]

53. **b** The first specimen should be drawn 30 minutes after the glucose load is administered, which is 8:00 AM in the example provided. If the patient follows a normal response curve, the highest level of plasma glucose will be achieved 30 minutes after the glucose load is administered.
[Garza 10e, p484, 487]

54. **d** The last specimen should be drawn 180 minutes after the glucose load is administered, which is 10:30 AM in the example provided. If the patient follows a normal response curve, glucose load, the plasma glucose levels will return to reference ranges 180 minutes after the glucose load is administered.
[Garza 10e, p484]

55. **d** During a routine GTT, a fasting specimen is collected prior to administration of the glucose load and at the following intervals after the glucose has been administered: 30, 60, 120, and 180 minutes totaling 5 blood collection procedures.
[McCall 7e, p352-353]

56. **c** The postprandial glucose test is a screening test for diabetes. Plasma glucose levels collected 120 minutes after a patient consumes a breakfast of 75-100 g of glucose are normally within reference ranges for glucose.
[Garza 10e, p487]

57. **b** Lactose tolerance is used to diagnose patients who have difficulty breaking down lactose, a sugar found in dairy products. Patients are given a dose of lactose and blood glucose levels are collected at timed intervals. Results are compared to the patient's GTT curve to assess lactose digestion.
[Garza 10e, p487-488]

58. **b** Lactose tolerance is used to diagnose patients who have difficulty breaking down lactose, a sugar found in dairy products. First, the patient submits to a GTT a day prior to the lactose tolerance test. Patients are given a dose of lactose and blood glucose levels are collected at timed intervals. Results are compared to the patient's GTT results to assess efficiency of lactose digestion. Symptoms associated with lactose intolerance include gastrointestinal discomfort and diarrhea, so it is important the patient has easy access to a lavatory during the test.
[Garza 10e, p488]

Specimen Handling, Transport & Processing — Explanations

59. **a** A noninvasive method to screen for lactose tolerance is using breath samples and measuring hydrogen content, produced by bacteria that breakdown lactose. Lactose tolerance is used to diagnose patients who have difficulty breaking down lactose, a sugar found in dairy products. Patients are given a dose of lactose and hydrogen levels in a patient's breath are collected at timed intervals. This procedure does not require comparison to a previously obtained GTT curve.
[Garza 10e, p488]

60. **a** Blood culture specimens are typically collected as a series of samples, usually 30-60 minutes apart, and timed to coincide with the next anticipated patient temperature spike to optimize the detection of pathogens in a patient's blood.
[McCall 7e, p343-344]

61. **d** Manufacturers recommend that phlebotomists select either a winged infusion needle or syringe to inoculate blood culture bottles to prevent back flow of media into the patient's vein (reflux).
[Garza 10e, p482]

62. **a** The aerobic bottle should be inoculated first because air from the tubing will be introduced into the bottle along with the specimen. Air introduced into an anaerobic bottle may destroy anaerobic microbes collected in the specimen, generating a false-negative result.
[Garza 10e, p480]

63. **c** Drugs included in a TDM program have a narrow therapeutic/toxic ranges, which are monitored through a TDM program. Inaccurate dosing may have serious clinical consequences for the patient.
[McCall 7e, p355-357]

64. **b** Aminoglycosides are characteristically incorporated into a TDM program. They belong in the antibiotic drug category. Aminoglycosides are characteristically prescribed to treat infections caused by antibiotic resistant bacteria.
[McCall 7e, p355-357]

65. **a** The most common reason a TDM specimen is rejected for analysis is incorrect collection times, based on the medication administration schedule. This is a preexamination/preanalytical error. Therapeutic drug monitoring programs confirm peak, trough, and random levels of drugs in the patient's serum. Timing of the draw is critically important to ensure that the appropriate specimen is collected for the drug level ordered by the patient's physician. Correct collection timing is most critical for drugs with short half-lives, most notably the aminoglycosides.
[Garza 10e, p494-495]

Explanations — Specimen Handling, Transport & Processing

66. b The time the last medication dose was administered must be verified before collecting the specimen to ensure that the appropriate specimen is collected for the drug level ordered by the patient's physician. Therapeutic drug monitoring programs confirm peak, trough, and random levels of drugs in the patient's serum.
[Garza 10e, p494]

67. a Trough specimens are collected prior to the next scheduled medication dose, ideally immediately before dose administration, but not more than 15 minutes before the scheduled medication dose.
[Garza 10e, p495]

68. d Trace metals are typically ordered by a physician to assess environmental exposure, nutritional deficiencies, or the metal-on-metal wear of artificial joints.
[McCall 7e, p358-359]

69. d Cobalt, chromium, and copper are trace metals. Aluminum, arsenic, copper, iron, lead, platinum, silver and zinc are also considered trace metals.
[McCall 7e, p358-359]

70. a Trace elements include dietary components such as copper and zinc and environmental trace elements such as lead present in minute amounts in patient specimens. Collection in standard evacuated tubes may contaminate specimens for trace element analysis because trace elements may be used in the manufacture of evacuated tubes. Collecting in a standard evacuated tube may result in a false elevation of the trace element being tested.
[Garza 10e, p495]

71. d Tan Hemogard evacuated tubes are certified to contain less than 0.01 µg/mL (ppm) lead. Tan Hemogard evacuated tubes are manufactured specifically for the collection of lead levels to minimize contamination of the specimen with lead introduced into the stopper or tube during manufacture.
[Garza 10e, p495; McCall 7e, p453-460, 476-479]

72. d Royal blue Hemogard evacuated tubes are specially formulated to contain low levels of trace elements, including zinc. Specific levels of trace elements in royal blue Hemogard evacuated tubes are specified with individual package inserts and are manufactured to minimize contamination of the specimen.
[Garza 10e, p495; McCall 7e, p453-460, 476-479]

73. c Certain hormone levels, including cortisol, fluctuate throughout the day. Cortisol, a hormone produced by the cortex of the adrenal gland, is active during stress and aids in metabolism. Highest levels of cortisol may be found in the morning (approximately 8:00 AM) and lower levels in the evening (8:00 PM). The evening sample may be decreased by as much as 1/3, compared to the morning specimen.
[Garza 10e, p202, 364, 590]

Specimen Handling, Transport & Processing — Explanations

74. **c** The highest levels of cortisol may be found in the morning (approximately 8:00 AM) and must be collected as close to 8:00 AM as possible so another phlebotomist should be paged and asked to attempt to obtain the specimen. If the second phlebotomist is not successful in securing the specimen, the physician should be notified. The physician may elect to reschedule the test for the next day.
[Garza 10e, p364]

75. **a** Aldosterone levels must be collected after a patient has been reclining for at least 30 minutes. Aldosterone is a hormone produced by the cortex of the adrenal gland and functions in sodium and potassium regulation.
[Garza 10e, p202, 364]

76. **a** Glass interferes with aldosterone analysis so the specimen must be collected in a plastic tube. Aldosterone levels must be collected after a patient has been reclining for at least 30 minutes. Aldosterone is a hormone produced by the cortex of the adrenal gland and functions in sodium and potassium regulation.
[Garza 10e, p202, 364]

77. **a** Newborn screening may detect a variety of genetic conditions, infections, and metabolic diseases using specimens collected on filter paper circles included on newborn screening cards. PKU is one of the most commonly ordered tests on newborns and screens for a genetic defect preventing the enzymatic breakdown of phenylalanine, which may ultimately accumulate in toxic levels leading to brain damage and mental retardation.
[Garza 10e, p324-328]

78. **b** Newborn screening specimens collected on filter paper must be dried in a horizontal position away from heat or sunlight at room temperature (22°C). If filter paper specimens are dried vertically, specimen migration to the low end of the filter paper may occur and erroneous results obtained.
[Garza 10e, p441, 639]

79. **c** Newborn screening specimens must be thoroughly dried before dispatch to the testing facility, which takes at least 3 hours at room temperature (22°C).
[McCall 7e, p326-328]

80. **c** Newborn screening specimens must dispatched to the testing facility within 24 hours of collection.
[Garza 10e, p441]

81. **c** Following skin puncture, the phlebotomist must wipe away the first drop of blood. The phlebotomist should use gentle pressure on the baby's heel to generate a large drop of blood, which is applied to the filter paper circle in one motion, using one side of the paper only. Pressure is maintained until the circle is completely saturated.
[Garza 10e, p44]

Explanations   **Specimen Handling, Transport & Processing**

82. **c**   Specimens for neonatal screening must be collected before the child is 72 hours old.
[Garza 10e, p439]

83. **a**   Specimens for neonatal screening must be obtained before an infant receives a blood transfusion for accurate results. Transfused blood cells contain the enzymes detected in the screening process and would invalidate the results.
[Garza 10e, p439]

84. **a**   Since 2009, all 50 states in the United States of America are required to screen for four genetic conditions, including cystic fibrosis. Screening for phenylketonuria, hypothyroidism, and galactosemia is also required.
[McCall 7e, p324-325]

85. **a**   Forensic (crime investigation) specimens require meticulous documentation of specimen accountability from the time the specimen is collected until the results are reported.
[Garza 10e, p541]

86. **a**   The Federal Drug Testing Custody and Control Form (CCF) is a component of the standards for drug testing prescribed by the Department of Transportation, Office of Drug and Alcohol Policy and Compliance.
[Garza 10e, p542]

87. **d**   The National Institute on Drug Abuse (NIDA) prescribes protocols to be followed when urine specimens are collected for drug screen, including patient preparation and specimen collection protocols.
[McCall 7e, p358]

88. **c**   To confirm results, urine specimens for drug screen are often split into an "A" specimen (minimum volume 30 mL) and a "B" specimen (minimum volume 15 mL) to total a required minimum volume of 45 mL.
[Garza 10e, p547-548]

89. **c**   Water is the most common substance used to adulterate drug screen urine specimens and, if used, may change the temperature of the specimen. Therefore, urine temperatures must be measured within 4 minutes after the specimen has been surrendered to the collector.
[Garza 10e, p547]

90. **a**   One indication of specimen tampering is urine temperature outside the range prescribed by the Department of Transportation. Specimen temperature must fall within the 32-38°C range to be acceptable.
[Garza 10e, p547]

Specimen Handling, Transport & Processing — Explanations

91. **a** The clinical laboratory may analyze hundreds, perhaps even thousands of blood specimens in a single day, depending on the size of the laboratory. Careful tracking of specimens ensures connection of the patient to the specimen and all of the laboratory processes and procedures used to analyze the specimen, including documentation procedures, is a process called accessioning.
[McCall 7e, p217-218]

92. **a** The clinical laboratory may analyze hundreds, perhaps even thousands of blood specimens in a single day, depending on the size of the laboratory. Accessioning of specimens ensures connection of the patient to the specimen and all of the laboratory processes and procedures used to analyze the specimen, including documentation procedures.
[McCall 7e, p217-218]

93. **c** An accession number is assigned by the laboratory information system and used to track specimens received in the laboratory. The accession number allows health care professionals to track multiple specimens from a single patient as well as track the status of a laboratory analysis ordered by a patient's physician.
[Garza 10e, p626]

94. **c** An accession number is assigned by the laboratory information system (LIS) and corresponds to each requisition. The accession number is assigned once the request is entered into the LIS and will correspond to the specimen as long as the specimen is in the laboratory.
[McCall 7e, p218, 378]

95. **a** Complete blood count (CBC) analysis is performed on whole blood specimens collected into EDTA evacuated tubes. To ensure quality results, the blood should be mixed with the tube additive by gently inverting the tube 5-10× immediately following collection. Once the specimen is delivered to the laboratory, it may be placed on a test tube rocker to ensure adequate mixing of blood with the additive before testing.
[Garza 10e, p407]

96. **a** Specimens must clot completely before centrifugation. Specimens collected in gel barrier tubes typically require at least 30 minutes to completely clot. Therefore, the specimen should be ready for centrifugation at 10:00 AM. Specimens from patients receiving anticoagulant therapy, such as heparin or Coumadin, may require longer clotting time. The phlebotomist should always ensure complete clotting of specimen before placing the specimen in the centrifuge.
[Garza 10e, p407; McCall 7e, p476-479]

Explanations

Specimen Handling, Transport & Processing

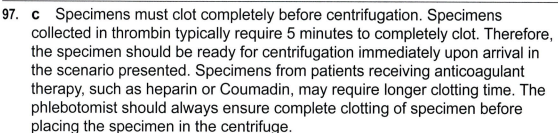

97. **c** Specimens must clot completely before centrifugation. Specimens collected in thrombin typically require 5 minutes to completely clot. Therefore, the specimen should be ready for centrifugation immediately upon arrival in the scenario presented. Specimens from patients receiving anticoagulant therapy, such as heparin or Coumadin, may require longer clotting time. The phlebotomist should always ensure complete clotting of specimen before placing the specimen in the centrifuge.
[Garza 10e, p407]

98. **c** Some laboratory professionals continue to adhere to a dated technique called "rimming." In this process, the collection tube stopper is removed and a wooden applicator stick is used to dislodge patient specimen from the walls of the collection tube and the stopper. This technique should never be employed because it presents the danger of aerosol formation, a hazard to the laboratory professional, and may cause specimen hemolysis, which may negatively impact patient results.
[Garza 10e, p407]

99. **c** Some laboratory professionals continue to adhere to a dated technique called "rimming." In this process, the collection tube stopper is removed and a wooden applicator stick is used to dislodge patient specimen from the walls of the collection tube and the stopper. This technique should never be employed because it presents the danger of aerosol formation, a hazard to the laboratory professional, and may cause specimen hemolysis, which may negatively impact patient results.
[Garza 10e, p407]

100. **a** If a specimen is not allowed to completely clot before centrifugation, fibrin may be retained in the serum which will interfere with test procedures. This may result in requiring the patient to be redrawn and a significant delay in reporting results.
[Garza 10e, p407]

101. **b** Specimens from patients receiving anticoagulant therapy, such as heparin or Coumadin, may require longer clotting time. The phlebotomist should always ensure complete clotting of specimen before placing the specimen in the centrifuge.
[Garza 10e, p407]

102. **d** Specimen labels are affixed after collecting the specimen and before leaving the patient. Labeling a specimen ahead of time increases the risk of selecting an incorrectly labeled tube for a venipuncture procedure. Labeling a tube after leaving a patient's bedside increases the risk of applying a label to an incorrect patient specimen.
[Garza 10e, p357]

Specimen Handling, Transport & Processing — Explanations

103. c The phlebotomist's initials are required on every specimen label in case there are questions regarding the specimen during the pre, post or examination processes of testing.
[Garza 10e, p357]

104. d Patient identification is always of paramount importance, but some facilities prescribe additional identification and labeling procedures when collecting blood specimens for type and screen or crossmatch analysis. As an added precaution, especially if a patient's identification cannot be confirmed due to emergency circumstances, the American Association of Blood Banks (AABB) requires an identification band or device attached to the patient that includes a name and temporary patient identification number matching the same information on the specimen label. A third component includes an identifier that may be affixed to the unit crossmatched using the patient's specimen.
[McCall 7e, p221-225]

105. b During a 3-hour glucose tolerance test (GTT), specimens are collected at 30 minutes, 1, 2, and 3 hours after the glucose load is administered. The sequence of specimen, ie, 30 minute, 1 hour, 2 hour, must also be included on the label of each specimen collected.
[Garza 10e, p484, 487]

106. d Blood culture specimens are often collected in a series which may typically range from 2-4 specimens, Additionally, the specimens are timed relative to the patient's next anticipated fever spike. Specimens should be collected from alternate venipuncture sites to increase the probability of recovering pathogens in the patient's bloodstream. To ensure multiple site selections and confirm results, specimens should also be labeled with the site selected for specimen collection, eg, right antecubital fossa.
[Garza 10e, p482]

107. d Specimen labels must contain complete first and last patient names. Since the label in this scenario included the patient's first name initial only, it should be rejected for testing and the patient's blood redrawn.
[McCall 7e, p404]

108. a Assuming all quality control parameters have been met, the result should be reported. If a hemoglobin of 5.8 g/dL is a critical (panic) value at this facility, the result should also be communicated to the physician immediately.
[Garza 10e, p418]

109. a The discrepancy in the two values occurred because the first specimen was clotted, significantly altering the results.
[McCall 7e, p391-392]

Explanations Specimen Handling, Transport & Processing

110. **c** The error that caused clotting in the EDTA evacuated tube and resulting disparity in patient results was preexamination/preanalytical. The specimen was not mixed adequately with the anticoagulant (EDTA) immediately following collection, resulting in specimen clotting before the specimen was delivered to the laboratory for analysis.
[McCall 7e, p391-392]

111. **c** Hemolysis in the plasma or serum of the specimen submitted for testing is the most common reason specimens are not accepted for analysis in the chemistry department of the laboratory.
[McCall 7e, p392]

112. **d** The second most common reason specimens are not accepted for analysis in the chemistry department of the laboratory is because the specimen is QNS (quantity not sufficient).
[McCall 7e, p387, 392]

113. **a** Clotting in the specimen submitted for testing is the most common reason specimens are not accepted for analysis in the hematology department of the laboratory.
[McCall 7e, p387, 392]

114. **a** If a specimen is hemolyzed, some analytes will be falsely elevated, including ammonia. Hemolysis occurs when red blood cell membranes are ruptured and the contents released into the plasma or serum. Some clinical conditions may cause hemolysis, but it is frequently due to collection error.
[Garza, p301-302]

115. **d** If a specimen is hemolyzed, some analytes will be falsely elevated, including potassium. Hemolysis occurs when red blood cell membranes are ruptured and the contents released into the plasma or serum. Some clinical conditions may cause hemolysis, but it is frequently due to collection error.
[Garza, p301-302]

116. **a** If a specimen is hemolyzed, some analytes will be falsely elevated, including amylase. Hemolysis occurs when red blood cell membranes are ruptured and the contents released into the plasma or serum. Some clinical conditions may cause hemolysis, but it is frequently due to collection error.
[McCall 7e, p294]

117. **c** If a specimen is hemolyzed, some analytes will be falsely elevated, including lactate dehydrogenase (LD). Hemolysis occurs when red blood cell membranes are ruptured and the contents released into the plasma or serum. Some clinical conditions may cause hemolysis, but it is frequently due to collection error.
[McCall 7e, p294]

Specimen Handling, Transport & Processing — Explanations

118. c If a specimen is hemolyzed, some analytes will be falsely elevated, including iron. Hemolysis occurs when red blood cell membranes are ruptured and the contents released into the plasma or serum. Some clinical conditions may cause hemolysis, but it is frequently due to collection error.
[Garza 10e, p301-302]

119. d Serum specimens collected into a red top or a gel barrier tube may be accepted for testing if there is no hemolysis (often caused by a traumatic venipuncture) and if there is sufficient specimen to run the analysis. Characteristically, specimens are composed of 45% cells and 55% plasma or serum. However, when the patient's hematocrit is elevated, the percentage of serum decreases, as is the case in this specimen. An underfilled evacuated tube combined with an abnormally high hematocrit most likely resulted in quantity not sufficient (QNS) to run the analysis. A QNS specimen is the second most common cause of specimen rejection in the chemistry department of the laboratory.
[Garza 10e, p230, 231, 363]

120. a Clotting in the specimen submitted for testing is the most common reason specimens are not accepted for testing in the hematology department of the laboratory. The specimen was likely not mixed adequately with the anticoagulant (EDTA) immediately following collection, resulting in specimen clotting before the specimen was delivered to the laboratory for analysis.
[McCall 7e, p391-392]

121. c Green top evacuated tubes contain heparin, either as lithium heparin or as sodium heparin. Electrolyte (Na, K, Cl, CO_2) analysis includes sodium level analysis. Heparanized specimens for electrolyte analysis must be collected in lithium heparin, not sodium heparin, to prevent specimen contamination with sodium. The phlebotomist should first examine the specimen tube label to confirm the additive in the collection tube. If the additive is sodium heparin, the specimen must be redrawn. If it is lithium heparin, the patient's physician must be notified of the critical (panic) value immediately
[McCall 7e, p199, 476-499]

122. c EDTA microcollection container tubes, when filled, contain 500 µL of specimen. The manual erythrocyte sedimentation rate (ESR) procedure will characteristically require at least 2 mL of blood. The ESR specimen collected in a microcollection container would be markedly less than required for the ESR analysis.
[McCall 7e, p388, 456]

123. a If a specimen for bilirubin analysis is exposed to the light, up to 50% of the bilirubin in the specimen may be destroyed in an hour.
[McCall 7e, p366, 454]

Explanations — Specimen Handling, Transport & Processing

124. d Many of the analyses performed in chemistry are performed on patient serum. Additionally, the inert polymer gel provides a physical barrier between serum and cells following centrifugation, minimizing the effects of metabolic processes, such as glycolysis. Therefore, the red and gray gel separator tube would be the best specimen for a chemistry analysis from the list provided. Additionally, the clot activator promotes clotting, contributing to a decrease in turnaround time.
[McCall 7e, p453-460, 476-479]

125. b Most of the analyses performed in hematology are performed on whole blood collected in EDTA using lavender top tubes. The EDTA additive generates a whole blood specimen. Additionally, EDTA preserves cellular morphology and inhibits platelet aggregation. Hematology analyses frequently involve an assessment of cellular morphology, including platelets, making EDTA the optimum additive for most hematology specimens.
[McCall 7e, p453-460, 476-479]

126. c Antistreptolysin-O (ASO) titers, cold agglutinin titers, and rapid plasma reagin analyses included in this question detect the presence of antibody and reagin levels in a patient's serum formed in response to infection. Typically these types of analyses are performed in the immunology department, sometimes referred to as the serology department.
[McCall 7e, p454-455, 459]

127. a Electrolytes, glucose, ALT, AST, BUN, calcium, and creatinine analyses included in this question refers to a panel of tests often referred to as a basic metabolic panel (BMP). The BMP is performed on either patient serum or heparinized plasma in the clinical chemistry department.
[McCall 7e, p24, 454]

128. b Prothrombin time (PT) assesses the effectiveness of a patient's extrinsic and common pathways, and partial thromboplastin time (PTT) measures the effectiveness of a patient's intrinsic and common coagulation pathways. PT is also used to monitor warfarin therapy and PTT is used to monitor heparin therapy. Both analyses are performed in the coagulation department on patient plasma collected in sodium citrate tubes. Additionally, sodium citrate preserves labile coagulation factors.
[McCall 7e, p24, 459]

129. d The microbiology department analyses primarily nonblood specimens for the presence of pathogens, usually bacteria. If a pathogenic bacteria is recovered in a patient's specimen, a sensitivity test may be performed to determine which antimicrobial therapy would be most effective.
[McCall 7e, p24]

Specimen Handling, Transport & Processing — Explanations

130. **d** The microbiology department analyses blood culture specimens to determine if a patient is suffering from bacteremia or septicemia. The yellow sodium polyanthole sulfonate (SPS) tube serves as an anticoagulant by binding calcium. Additionally, it inhibits complement and the phagocytic activity of white cells, thereby increasing recovery rates of bacteria in the patient's bloodstream.
[McCall 7e, p476-479]

131. **d** The immunohematology or blood bank department collects, screens, and prepares blood products for transfusion. Additionally, crossmatch or compatibility tests including ABO blood typing and antibody screens are performed in the immunohematology department.
[McCall 7e, p28-29]

132. **a** The immunohematology or blood bank department collects, screens, and prepares blood products for transfusion. Testing may be performed on pink, plastic evacuated tubes spray-coated with EDTA.
[McCall 7e, p476-479]

133. **c** Many of the analyses performed in the coagulation department are performed on patient plasma collected in sodium citrate (light blue) tubes. Sodium citrate acts as an anticoagulant by binding calcium. Additionally, sodium citrate preserves labile coagulation factors.
[McCall 7e, p476-479]

134. **a** Arterial blood gas (ABG) specimens should be analyzed within 15 minutes of collection for optimal results. Blood cells continue to metabolize glucose, oxygen, and nutrients generating waste products such as carbon dioxide and acid. Several analytes will be altered by clinically significant margins if an ABG sample is allowed to remain at room temperature (22°C) longer than 30 minutes.
[Garza 10e, p401, 493]

135. **d** Blood cells continue to metabolize glucose, oxygen, and nutrients generating waste products such as carbon dioxide and acid. Several analytes, including pH and blood gases, will be altered by clinically significant margins if an ABG sample is allowed to remain at room temperature (22°C) longer than 30 minutes.
[McCall 7e, p439-440]

136. **a** If the pneumatic tube system meets operational benchmarks and the specimen is packed properly, the pneumatic tube system serves as an efficient mechanism for transporting specimens to the laboratory for analysis, resulting in decreased specimen delivery time. Specimens must be loaded into pneumatic tube systems using plastic bags to house the specimens and shock absorbent inserts to minimize breakage.
[Garza 10e, p405]

Explanations   Specimen Handling, Transport & Processing

137. c Complete blood count (CBC) specimens collected in EDTA microcollection containers should be analyzed within 4 hours of collection.
[McCall 7e, p455]

138. d Complete blood count (CBC) specimens collected in EDTA evacuated tubes are stable for 24 hours following collection if stored at room temperature (22°C).
[McCall 7e, p453-460]

139. b Erythrocyte sedimentation rate (ESR) specimens collected in EDTA evacuated tubes are stable for 4 hours following collection if stored at room temperature (22°C).
[McCall 7e, p453-460]

140. c Erythrocyte sedimentation rate (ESR) specimens collected in EDTA evacuated tubes are stable for 12 hours following collection if stored at refrigerator temperatures.
[McCall 7e, p453-460]

141. d Glucose specimens collected in sodium fluoride evacuated tubes are stable for 24 hours following collection if stored at room temperature (22°C).
[McCall 7e, p453-460]

142. d Prothrombin time (PT) specimens collected in sodium citrate evacuated tubes are stable for 24 hours following collection if stored at room temperature (22°C).
[McCall 7e, p453-460]

143. b Partial thromboplastin time (PTT) specimens collected in sodium citrate evacuated tubes are stable for 4 hours following collection if stored at room temperature (22°C).
[McCall 7e, p453-460]

144. c Specimens for cold agglutinin titer testing must be collected in an evacuated tube prewarmed, transported, and stored at 37°C until the serum is separated from the cells. The antibody detected in a cold agglutinin titer is indicative of primary atypical pneumonia, caused by the pathogen *Mycoplasma pneumoniae*.
[McCall 7e, p453-460]

145. c Specimens for cold agglutinin titer testing must be collected in an evacuated tube prewarmed, transported, and stored at 37°C until the serum is separated from the cells. The antibody detected in a cold agglutinin titer is indicative of primary atypical pneumonia, caused by the pathogen *Mycoplasma pneumoniae*.
[McCall 7e, p453-460]

Specimen Handling, Transport & Processing — Explanations

146. d Specimens for cryoglobulin testing must be drawn into specimen tubes (serum or EDTA) prewarmed, transported, and stored at 37°C until the serum or plasma is separated from the cells. Cryoglobulin testing screens for immunologic diseases such as rheumatoid arthritis.
[McCall 7e, p453-460]

147. d Specimens for cryofibrinogen testing must be drawn into specimen tubes prewarmed, transported, and stored at 37°C until the specimen is processed. Cryofibrinogen analysis screens for clotting disorders.
[McCall 7e, p389-390]

148. b Portable heat blocks may be placed in an incubator to reach 37°C and used to transport specimens at 37°C. Alternatively, commercially prepared heat sources, such as infant heel warmers, may be used to transport thermolabile specimens.
[Garza 10e, p401]

149. c Some specimens are thermolabile and must be chilled immediately after collection and labeling. Thermolabile specimens should be transported in a mixture of ice and water, also called an ice slurry. Transporting thermolabile specimens using ice cubes is not appropriate because the specimen may not be chilled uniformly, ranging from freezing the specimen adjacent to the ice and inadequate chilling of the specimen distal to the ice cubes. Both situations may negatively impact the integrity of the specimen.
[Garza 10e, p401-402]

Please consult the explanation below for questions 150-159 regarding transport of thermolabile specimens.

Questions 150-159 address the correct method for transporting thermolabile specimens. Thermolabile specimens are sensitive to higher temperatures and must be chilled immediately following collection. Thermolabile specimens should be transported in an ice slurry to slow down metabolic processes that could compromise specimen integrity. Correct transport of thermolabile specimens is a task associated with the preexamination/preanalytical process of laboratory workflow, which falls in the domain of the phlebotomist.

150. b Ammonia specimens are thermolabile and must be chilled immediately after collection and labeling. Ammonia levels are requested to assist in evaluating liver function.
[Garza 10e, p401-402]

151. b Adrenocorticotropic hormone (ACTH) specimens are thermolabile and must be chilled immediately after collection and labeling. ACTH levels are requested to assist in the evaluation of adrenal gland function.
[McCall 7e, p389-390]

Explanations Specimen Handling, Transport & Processing

152. d Parathyroid hormone (PTH) specimens are thermolabile and must be chilled immediately after collection and labeling. PTH levels are requested to assist in the evaluation of parathyroid gland function.
[McCall 7e, p389-390]

153. c Angiotensin-converting enzyme (ACE) specimens are thermolabile and must be chilled immediately after collection and labeling. ACE functions in constricting blood vessels, which may lead to elevated blood pressure.
[McCall 7e, p389-390]

154. a Acetone specimens are thermolabile and must be chilled immediately after collection and labeling. Acetone analysis is requested to assist in managing diabetes.
[McCall 7e, p389-390]

155. a Catecholamine specimens are thermolabile and must be chilled immediately after collection and labeling. Catecholamine analysis is requested to assist in assessing adrenal gland function.
[McCall 7e, p389-390]

156. a Lactic acid specimens are thermolabile and must be chilled immediately after collection and labeling. Lactic acid analysis is requested to assess anaerobic glycolysis following strenuous exercise and may also be used to assess liver disease.
[McCall 7e, p389-390]

157. d Homocysteine specimens are thermolabile and must be chilled immediately after collection and labeling. Homocysteine analysis is requested to assess risk of cardiovascular disease.
[McCall 7e, p389-390]

158. a Gastrin specimens are thermolabile and must be chilled immediately after collection and labeling. Gastrin analysis is requested to assess digestive disorders, particularly of the stomach.
[McCall 7e, p389-390]

159. b Renin specimens are thermolabile and must be chilled immediately after collection and labeling. Renin analysis is requested to assess hypertensive disorders.
[McCall 7e, p389-390]

160. b According to the Clinical & Laboratory Standards Institute (CLSI) guideline GP44-A4, blood specimens collected in gel barrier evacuated tubes must be centrifuged within 2 hours of collection to ensure specimen integrity. Placing the specimen in the refrigerator will not preserve the potassium level. In fact, storing the specimen in the refrigerator without centrifugation will result in a false elevation of the potassium level.
[McCall 7e, p393-395, 453-460]

Specimen Handling, Transport & Processing — **Explanations**

161. d The specimen was processed within the guidelines for processing specimens for prothrombin time analysis. Prothrombin time (PT) specimens collected in sodium citrate evacuated tubes are stable for 24 hours following collection if stored at room temperature (22°C).
[McCall 7e, p390]

162. a Photosensitive specimen analytes decompose when exposed to light and exposing these specimens to light during transport and handling may result in a falsely lowered value during analysis. To prevent this, photosensitive specimens must be protected from the light. Wrapping the specimen in aluminum foil is one of the most common methods for protecting the specimen from light.
[Garza 10e, p401-402]

163. b Bilirubin, a liver function test, is the most commonly ordered photosensitive analyte and may decrease by as much as 50% if exposed to light for an hour. To prevent this, photosensitive specimens must be protected from the light.
[Garza 10e, p401-402]

164. b β-carotene, a test used to screen for carotenemia, is photosensitive. Photosensitive specimen analytes decompose when exposed to light and exposing these specimens to light during transport and handling may result in a falsely lowered value during analysis. To prevent this, carotene specimens must be protected from the light.
[Garza 10e, p401-402]

165. d Folate levels, which may be used to assess anemia, are photosensitive. Photosensitive specimen analytes decompose when exposed to light and exposing these specimens to light during transport and handling may result in a falsely lowered value during analysis. To prevent this, specimens collected for folate levels must be protected from the light.
[Garza 10e, p401-402]

166. d Vitamin B_{12} levels, which may be used to assess vitamin deficiency and certain anemias, are photosensitive. Photosensitive specimen analytes decompose when exposed to light and exposing these specimens to light during transport and handling may result in a falsely lowered value during analysis. To prevent this, specimens collected for B_{12} levels must be protected from the light.
[McCall 7e, p389-390]

167. d Vitamin B_6 levels, which may be used to assess vitamin deficiency, are photosensitive. Photosensitive specimen analytes decompose when exposed to light. Exposing photosensitive specimens to light during transport and handling may result in a falsely lowered value during analysis. To prevent this, specimens collected for B_6 levels must be protected from the light.
[Garza 10e, p401-402]

Explanations   Specimen Handling, Transport & Processing

168. d   Vitamin C levels, which may be used to assess vitamin deficiency are photosensitive. Photosensitive specimen analytes decompose when exposed to light and exposing these specimens to light during transport and handling may result in a falsely lowered value during analysis. To prevent this, specimens collected for vitamin C levels must be protected from the light.
[McCall 7e, p389-390]

Please consult the explanation below for questions 169 & 170 and 173-180 regarding centrifugation of specimens collected in gel barrier tubes.

Clinical & Laboratory Standards Institute (CLSI) guideline GP44-A4 requires separation of serum from cells within 2 hours of specimen collection. Analytes may be falsely decreased or increased if more than 2 hours elapses between collection and centrifugation, as noted in the questions specified.

169. b   Placing the specimen in the refrigerator without centrifugation will not preserve the phosphorous level. In fact, storing the specimen in the refrigerator without centrifugation will result in a false elevation of the phosphorous level. .
[McCall 7e, p393-395]

170. d   Specimen transport to the laboratory should occur as soon as possible following specimen collection. However, Clinical & Laboratory Standards Institute (CLSI) guideline GP44-A4 requires separation of serum from cells within 2 hours of specimen collection.
[McCall 7e, p387, 393, 453-460]

171. c   Unless a specimen is collected in an antiglycolytic agent such as sodium fluoride, the red cells continue to metabolize glucose in the plasma or serum which may falsely decrease glucose levels in a patient's serum or plasma over time.
[McCall 7e, p388]

172. d   The specimen values will be unaffected because the specimen was centrifuged within 2 hours of collection. Following centrifugation, the inert polymer gel arrives at a position between the cells and serum, forming a physical barrier. This prevents the cells from metabolizing analytes in the patient's serum. Therefore, the results are unaffected.
[McCall 7e, p388]

173. c   Ionized calcium will falsely decrease with prolonged exposure to blood cells.
[McCall 7e, p387, 393, 453-460]

174. d   Lactate dehydrogenase (LD) will falsely increase with prolonged exposure to blood cells.
[McCall 7e, p387, 393, 453-460]

175. a   Folate will falsely decrease with prolonged exposure to blood cells.
[McCall 7e, p387, 393, 453-460]

Specimen Handling, Transport & Processing — Explanations

176. **d** Potassium will falsely increase with prolonged exposure to blood cells.
[McCall 7e, p387, 393, 453-460]

177. **a** Bicarbonate (CO_2) will falsely decrease with prolonged exposure to blood cells.
[McCall 7e, p387, 393, 453-460]

178. **a** Aspartate aminotransferase (AST) will falsely increase with prolonged exposure to blood cells.
[McCall 7e, p387, 393, 453-460]

179. **a** Alanine aminotransferase (ALT) will falsely increase with prolonged exposure to blood cells.
[McCall 7e, p387, 393, 453-460]

180. **a** Aldosterone will falsely increase with prolonged exposure to blood cells. The remaining tests listed are related to cell-associated measures in the blood. WBC is a white cell count and MCHC and MCV are measures of red cell hemoglobin concentration and size.
[Garza 10e, p399]

181. **d** Blood cells in the patient's specimen continue metabolic activities until cells are separated from serum or plasma. In this instance, the specimen was appropriately centrifuged within 2 hours of collection. Following centrifugation, the inert polymer gel arrives at a position between the cells and serum, forming a physical barrier. This prevents the cells from metabolizing analytes in the patient's serum. Therefore, the results are unaffected.
[McCall 7e, p387-388]

182. **b** Potassium is highly concentrated in red cells, compared to levels of potassium in plasma. If the plasma is allowed to remain in contact with patient red cells, the potassium will move out of the red cells into the plasma to achieve ionic equilibrium, causing a false elevation of potassium levels. In this instance, the specimen was appropriately centrifuged immediately upon arrival in the laboratory but this is a heparinized evacuated tube (dark green instead of mint green). It did not contain inert polymer gel so the cells remained in contact with the plasma and potassium moved from the red cells into the plasma, falsely elevating the plasma potassium levels. Therefore, the results are falsely increased.
[Garza 10e, p420, 620, 654-655]

Explanations
Specimen Handling, Transport & Processing

183. b Lactate dehydrogenase (LD) is highly concentrated in red cells, compared to levels of LD in serum. If the serum is allowed to remain in contact with patient red cells, the LD will move out of the red cells into the serum to achieve equilibrium, causing a false elevation of LD levels. Blood cells in the patient's specimen continue metabolic activities until cells are separated from serum. In this instance, the specimen was appropriately centrifuged within 2 hours of collection. However, the red top evacuated tube does not contain inert polymer gel. Since there is no barrier between the cells and serum, the LD will likely be falsely elevated.
[McCall 7e, p387-388]

184. d Specimen transport to the laboratory should occur as soon as possible following specimen collection. The specimen values will be unaffected because the specimen was centrifuged within 2 hours of collection. Following centrifugation, the inert polymer gel arrives at a position between the cells and serum, forming a physical barrier. This prevents the cells from metabolizing analytes in the patient's serum. Therefore, the results are unaffected.
[McCall 7e, p387-388, 396]

185. d The specimen values will be unaffected because the specimen was collected in sodium fluoride, a glycolytic inhibitor. Consequently, the specimen is stable at room temperature (22°C) for up to 24 hours. Therefore, the results are unaffected.
[McCall 7e, p387-388, 396]

186. b Potassium is highly concentrated in red cells, compared to levels of potassium in plasma. If the specimen is hemolyzed, red cells contents, including hemoglobin and potassium, are liberated into patient plasma, falsely elevating the results. The specimen should be redrawn.
[McCall 7e, p387-388]

187. a Specimens collected in an anticoagulant, such as heparin, may be centrifuged immediately following collection.
[Garza 10e, p407]

188. c Specimens collected in a gold Hemogard tube must be allowed to clot completely before centrifugation, which characteristically takes approximately 30 minutes to complete.
[Garza 10e, p407]

Specimen Handling, Transport & Processing — Explanations

189. a Reticulocyte counts are performed on whole blood specimens which should not be centrifuged. Specimens for reticulocyte counts should be placed on test tube rockers to ensure adequate mixing of the specimen prior to analysis.
[Garza 10e, p407]

190. a When blood specimens are transported to a laboratory by automobile, the specimens should be maintained in an upright position in an enclosed or lockable, leakproof container.
[Garza 10e, p403]

191. c When blood specimens are transported to a laboratory by automobile, the specimens should be maintained in an upright position in an enclosed or lockable, leakproof container.
[Garza 10e, p403]

192. b Specimens transported via a pneumatic tube system must be encased in shock absorbent material to prevent breakage.
[Garza 10e, p405]

193. b The primary specimen container, which is characteristically the evacuated tube containing the specimen, must be watertight.
[Garza 10e, p414-417]

194. a A layer of absorbent material sufficient to accommodate the volume of specimen in the primary container must be positioned between the primary and secondary shipping containers.
[Garza 10e, p414-417]

195. c The Department of Transportation (DOT) is the primary source for regulations governing specimen and biological shipments in the United States.
[Garza 10e, p413]

196. d Specimens must be placed in a centrifuge so the centrifuge is balanced. Specimens of similar size & volume must be placed directly across from each other.
[Garza 10e, p408-409]

197. a In a properly operated centrifuge, specimens are balanced. Specimens of equal volume and weight are located opposite each other in the centrifuge. When centrifuges are unbalanced, the centrifuge begins to vibrate and make an uncharacteristically loud noise, much like an unbalanced washing machine.
[Garza 10e, p408-409]

Explanations
Specimen Handling, Transport & Processing

198. d When centrifuges are unbalanced, the centrifuge begins to vibrate and make an uncharacteristically loud noise, much like an unbalanced washing machine. The appropriate course of action is to immediately turn off the centrifuge and allow it to stop completely. Once the centrifuge has completely stopped, the phlebotomist should inspect the evacuated tubes, moving them to a balanced placement and complete the centrifugation process. Allowing an unbalanced centrifuge to operate may result in tube breakage and aerosol formation. In a properly operated and balanced centrifuge, specimens of equal volume and weight are located opposite each other in the centrifuge.
[Garza 10e, p408-409]

199. a If testing is delayed by more than 48 hours, the specimen may be frozen and stored at –20°C. Specimens may be frozen once and then analyzed. Specimens should not be frozen and thawed multiple times.
[Garza 10e, p410]

200. c Stopper removal carries the potential of aerosol formation. OSHA states, "All procedures involving blood or potentially infectious materials shall be performed in such a manner as to minimize splashing, spraying, splattering, and generation of droplets of these substances". To comply with this mandate, stopper removal must occur behind a splash shield or a full length face shield.
[McCall 7e, p393, 397-399]

201. b Specimens should be placed in a centrifuge with the stoppers intact.
[McCall 7e, p393]

202. b When a specimen containing an inert polymer gel is centrifuged in an unbalanced centrifuge, the gel interface between cells and serum or plasma will be slanted.
[Garza 10e, p411]

203. a Basal state is when a patient is resting and fasting for at least 12 hours. Most specimens for laboratory tests are collected from hospital inpatients while the patient is in basal state, usually early in the morning.
[Garza 10e, p289]

204. b Diurnal rhythms, sometimes referred to as circadian rhythms, are fluctuations in the body's functions or fluids that occur daily or during the daytime hours. For example, cortisol levels may be as much as 50% higher in the morning (8:00 AM) than in the evening, but eosinophil counts may be higher in the evening.
[Garza 10e, p292-293, 364]

205. d Reference ranges refer to normal laboratory value ranges for healthy individuals. The values are calculated to include a high and a low range of values. Physicians use reference ranges as a point of comparison for patient results.
[Garza 10e, p239-241, 635]

Specimen Handling, Transport & Processing — Explanations

206. a Hemoconcentration results when the fluid content of the blood is decreased, resulting in increased concentration of large molecule blood components including proteins, coagulation factors, and blood cells. Prolonged tourniquet application (more than 1 minute), drawing through an occluded vein, or probing with a needle may cause hemoconcentration of the specimen.
[Garza 10e, p300, 340, 631]

207. d The suffix, *-emia* means "blood"' the word root *lip* refers to "fat" so literally translated, *lipemia* means fat, or lipid, in the blood. Lipemic specimens have a high lipid content and appear cloudy or milky, usually transient in nature and following ingestion of a fatty meal including substances such as butter, cream, cheese, or meat.
[Garza 10e, p165, 290, 411-412, 632]

208. b Reference laboratories accept and analyze specimens from a wide variety of facilities that may be local, regional, or interstate. Reference laboratories work with very high volumes of specimens and offer fast turnaround times and reduced costs as advantages.
[McCall 7e, p29]

209. d Trough specimens are collected prior to the next scheduled dose of medication when the drug is at the lowest concentration in the patient's bloodstream. Trough levels are collected to confirm that drug levels are within therapeutic range.
[Garza 10e, p495, 637]

210. d "STAT" is from the Latin *statim,* which means "immediately." Physicians order blood tests STAT because the patient is an emergency situation requiring immediate attention and blood tests assist with decision making in those circumstances. Tests ordered STAT should be given the highest priority.
[Garza 10e, p52, 636]

211. b *Hemat* is the word root which means "blood" and *-logy* is the suffix that means "study of." *Hematology* is the "study of blood" and the hematology department in the laboratory identifies disease and monitors treatment of the blood forming tissues. Examples of tests performed in the hematology department are complete blood count (CBC), erythrocyte sedimentation rate (ESR), reticulocyte count, and platelet count.
[Garza 10e, p6, 168, 248, 266-267, 631]

212. b Coagulation tests measure the patient's ability to form and dissolve clots and also to monitor anticoagulant therapy. The most common tests performed by the coagulation department are prothrombin time and activated partial thromboplastin time.
[McCall 7e, p25, 361-362]

Explanations

Specimen Handling, Transport & Processing

213. c *Micro-* is the prefix which means "small," *bio-* is the prefix that means "life" and *-logy* is the suffix that means "study of." *Microbiology* is the "study of small life forms." The microbiology department primarily uses the methods of culture and sensitivity to identify the presence of microorganisms in blood and body fluids and the antimicrobial therapy that would best combat them. The most common blood test analyzed by the microbiology department is blood culture and the most common body fluid specimen analyzed is urine.
[McCall 7e, p25, 27]

214. b The immunohematology department, or blood bank, prepares blood products for transfusion. Blood bank personnel are responsible for testing donor and patient blood to prevent transfusion reactions. The most common tests performed by this department are ABO and Rh typing, antibody screen, type and screen, and type and crossmatch.
[McCall 7e, p28]

215. d The immunology, or serology, department studies patient antigen-antibody responses to determine the patient's immune response to an antigen and also screens for autoimmune diseases. Common tests performed in the immunology department are antistreptolysin-O (ASO) testing, cold agglutinin titers, and rapid plasma reagin (RPR).
[McCall 7e, p25]

216. b The word root *cyt* means "cell" and the suffix *-logy* means "study of." Cytology, therefore, means "the study of cells." The cytology department examines cells in tissue and body fluids to identify premalignant and malignant conditions on the cellular level. The most common test performed in the cytology department is the Pap test.
[McCall 7e, p29]

217. d The word root *hist* means "tissue" and the suffix *-logy* means "study of." *Histology*, therefore, means "the study of tissue." The histology department examines tissue obtained through surgeries and autopsies to determine the presence or absence of disease. The histology department commonly employs the techniques of biopsy and frozen section to examine specimens.
[McCall 7e, p29-30; 28-29]

218. b Oftentimes, only a portion of a patient's specimen is used for testing. The process of separating the component of the specimen required for testing is "to aliquot" and the sub-specimen is an aliquot.
[Garza 10e, p34, 406, 410, 626]

219. b Blood cultures are used to assist physicians in diagnosing septicemia, the presence of microorganisms and/or toxins in the patient's bloodstream, a very serious condition and a leading cause of death in the United States.
[Garza 10e, p474, 589, 627]

Specimen Handling, Transport & Processing — Explanations

220. d Blood cultures are used to confirm the presence of microorganisms and/or toxins in the patient's bloodstream, a very serious condition often manifested in patients as fevers of unknown origin (FUO). Specimen collections are frequently timed to occur before the next anticipated temperature spike.
[Garza 10e, p474, 482, 589, 627]

221. a Half-life refers to the time required for a patient to metabolize half of the drug administered. Drugs with short half-lives such as the aminoglycosides required strict adherence to prescribed specimen collection times for therapeutic drug monitoring.
[Garza 10e, p495]

222. b Thermolabile specimens are sensitive to higher temperatures and must be chilled immediately following collection. Thermolabile specimens should be transported in an ice slurry to slow down metabolic processes that could compromise specimen integrity. Examples of tests requiring chilled transport are adrenocorticotropic hormone (ACTH), acetone, ammonia, gastrin, homocysteine, lactic acid, and renin.
[McCall 7e, p389-390]

223. c Photosensitive analytes decompose if exposed to bright lights following collection, potentially altering the results of the analysis. In these cases, the specimen must be shielded from light immediately, often by wrapping in aluminum foil to prevent compromise of specimen integrity. Examples of tests requiring chilled transport are bilirubin, carotene, and vitamins B_2, B_6, B_{12} and C.
[McCall 7e, p390-391]

224. c A patient value so far outside the reference range it may be considered life threatening is a critical (panic) value. Health care workers are required to report critical (panic) values to a patient's physician immediately.
[Garza 10e, p418, 629]

225. d The turnaround time (TAT) is the time required to complete a laboratory analysis from the time the analysis is ordered by the patient's physician to the time a result is reported to the physician and includes specimen collection, transport, processing, analysis, and reporting of results.
[Garza 10e, p397, 637]

226. c The pneumatic tube system serves as an efficient mechanism for transporting specimens to the laboratory for analysis. Prior to use, the pneumatic tube system is evaluated to be sure it meets established parameters for breakage rates, carrier size, distance, shock absorbency, and speed.
[Garza 10e, p405]

227. a Specimens should remain stoppered when awaiting centrifugation and during centrifugation. Removing stoppers before or during centrifugation can lead to aerosol formation, which represents a hazard for the health care worker.
[McCall 7e, p393-399]

Explanations   Specimen Handling, Transport & Processing

228. **d**   The specimen shown represents normal serum, which is clear and yellow.
[McCall 7e, p169-170]

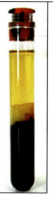

229. **c**   The specimen shown is a lipemic specimen. The suffix, -*emia* means "blood" the word root *lip* refers to "fat" so literally translated, *lipemia* means fat, or lipid, in the blood. Lipemic specimens have a high lipid content and appear cloudy or milky, usually transient in nature and following ingestion of a fatty meal including substances such as butter, cream, cheese, or meat.
[Garza 10e, p165, 290, 411-412, 632]

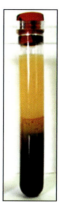

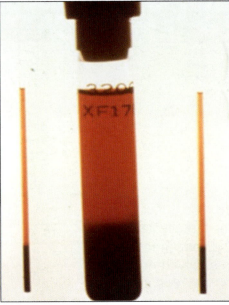

230. **a** The specimen shown is a hemolyzed specimen. Hemolysis occurs when red blood cell membranes are ruptured and the contents released into the plasma or serum turning the plasma or serum from yellow to pink or red. Some clinical conditions may cause hemolysis, but it is frequently due to collection error. If a specimen is hemolyzed, some analytes will be falsely elevated.
[Garza 10e, p301]

Waived & Point-of-Care Testing

The following items have been identified as appropriate for those preparing for the PBT examination.

1. Which of the following point-of-care testing procedures does not typically use instrumentation at the patient's bedside?
   a   blood gas
   b   hemoglobin & hematocrit
   c   troponin
   d   urine dipstick

2. What kind of quality control procedures may be required for urine dipstick analysis when using the manual method?
   a   delta checks & electronic QCs
   b   electronic QCs & relative centrifugal force
   c   low & high external control solutions
   d   relative centrifugal force

3. How frequently should quality control procedures required for urine dipstick analysis be performed?
   a   daily
   b   every shift
   c   monthly
   d   weekly

4. Which of the following personnel are authorized to complete a microscopic examination as part of a urinalysis?
   a   certified medical assistant
   b   certified phlebotomist
   c   medical laboratory assistant
   d   medical laboratory technician

5. Which of the following may be detected using a reagent strip on a urine specimen?
   a   bacteria, blood & protein
   b   bacteria, blood & casts
   c   blood, crystals & protein
   d   blood, protein & yeast

Waived & Point-of-Care Testing — Questions

6. Which of the following may be detected using a reagent strip on a urine specimen?
   a   bacteria, blood & casts
   b   blood, crystals & protein
   c   glucose, leukocytes, urobilinogen
   d   glucose, leukocytes & yeast

7. How should urinalysis reagent strips for point-of-care testing be stored?
   a   4°C in a clear plastic bag labeled with the biohazard label
   b   4°C in the original container with the cap securely fastened
   c   22°C in a clear plastic bag labeled with the biohazard label
   d   22°C in the original container with the cap securely fastened

8. Which of the following point-of-care analyses screens for anemia?
   a   glycosylated hemoglobin & occult blood
   b   hemoglobin & hematocrit
   c   prothrombin time & partial thromboplastin time
   d   troponin T&I

9. Which of the following methods may be used to obtain a hematocrit value?
   a   cell counter
   b   centrifugation
   c   comparing color to a reagent strip
   d   standardized incision

10. According to the American Medical Association (AMA), which of the following analyses is most accurate for diagnosis and treatment of anemia?
    a   glycosylated hemoglobin
    b   hemoglobin
    c   hematocrit
    d   prothrombin time

11. Which of the following point-of-care instruments may be used to measure hemoglobin?
    a   AccuChek
    b   DCA Vantage
    c   HemoCue system
    d   CritSpin

12. Which of the following point-of-care testing procedures does not use instrumentation?
    a   bleeding time
    b   blood gas
    c   hemoglobin and hematocrit
    d   troponin

Questions
Waived & Point-of-Care Testing

13. The purpose of a bleeding time (BT) test is to assess:
    a capillary integrity & platelet function
    b capillary integrity & coagulation factor deficiencies
    c effectiveness of heparin therapy
    d effectiveness of warfarin therapy

14. A phlebotomist receives a requisition for a bleeding time (BT) test on a patient scheduled for cardiac surgery. What site should she use for the test?
    a antecubital fossa
    b earlobe
    c lateral aspect of the volar surface of the forearm
    d medial aspect of the volar surface of the forearm

15. What are the dimensions of the blade used during a bleeding time (BT) test?
    a 1.0 mm wide & 2.5 mm deep
    b 1.0 mm wide & 5.0 mm deep
    c 2.5 mm wide & 1.0 mm deep
    d 5.0 mm wide & 1.0 mm deep

16. During a bleeding time (BT) test, the blood pressure cuff should be inflated to:
    a 20 mm/Hg
    b 40 mm/Hg
    c 60 mm/Hg
    d 80 mm/Hg

17. After the blood pressure cuff has been inflated during a bleeding time (BT) test, the incision must be made within:
    a 30-60 seconds
    b 45-90 seconds
    c 1-2 minutes
    d 2-3 minutes

18. What medication will interfere with a bleeding time test?
    a aminoglycosides
    b lisinopril
    c lithium
    d salicylate

19. While a phlebotomist is performing a bleeding time (BT) test, she notices that the drops of blood on the filter paper diminished in size and then became larger again. What could account for this change?
    a absorbent filter paper
    b dislodging the platelet plug
    c incorrect incision depth
    d incorrect incision width

Waived & Point-of-Care Testing — Questions

20. While a phlebotomist is performing a bleeding time (BT), she notices that the drops of blood on the filter paper diminished in size and then became larger again. How will this impact bleeding time results? The time will be:
    a accurate
    b falsely decreased
    c falsely increased
    d unaffected

21. The bleeding time (BT) is being replaced with:
    a coagulation factor assays
    b platelet count
    c platelet function assays
    d PT/PTT analyses

22. Which of the following point-of-care tests may be used to monitor warfarin therapy?
    a partial thromboplastin times (PTT) & international normalized ratio (INR)
    b partial thromboplastin times (PTT) & prothrombin time (PT)
    c platelet count & international normalized ratio (INR)
    d prothrombin time (PT) & international normalized ratio (INR)

23. What is the reference range for blood glucose levels obtained by point-of-care testing?
    a 12-14 g/dL
    b 14-16 g/dL
    c 70-110 mg/dL
    d 96-103 mmol/L

24. Which of the following conditions is frequently monitored using a point-of-care instrument?
    a chronic obstructive pulmonary disease (COPD)
    b diabetes mellitus
    c renal failure
    d septicemia

25. What specimen is used for a glucose analysis completed by point-of-care testing?
    a whole blood obtained by venipuncture
    b whole blood obtained by skin puncture
    c plasma obtained by skin puncture
    d serum obtained by venipuncture

26. To prevent the spread of infection by point-of-care glucose instruments, the instruments may be cleaned with a:
    a 1:10 bleach solution, mixed fresh daily
    b 1:10 bleach solution, mixed weekly
    c hydrogen peroxide solution
    d tincture of iodine

Questions

Waived & Point-of-Care Testing

27. To prevent the spread of infection by point-of-care testing (POCT) glucose instruments, the instruments may be cleaned with:
    a   CDC-registered bleach wipes, prepared for POCT instruments
    b   EPA-registered bleach wipes, prepared for POCT instruments
    c   NIOSH-75 registered bleach wipes, prepared for POCT instruments
    d   NIOSH-95 registered bleach wipes, prepared for POCT instruments

28. Advantages of point-of-care testing include:
    a   patient convenience & increased oversight controls
    b   patient convenience & decreased turnaround times
    c   increased accuracy & decreased turnaround times
    d   increased accuracy & oversight controls

29. Which of the following may act as a fomite?
    a   point-of-care testing instruments
    b   quality control solutions
    c   reagent strips
    d   reverse air flow

30. Which of the following infections have been transmitted through point-of-care testing instruments?
    a   antibiotic resistant organisms & hepatitis B
    b   antibiotic resistant organisms & hepatitis A
    c   hepatitis A & hepatitis B
    d   hepatitis A & tuberculosis

31. Personnel who perform point-of-care testing must meet testing requirements prescribed by:
    a   American Society for Clinical Pathology (ASCP)
    b   Centers for Medicare & Medicaid Services (CMS)
    c   Clinical Laboratory Improvement Amendments of 1988 (CLIA)
    d   state or local personnel regulations

32. Personnel who perform point-of-care testing must meet specimen handling requirements prescribed by:
    a   American Society for Clinical Pathology (ASCP)
    b   Centers for Medicare & Medicaid Services (CMS)
    c   Clinical Laboratory Improvement Amendments of 1988 (CLIA)
    d   Occupational Safety & Health Administration (OSHA)

33. What type of specimens are approved for use with waived tests?
    a   processed by centrifugation
    b   unprocessed, requiring additional handling by the technician
    c   unprocessed, requiring no additional handling by the technician
    d   shielded from light & transported at 37°C

Waived & Point-of-Care Testing — **Questions**

34. Patient results obtained by point-of-care testing must correlate with results generated by:
    a   an approved or accredited laboratory
    b   confirmatory testing
    c   delta checks
    d   standard deviation

35. How many types of quality control procedures are typically found associated with point-of-care instruments?
    a   1
    b   2
    c   3
    d   4

36. Quality control procedures for point-of-care instrumentation manufactured into the test system and performed electronically are:
    a   built-in quality control
    b   external quality control
    c   mandated by Occupational Safety & Health Administration (OSHA)
    d   recommended by the Centers for Disease Control (CDC)

37. Quality control procedures for point-of-care instrumentation using materials similar to patient specimens with validated results are:
    a   electronic
    b   external
    c   mandated by Occupational Safety & Health Administration (OSHA)
    d   recommended by the Centers for Disease Control (CDC)

38. Quality checks on point-of-care instruments must be performed:
    a   according to Centers for Disease Control recommendations
    b   according to manufacturer recommendations
    c   daily
    d   monthly

39. A phlebotomist is performing a glucose analysis using a point-of-care instrument. She realizes the physician's office laboratory has run out of reagent strips for the available instrument. What may she use instead?
    a   nothing; she must notify the physician of the situation
    b   outdated reagent strips from a neighboring physician's office
    c   quality control calibration strips
    d   reagent strips from a different brand of glucose analyzer

40. Point-of-care testing personnel are required to obtain:
    a   certification
    b   documentation of on-the-job training completion
    c   licensure
    d   malpractice insurance

Questions — Waived & Point-of-Care Testing

41. On-the-job training for point-of-care testing personnel requires the trainee to:
    a process the specimen, demonstrate the test, perform the test, including delta checks
    b process the specimen, read the test instructions, demonstrate the test
    c read the test instructions, demonstrate the test, perform the test, document the training
    d read the test instructions, demonstrate the test, perform delta checks

42. What qualifications are required for a trainer of personnel on point-of-care testing procedures?
    a baccalaureate degree
    b certification
    c knowledge of test procedures
    d licensure

43. What qualifications are required for a trainer of personnel on point-of-care testing procedures?
    a baccalaureate degree
    b certification
    c good laboratory practices
    d licensure

44. A phlebotomist performs a skin puncture prior to point-of-care testing. What protocols for patient confidentiality must she adhere to?
    a Americans with Disabilities Act
    b Employee Right to Know
    c Health Information Portability & Accountability Act (HIPAA)
    d Patient's Bill of Rights

45. A phlebotomist performs a skin puncture prior to point-of-care testing. What OSHA protocols for infection control must she adhere to?
    a Bloodborne Pathogen Standard
    b Employee Right to Know
    c HazMat Standard
    d Health Information Portability & Accountability Act (HIPAA)

46. A phlebotomist performs a skin puncture prior to point-of-care testing. What OSHA protocols must she adhere to?
    a Employee Right to Know
    b HazMat Standard
    c Needle Safety & Prevention Act
    d Health Information Portability & Accountability Act (HIPAA)

47. On-the-job training for point-of-care testing personnel requires the trainer to:
    a evaluate the trainee on test performance & document the training
    b evaluate the trainee on test performance, including delta checks
    c demonstrate specimen processing, demonstrate the test, perform the test
    d process the specimen, perform the test, including delta checks

Waived & Point-of-Care Testing — **Questions**

48. Specimens for point-of-care testing are commonly collected by:
    a   arterial puncture
    b   skin puncture
    c   sweat analysis
    d   venipuncture

49. Which of the following is a common error associated with specimen collection for point-of-care testing?
    a   alcohol is not allowed to dry completely prior to puncture
    b   hemoconcentration
    c   lipemia
    d   quantity not sufficient

50. Which of the following is a common error associated with specimen collection for point-of-care testing?
    a   hemoconcentration
    b   incorrect timing of procedure
    c   lipemia
    d   quantity not sufficient

51. Terms also used for point-of-care testing are:
    a   alternate site & off-site
    b   alternate site & centralized
    c   decentralized laboratory & patient-focused
    d   decontamination processes & nonwaived

52. Terms also used for point-of-care testing are:
    a   alternate site & bedside
    b   alternate site & centralized
    c   off-site & patient-focused
    d   decontamination processes & nonwaived

53. Which of the following categorizes laboratory test procedures according to levels of complexity?
    a   Centers for Disease Control & Prevention (CDC)
    b   Clinical Laboratory Improvement Amendments of 1988 (CLIA)
    c   College of American Pathologists (CAP)
    d   Patient's Bill of Rights (PBR)

54. Which of the following categories of laboratory testing defined by the Clinical Laboratory Improvement Amendments (CLIA) is associated with a low risk to patients?
    a   high complexity
    b   moderate complexity
    c   nonwaived
    d   waived

Questions — Waived & Point-of-Care Testing

55. Which of the following laboratory test categories defined by the Clinical Laboratory Improvement Amendments (CLIA) is easiest to perform?
    a   high complexity
    b   moderate complexity
    c   nonwaived
    d   waived

56. Which of the following laboratory test categories defined by the Clinical Laboratory Improvement Amendments (CLIA) is associated with a low error rate?
    a   high complexity
    b   moderate complexity
    c   nonwaived
    d   waived

57. A home pregnancy test kit approved by the Food & Drug Administration (FDA) is an example of a:
    a   high-complexity test
    b   moderate-complexity test
    c   nonwaived test
    d   waived test

58. To conduct waived testing, a physician's office laboratory must:
    a   be accredited by The Joint Commission (TJC)
    b   be accredited by the College of American Pathologists (CAP)
    c   obtain a Clinical Laboratory Improvement Amendments (CLIA) Certificate of Waiver (CW)
    d   obtain Clinical Laboratory Improvement Amendments (CLIA) certification

59. A process used to document instrumentation function and accuracy of results is called:
    a   calibration check
    b   control value
    c   critical (panic) value
    d   reference range

60. Complex tests that require specimen processing after collection, quality control procedures and training requirements for personnel conducting the analyses are:
    a   confirmatory
    b   Food & Drug Administration (FDA) approved
    c   nonwaived tests
    d   waived tests

Waived & Point-of-Care Testing — **Questions**

61. The legislation that categorizes medical laboratory tests according to the complexity of the test and potential risk to the patient if an error is made in performing the test is the:
    a   Clinical Laboratory Improvement Amendments of 1988
    b   Hazard Communications Standard
    c   Needlestick Safety and Prevention Act 2001
    d   OSHA's Bloodborne Pathogen Standard

62. Laboratory analyses that are easy to perform, have little risk of error, and are least risky for the patient if an error is made are classified as:
    a   send-out tests
    b   tests of moderate complexity
    c   tests of high complexity
    d   waived tests

63. Which of the following analyses may be performed as a waived test?
    a   arterial blood gases
    b B_{12}/folate analysis
    c   hemoglobin electrophoresis
    d   urine pregnancy test

64. The most common specimen used in a waived test kit to screen for pregnancy is:
    a   amniotic fluid
    b   cerebrospinal fluid
    c   urine
    d   whole blood

65. What type of urine specimen is most suitable for a waived kit test for pregnancy screening?
    a   clean catch
    b   first morning
    c   midstream collection
    d   sterile

66. Which of the following analytes is detected in a qualitative screen using a waived kit test?
    a   homocysteine
    b   human chorionic gonadotropin
    c   human leukocyte antigen
    d   humoral immunity

67. Which of the following tests is a waived test?
    a   arterial blood gases
    b   osmotic fragility
    c   protein electrophoresis
    d   rapid group A strep test

Questions

68. Which specimen is most often used in a waived test kit to screen for group A *Streptococcus*?
    - a amniotic fluid
    - b cerebrospinal fluid
    - c throat swab
    - d whole blood

69. Which of the following analyses may be performed as a qualitative screen using a waived kit test?
    - a direct antiglobulin test (DAT)
    - b indirect antiglobulin test (IAT)
    - c malarial blood smear screen (MBS)
    - d rapid influenza diagnostic test (RIDT)

70. Which specimen is most often used in a waived test kit to screen for influenza?
    - a amniotic fluid
    - b nasal swab
    - c throat swab
    - d urine, first morning

Waived & Point-of-Care Testing — Explanations

The following items have been identified as appropriate for those preparing for the PBT examination.

1. **d** One point-of-care testing procedure that may not use instrumentation at the patient's bedside is the urine dipstick procedure, which involves dipping a set of reagent pads on a plastic strip into a urine specimen and reading the results off the color-coded result chart on the side of the reagent strip bottle. Since there are no internal control mechanisms associated with an instrument in this procedure, daily external liquid quality control must be performed and documented.
   [McCall 7e, p411-412]

2. **c** The point-of-care testing procedure that may not use instrumentation at the patient's bedside is the urine dipstick procedure. Since there are no internal control mechanisms associated with an instrument in this procedure, daily external liquid quality control using low and high values must be performed and documented.
   [McCall 7e, p404]

3. **a** The point-of-care testing procedure that may not use instrumentation at the patient's bedside is the urine dipstick procedure. Since there are no internal control mechanisms associated with an instrument in this procedure, daily external liquid quality control using low and high values must be performed and documented. Quality control procedures must also be performed whenever a new lot number of reagent strips is opened for use.
   [McCall 7e, p411-412]

4. **d** Routine urinalysis includes a physical, chemical, and microscopic examination of the specimen. The microscopic examination of urine is a moderate complexity test and must be performed by trained personnel, including medical laboratory technicians.
   [McCall 7e, p412]

5. **a** Chemical testing on a urine specimen using a reagent strip typically includes the following analyses: pH, specific gravity, bacteria, blood, bilirubin, glucose, ketones, leukocytes, nitrites, protein, and urobilinogen. Casts, crystals, and yeast are typically identified during the microscopic phase of urinalysis, a moderate complexity test.
   [McCall 7e, p412]

6. **c** Chemical testing on a urine specimen using a reagent strip typically includes the following analyses: pH, specific gravity, bacteria, blood, bilirubin, glucose, ketones, leukocytes, nitrites, protein, and urobilinogen. Casts, crystals, and yeast are typically identified during the microscopic phase of urinalysis, a moderate complexity test.
   [McCall 7e, p412]

7. **d** Urinalysis reagent strips should be stored at room temperature (22°C) in the original container with the cap securely fastened.
   [McCall 7e, p412]

Explanations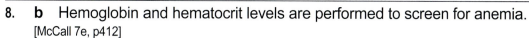

8. **b** Hemoglobin and hematocrit levels are performed to screen for anemia.
[McCall 7e, p412]

9. **b** Centrifugation may be employed to measure hematocrit levels.
[McCall 7e, p412]

10. **b** According to the American Medical Association, hemoglobin is the most accurate measure for the diagnosis and treatment of anemia.
[McCall 7e, p412]

11. **c** The HemoCue β-hemoglobin analyzer may be used to measure hemoglobin. AccuChek is used to monitor glucose, DCA Vantage measures glycosylated hemoglobin and the CritSpin centrifuge measures hematocrit levels.
[McCall 7e, p24-25]

12. **a** The bleeding time (BT) test is a point-of-care testing procedure that does not use instrumentation.
[McCall 7e, p351]

13. **a** The purpose of the bleeding time (BT) test is to measure capillary integrity and platelet function.
[McCall 7e, p351]

14. **c** Bleeding time procedures are performed on the lateral aspect of the volar surface of the forearm.
[McCall 7e, p24-25]

15. **d** The dimensions of the standardized blade used to perform a bleeding time (BT) test are 5.0 mm wide and 1.0 mm deep.
[McCall 7e, p362]

16. **b** The blood pressure cuff should be inflated to 40 mm/Hg during the bleeding time (BT) test.
[McCall 7e, p351]

17. **a** The incision must be made within 30-60 seconds after inflation of the blood pressure cuff during a bleeding time (BT) test.
[McCall 7e, p351]

18. **d** Salicylate (aspirin) will interfere with the results of a bleeding time (BT) test because it interferes with platelet function.
[McCall 7e, p351]

19. **b** The pattern suggests that the platelet plug was disrupted and consequently the bleeding time (BT) may be falsely prolonged.
[McCall 7e, p351]

20. **c** The pattern suggests that the platelet plug was disrupted and consequently the bleeding time (BT) may be falsely prolonged.
[McCall 7e, p351]

21. **c** The bleeding time test (BT) is an indirect measure of platelet function compared to platelet function assays performed on specimens obtained by venipuncture. BT tests are still performed in some facilities.
[McCall 7e, p351]

Waived & Point-of-Care Testing — Explanations

22. **d** The prothrombin (PT) and international normalized ratio (INR) are used to monitor patient warfarin therapy.
[McCall 7e, p362-363]

23. **c** The reference range for blood glucose levels are 70-110 mg/dL. Glucose levels in specimens collected by skin puncture will be higher than glucose specimens collected by venipuncture. For this reason, it must be noted that specimens for point-of-care testing were collected by skin puncture so the physician may interpret the result within that context.
[McCall 7e, p367-368]

24. **b** Patients with diabetes mellitus are frequently monitored using a point-of-care testing program.
[McCall 7e, p367-369]

25. **b** The specimen used for glucose analysis completed by point-of-care testing is whole blood obtained by skin puncture.
[McCall 7e, p367]

26. **a** A 1:10 bleach solution prepared fresh daily may be used to clean point-of-care glucose instruments to prevent the spread of infection.
[McCall 7e, p86, 187]

27. **b** Environmental Protection Agency (EPA)-registered bleach wipes may be used to clean point-of-care glucose instruments to prevent the spread of infection.
[McCall 7e, p86, 187]

28. **b** Advantages associated with point-of-care testing procedures include patient convenience and decreased turnaround times.
[McCall 7e, p360]

29. **a** Point-of-care testing instruments may act as fomites (ie, inanimate items that may be contaminated with infectious agents).
[McCall 7e, p361]

30. **a** Antibiotic resistant organisms and hepatitis B have been transmitted through point-of-care testing instruments. Point-of-care instruments should be routinely cleaned to prevent the spread of infection, following manufacturer's recommendations.
[McCall 7e, p361]

31. **d** No personnel requirements are prescribed by the Clinical Laboratory Improvement Amendments of 1988 (CLIA) for persons conducting waived testing. Personnel who perform point-of-care testing may be required to meet requirements prescribed by state and local regulations.
[McCall 7e, p37-38]

32. **d** Personnel who perform point-of-care testing must adhere to standard precautions mandated by the Occupational Safety & Health Administration (OSHA).
[McCall 7e, p360-361]

Explanations

Waived & Point-of-Care Testing

33. **c** To qualify as a waived test, the specimen used must be unprocessed, requiring no additional handling by the technician.
[McCall 7e, p361]

34. **a** Patient results obtained by point-of-care testing must correlate with results generated by an approved or accredited laboratory.
[McCall 7e, p360-361]

35. **b** Two types of quality control procedures are typically found associated with point-of-care instruments: 1) electronic built-in controls internal to the testing instrument designed to confirm that the test system is operating correctly and 2) external quality control materials similar to patient specimens to confirm accurate analyte measurement. Quality control procedures must be completed in strict adherence to manufacturer recommendations and consistent with the policies and procedures of the institution.
[McCall 7e, p361]

36. **a** Two types of quality control procedures are typically found associated with point-of-care instruments: 1) electronic built-in controls internal to the testing instrument designed to confirm that the test system is operating correctly and 2) external quality control materials similar to patient specimens to confirm accurate analyte measurement. Quality control procedures must be completed in strict adherence to manufacturer recommendations and consistent with the policies and procedures of the institution.
[McCall 7e, p361]

37. **b** Two types of quality control procedures are typically found associated with point-of-care instruments: 1) electronic built-in controls internal to the testing instrument designed to confirm that the test system is operating correctly and 2) external quality control materials similar to patient specimens to confirm accurate analyte measurement. Quality control procedures must be completed in strict adherence to manufacturer recommendations and consistent with the policies and procedures of the institution.
[McCall 7e, p361]

38. **b** Two types of quality control procedures are typically found associated with point-of-care instruments: 1) electronic built-in controls internal to the testing instrument designed to confirm that the test system is operating correctly and 2) external quality control materials similar to patient specimens to confirm accurate analyte measurement. Quality control procedures must be completed in strict adherence to manufacturer recommendations and consistent with the policies and procedures of the institution.
[McCall 7e, p361]

39. **a** The phlebotomist must notify the physician or testing site supervisor of the situation and ask for direction. The phlebotomist must only use reagent strips manufactured specifically for the instrument used to obtain patient results. Outdated reagent strips, reagent strips from another analyzer, or calibration strips should never be used to obtain a patient result.
[McCall 7e, p367-368]

Waived & Point-of-Care Testing — Explanations

40. **b** Point-of-care testing personnel are required to create and obtain documentation of on-the-job training completion, which requires the trainee to: 1) read the test instructions; 2) demonstrate the test; 3) perform the test; 4) document the training.
[McCall 7e, p30-31, 360-361]

41. **c** Point-of-care testing personnel are required to create and obtain documentation of on-the-job training completion, which requires the trainee to: 1) read the test instructions; 2) demonstrate the test; 3) perform the test; 4) document the training.
[McCall 7e, p30-31, 360-361]

42. **c** The trainer of point-of-care testing personnel is required to have knowledge of 1) good laboratory practices; 2) the specific test procedure including the ability to assess the effectiveness of training processes and procedures; 3) OSHA's Bloodborne Pathogen Standard and Needle Safety & Prevention Act; and 4) quality control.
[McCall 7e, p360-361]

43. **c** The trainer of point-of-care testing personnel is required to have knowledge of 1) good laboratory practices; 2) the specific test procedure including the ability to assess the effectiveness of training processes and procedures; 3) OSHA's Bloodborne Pathogen Standard and Needle Safety & Prevention Act; and 4) quality control.
[McCall 7e, p30-31]

44. **c** Anyone performing laboratory testing (including point-of-care testing) must maintain patient confidentiality consistent with the Health Information Portability & Accountability Act (HIPAA).
[McCall 7e, p8-9]

45. **a** Point-of-care testing personnel are required to have knowledge of good laboratory practices, which include OSHA's Bloodborne Pathogen Standard and Needle Safety & Prevention Act.
[McCall 7e, p360-361]

46. **c** Point-of-care testing personnel are required to have knowledge of good laboratory practices; which include OSHA's Bloodborne Pathogen Standard and Needle Safety & Prevention Act.
[McCall 7e, p84]

47. **a** The trainer responsible for providing on-the-job training for point-of-care testing personnel is required to evaluate the trainee on test performance and document the training.
[McCall 7e, p30-31]

48. **b** Specimens for point-of-care testing are frequently collected by skin puncture.
[McCall 7e, p361]

49. **a** A common error associated with specimen collection for point-of-care testing is not allowing the alcohol to air dry completely prior to puncture.
[McCall 7e, p235-236, 247]

Explanations   **Waived & Point-of-Care Testing**

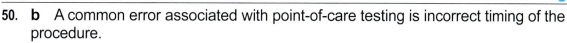

50. **b** A common error associated with point-of-care testing is incorrect timing of the procedure.
[McCall 7e, p361]

51. **c** Synonymous terms for point-of-care testing include alternate site, bedside, decentralized laboratory and patient-focused testing.
[McCall 7e, p360]

52. **a** Synonymous terms for point-of-care testing include alternate site, bedside, decentralized laboratory and patient-focused testing.
[McCall 7e, p360]

53. **b** The Clinical Laboratory Improvement Amendments of 1988 (CLIA) categorizes laboratory test procedures according to levels of complexity.
[McCall 7e, p38]

54. **d** The Clinical Laboratory Improvement Amendments of 1988 (CLIA) categorizes tests according to complexity. Waived tests are characterized by ease of completion, a low error rate, and low risk to patients in the event of an erroneous result.
[McCall 7e, p38]

55. **d** The Clinical Laboratory Improvement Amendments of 1988 (CLIA) categorizes tests according to complexity. Waived tests are characterized by ease of completion, a low error rate, and low risk to patients in the event of an erroneous result.
[McCall 7e, p38]

56. **d** The Clinical Laboratory Improvement Amendments of 1988 (CLIA) categorizes tests according to complexity. Waived tests are characterized by ease of completion, a low error rate, and low risk to patients in the event of an erroneous result.
[McCall 7e, p38]

57. **d** A home pregnancy test kit approved by the Food & Drug Administration (FDA) is an example of a waived test.
[McCall 7e, p361]

58. **c** In order to conduct waived testing, a physician's office must obtain a Clinical Laboratory Improvement Amendments (CLIA) Certificate of Waiver (CW).
[McCall 7e, p38]

59. **a** A process used to document instrumentation function and accuracy of results is called a calibration check or control check.
[McCall 7e, p46-48]

60. **c** Complex tests that require specimen processing after collection, training requirements for personnel, and specific quality measures are called nonwaived tests.
[McCall 7e, p38]

Waived & Point-of-Care Testing — Explanations

61. **a** The Clinical Laboratory Improvement Amendment of 1988 was enacted to establish quality standards that apply to all facilities performing laboratory analyses. Laboratory analyses are classified as waived, moderate complexity, or high complexity.
[Garza 10e, p99-100]

62. **d** The Clinical Laboratory Improvement Amendments of 1988 identifies waived tests as analyses that are easy to perform, have little risk of error, and are least risky for the patient if an error is made.
[Garza 10e, p637]

63. **d** The urine pregnancy test may be completed as a qualitative screen, waived test, using a commercially manufactured kit test. The remaining tests listed are tests of either moderate or high complexity.
[Garza 10e, p100, McCall 7e, p416]

64. **c** The specimen used most commonly in a waived kit test for pregnancy is urine. Serum, not whole blood, sometimes is also an acceptable specimen.
[McCall 7e, p416]

65. **b** The first morning urine specimen is preferred because it is the most concentrated and would have the highest levels of human chorionic gonadotropin (hCG).
[McCall 7e, p416]

66. **b** Pregnancy may be confirmed using a waived test kit. Test kits screen for the presence of human chorionic gonadotropin (hCG), which appears in the urine approximately 8-10 days after fertilization.
[McCall 7e, p416]

67. **d** Rapid group A strep test may be completed as a waived test, using a commercially manufactured kit test. The remaining tests are either tests of moderate or high complexity.
[Garza 10e, p100, McCall 7e, p430]

68. **c** The most common specimen used in a waived kit test to screen for group A *Streptococcus* is a throat swab.
[McCall 7e, p430-431]

69. **d** Rapid influenza diagnostic tests (RIDTs) are qualitative screening waived test kits that may be used to detect influenza infection. RIDTs may detect both influenza A and B antigens, although some test kits may not be able to distinguish between the two strains.
[McCall 7e, p421-422]

70. **b** The specimen used most commonly used in a waived kit test for influenza is a nasal or nasopharyngeal swab.
[McCall 7e, p421-422]

Nonblood Specimens

The following items have been identified as appropriate for those preparing for the PBT examination.

1. Which body system functions in homeostasis by maintaining pH balance through the excretion of waste products of protein metabolism?
   a   digestive system
   b   endocrine system
   c   respiratory system
   d   urinary system

2. Which of the following analytes are capable of conducting electricity when in solution with water *in vitro* and functions in maintaining acid-base balance *in vivo*?
   a   electrolytes
   b   enzymes
   c   hormones
   d   vitamins

3. Which of the following anatomic structures is/are normally found in the urinary system?
   a   1 ureter
   b   1 urethra
   c   2 bladders
   d   3 kidneys

4. Which anatomic structure filters water, electrolytes, and waste products from the bloodstream?
   a   Bowman capsule
   b   glomerulus
   c   nephron
   d   prostate gland

5. Nephrons are located in the:
   a   kidney
   b   plasma
   c   serum
   d   urethra

Nonblood Specimens — Questions

6. Which of the following organs produce erythropoietin?
   a   bladder
   b   kidney
   c   ureter
   d   urethra

7. The presence of leukocytes in urine indicates:
   a   anemia
   b   infection
   c   leukemia
   d   within reference range

8. The presence of ketones in the urine indicates:
   a   anemia
   b   infection
   c   liver disease
   d   starvation

9. The term meaning the study of poisons is:
   a   taxidermy
   b   toxicology
   c   toxicophobia
   d   toxuria

10. The type of drug screen procedure that generates either a positive or negative result is:
    a   inaccurate
    b   qualitative
    c   quantitative
    d   unreliable

11. The type of drug screen procedure that reports a specific amount of drug present in the specimen is:
    a   inaccurate
    b   qualitative
    c   quantitative
    d   unreliable

12. The following form of alcohol is measured in a blood alcohol concentration (BAC):
    a   ethanol
    b   glycerol
    c   methanol
    d   propanol

Questions
Nonblood Specimens

13. The National Collegiate Athletic Association (NCAA) prohibits athletes from using the following substance:
    a erythroplastid
    b erythropoietin
    c ethylene
    d ethylenediaminetetraacetic acid

14. Which of the following body fluids is the specimen most commonly used for drug screen procedures:
    a blood
    b feces
    c saliva
    d urine

15. A college student uses marijuana approximately once a month. How long after using can it be detected in his urine?
    a days
    b months
    c only a few hours
    d years

16. Which of the following laboratory tests may be performed on a random urine specimen?
    a 12 hour urine collection
    b 24-hour urine collection
    c routine urinalysis
    d urine culture and sensitivity

17. Requisitions for routine urinalysis originate with the:
    a employer
    b nurse
    c patient
    d physician

18. Which of the following procedures is commonly used to collect a specimen for routine urinalysis?
    a 24-hour urine collection
    b 48 hour urine collection
    c catheterization
    d random urine collection

19. The patient is routinely provided with the following information prior to urine specimen collection:
    a date of the last survey by The Joint Commission (TJC)
    b the manufacturer of the collection container
    c phlebotomist's name
    d reference ranges

Nonblood Specimens — Questions

20. Prior to collecting a specimen for routine urinalysis, the phlebotomist is required to:
    - a ask the patient to state his name
    - b confirm the patient's identity by asking, "Are you Mr. Smith"?
    - c determine if the patient has been fasting
    - d instruct the patient to drink a full, 8 ounce glass of water

21. Which of the following collection containers is appropriate to use to collect a urine specimen for routine analysis?
    - a chemistry urine strip
    - b clean, dry plastic container
    - c osmolality meter
    - d sterile swab

22. Which of the following collection containers may be used by a phlebotomist to collect a urine sample from a baby?
    - a catheter
    - b clean, dry plastic container
    - c disposable bag with hypoallergenic skin adhesive
    - d sterile container

23. Which of the following collection containers is used to collect a routine urine sample from a 90-year-old male?
    - a clean, dry amber container
    - b clean, dry plastic container
    - c disposable bag with hypoallergenic skin adhesive
    - d sterile container

24. A phlebotomist must instruct a male patient in the proper technique for collecting a midstream urine specimen. The phlebotomist should provide the patient with an appropriate container and instruct the patient to:
    - a begin to void into the toilet, momentarily interrupt the urine flow, position the collection container underneath the anticipated urine stream, resume voiding, and collect the remaining specimen
    - b cleanse the end of the penis with a prepackaged cleansing agent and void into the container provided
    - c cleanse the end of the penis with a prepackaged cleansing agent, begin to void into the toilet; momentarily interrupt the urine flow, position the collection container underneath the anticipated urine stream, resume voiding, and collect the remaining specimen
    - d void into the container provided followed by cleansing the tip of the penis with the cleansing agent provided

Questions

Nonblood Specimens

25. A patient prefers to collect a first morning urine sample at home. After voiding, the patient must deliver the specimen within what time frame?
    a 15 minutes
    b 30 minutes
    c 45 minutes
    d 60 minutes

26. A patient collects a first morning specimen at home using the collection container provided by her physician's office. How quickly must the specimen be delivered to the laboratory?
    a at the patient's convenience
    b anytime during business hours
    c within 60 minutes of voiding the specimen
    d within 3 hours of voiding the specimen

27. Labels for first morning urine samples should be affixed to the specimen:
    a container
    b lid
    c requisition
    d transport bag

28. What personal protective equipment should a phlebotomist wear when handling urine specimens from outpatients?
    a gloves
    b gown & mask
    c N95 fit mask
    d gowns, gloves & mask

29. What information must be included on a urine specimen label in addition to the patient's name and identification number?
    a date & time of collection, initials of the person supervising the collection, type of specimen
    b date & time of collection, type of specimen
    c date of collection, initials of the person supervising the collection
    d date & time of collection, initials of the person supervising the collection

30. A urine sample was collected in a physician's office at 9:00 AM. The laboratory's courier service is scheduled to pick up specimens at 11:30 AM. At what temperature should the specimen be stored?
    a −20°C
    b 4°C
    c 22°C
    d 37°C

Nonblood Specimens — Questions

31. Requisitions for urine culture and sensitivity originate with the:
    a   insurance company
    b   nurse
    c   patient
    d   physician

32. Which of the following procedures is commonly used to collect a specimen for urine culture and sensitivity?
    a   routine void
    b   midstream
    c   midstream clean-catch
    d   postprandial

33. The patient is routinely provided with the following information prior to urine collection for culture and sensitivity:
    a   expiration date of the reagents
    b   manufacturers of the collection container
    c   phlebotomist's name
    d   reference ranges

34. Prior to collecting a specimen for urine culture and sensitivity, the phlebotomist is required to:
    a   ask the patient to state his name
    b   confirm the patient's identity by asking, "Are you Mr. Smith?"
    c   determine if the patient has been fasting
    d   instruct the patient to drink a full, 8 ounce glass of water

35. Which of the following collection containers is appropriate to use to collect a urine specimen for culture and sensitivity?
    a   chemistry urine strip
    b   clean, dry plastic container, shipped in bulk
    c   sterile plastic container, individually wrapped
    d   sterile swab

36. A patient asks the phlebotomist why the clean-catch specimen collection procedure is necessary, the phlebotomist should respond:
    a   "I don't know. Please ask your physician."
    b   "Because you might have diabetes."
    c   "The requisition indicates this additional step is necessary."
    d   "To prevent specimen contamination."

37. Which of the following collection containers is used to collect a urine sample for culture and sensitivity from a 30-year-old pregnant woman?
    a   clean, dry amber container
    b   clean, dry plastic container
    c   disposable bag with hypoallergenic skin adhesive
    d   sterile specimen container

Questions

Nonblood Specimens

38. A phlebotomist must instruct a 55-year-old female patient in the proper technique for collecting a midstream clean-catch urine specimen. The phlebotomist should instruct the patient to first:
   - a begin to void into the toilet, momentarily interrupt the urine flow, position the collection container underneath the anticipated urine stream, resume voiding, and collect the remaining specimen
   - b separate the skin folds around the urethra and cleanse the area using a prepackaged cleansing agent in the direction front to back
   - c separate the skin folds around the urethra and cleanse the area a prepackaged cleansing agent in the direction back to front
   - d wash her hands

39. A phlebotomist must instruct a 25-year-old male patient in the proper technique for collecting a midstream clean-catch urine specimen. The phlebotomist should provide the patient with a prepackaged cleansing agent and instruct the patient to:
   - a void into the toilet, momentarily interrupt the urine flow, position the collection container underneath the anticipate urine stream, resume voiding, and collect the remaining specimen
   - b position the collection container underneath the anticipated urine stream, void into the container, and collect the specimen
   - c wash his hands and then, using the prepackaged cleansing agent provided, cleanse the tip of his penis in concentric circles beginning at the periphery and moving toward the middle
   - d wash his hands and then, using the prepackaged cleansing agent provided, cleanse the tip of his penis in concentric circles beginning at the middle and moving outward

40. A phlebotomist must instruct an uncircumcised male patient in the proper technique for collecting a midstream clean-catch urine specimen. The phlebotomist should provide the patient with a prepackaged cleansing agent and instruct the patient to:
   - a after cleansing the collection container, begin to void into the toilet, momentarily interrupt the urine flow, position the collection container underneath the anticipated urine stream, resume voiding, and collect the remaining specimen
   - b position the collection container underneath the anticipated urine stream, void into the container, and collect the specimen
   - c retract the foreskin and cleanse the tip of his penis using the cleansing agent provided in concentric circles beginning at the periphery and moving toward the middle
   - d retract the foreskin and cleanse the tip of his penis using the prepackaged cleansing agent provided in concentric circles beginning at the middle and moving outward

41. A 16-year-old male patient was instructed in the procedure to collect a midstream clean-catch urine sample. When the patient handed the specimen to the phlebotomist he stated, "I accidentally dropped the container in the sink before collecting the specimen." The phlebotomist determined the patient touched the edges of the container onto the surface of the sink. What is the appropriate course of action?

    a   discard the specimen and recollect
    b   label the specimen container and submit for testing
    c   label the specimen lid and submit for testing
    d   notify the patient's physician and submit for testing

42. A urine specimen for culture and sensitivity should be stored immediately after collection at:

    a   4°C
    b   22°C
    c   37°C
    d   56°C

43. Labels for urine culture and sensitivity urine samples should be affixed to the specimen:

    a   container
    b   lid
    c   requisition
    d   transport bag

44. What personal protective equipment should a phlebotomist wear when handling urine specimens from outpatients?

    a   gloves
    b   gown and mask
    c   N95 fit mask
    d   gown, gloves and mask

45. What information must be included on the label of a urine specimen for culture and sensitivity in addition to the patient's name and identification number?

    a   date & time of collection, initials of the person supervising the collection, type of specimen
    b   date & time of collection, patient initials, type of specimen
    c   date of collection, initials of the person supervising the collection
    d   date & time of collection, initials of the person supervising the collection

46. What is the minimum volume of specimen required to complete a urine culture and sensitivity analysis?

    a   10 mL
    b   15 mL
    c   20 mL
    d   30 mL

Questions
Nonblood Specimens

47. Which of the following urine collection containers may be equipped with a caustic chemical as a preservative?
    a 12 hour
    b 24-hour
    c drug screen
    d sterile plastic

48. A 24-hour urine collection procedure typically begins in the:
    a afternoon
    b evening
    c midnight
    d morning

49. When providing a patient with instructions for 24-hour urine collection, the phlebotomist should emphasize the importance of:
    a handwashing
    b remaining in a supine position
    c voiding as frequently as possible
    d voiding as infrequently as possible

50. Instructions for a 24-hour urine collection should be provided:
    a at least 1 week ahead of the collection date
    b only by the patient's physician
    c using diagrams
    d verbally & written

51. Which of the following quantitative urine collection procedures requires a blood specimen collection at midpoint?
    a creatinine clearance
    b glucose tolerance
    c hormone studies
    d urobilinogen

52. Preservatives required for a 24-hour urine should be added by the:
    a patient before every void
    b patient after every void
    c phlebotomist before issuing the collection container to the patient
    d phlebotomist immediately upon receipt of the specimen from the patient

53. Which of the following analysis require dietary restrictions including no avocados, bananas, tomatoes, or walnuts for several days prior to specimen collection?
    a 5-hydroxyindoleacetic acid (5-HIAA)
    b creatinine clearance
    c urate
    d urobilinogen

Nonblood Specimens — Questions

54. A 24-hour urine container typically has a volume of at least:
    a   30 mL
    b   50 mL
    c   3,000 mL
    d   5,000 mL

55. To begin a 24-hour urine collection, the patient should void into the:
    a   collection container
    b   evacuated tube
    c   sterile collection container
    d   toilet

56. Once a 24-hour urine collection procedure has been initiated, the patient should collect:
    a   all urine voided
    b   only urine voided at home
    c   the first and last specimens only
    d   urine generated every other void

57. To complete a 24-hour urine collection, the patient should void into the:
    a   collection container
    b   evacuated tube
    c   sterile collection container
    d   toilet

58. Unless otherwise directed by the patient's physician, patient fluid intake during a 24-hour urine collection should be:
    a   decreased
    b   increased
    c   normal
    d   recorded

59. What information must be included on a 24-hour urine specimen label in addition to the patient's name and identification number?
    a   24-hour urine
    b   date and time of each fluid intake
    c   date and time of each void
    d   total number of times the patient voided a specimen

60. What information must be included on a 24-hour urine specimen label in addition to the patient's name and identification number?
    a   start & end time of the collection
    b   date & time of each fluid intake
    c   date & time of each void
    d   total number of times the patient voided a specimen

Questions

Nonblood Specimens

61. What temperature are 24-hour urine specimens typically stored at?
    - a −20°C
    - b 4°C
    - c 22°C
    - d 37 °C

62. Labels for 24-hour urine specimens should be affixed to the specimen:
    - a container
    - b lid
    - c requisition
    - d transport cooler

63. What kind of protocol must be followed for forensic specimens?
    - a chain of command
    - b chain-of-custody
    - c incident report
    - d respondeat superior

64. Individuals requiring a drug screen will be asked to:
    - a eat a meal of at least 100 g of glucose 2 hours before specimen collection
    - b eat a meal of at least 100 g of lactose 2 hours before specimen collection
    - c sign a consent form
    - d sign a consent form in the presence of a witness

65. Individuals requiring a drug screen will be asked to submit:
    - a identification including a photo
    - b identification including proof of residence
    - c list of prescription drugs they are currently taking
    - d physician's order

66. Which of the following identification methods are acceptable when identifying an individual for a drug screen:
    - a identification by a coworker
    - b identification by a safety officer
    - c passport
    - d voter's card

67. Why would an individual be required to submit to a drug screen procedure?
    - a comply with College of American Pathologists guidelines
    - b comply with Centers for Disease Control guidelines
    - c establish a baseline
    - d pre-employment testing

Nonblood Specimens — Questions

68. What cleansing agent should a phlebotomist use to prepare a venipuncture site prior to the collection of a blood alcohol level?
    a   70% isopropyl alcohol
    b   90% isopropyl alcohol
    c   aqueous povidone iodine
    d   tincture of iodine

69. Which of the following evacuated tubes should be used to collect a blood alcohol level?
    a   glass gray top sodium fluoride tube
    b   plastic grey top sodium fluoride tube
    c   glass lavender top EDTA tube
    d   plastic lavender top EDTA tube

70. A phlebotomist accepted a urine specimen from an individual for a random drug screen. She noticed the specimen appeared markedly turbid. The appropriate course of action is to:
    a   accept the specimen for testing
    b   collect another specimen per the policy at the facility
    c   notify the individual's physician immediately
    d   notify NIDA immediately

71. A phlebotomist receives a urine specimen at 0906 (military time) from an individual for a pre-employment drug screen. The temperature of the urine must be taken no later than:
    a   0910
    b   0911
    c   0926
    d   0936

72. A phlebotomist receives a urine specimen for random drug testing from a pilot. What temperature range must the urine temperature fall in to be acceptable for testing?
    a   89-102°F
    b   90-100°F
    c   98-102°F
    d   95-99°F

73. What type of urine sample is required for confirmation drug testing?
    a   clean-catch
    b   postprandial
    c   random
    d   split specimen

Questions
Nonblood Specimens

74. Which of the following security measures is routinely performed by collection sites for urine drug testing to ensure specimen integrity?
    a accept catheterized specimens only
    b collect in a sterile container
    c label using a Typenex band
    d place bluing material in the toilet

75. The process maintaining accountability of a specimen from collection to disposition, including the identity of each person handling the specimen and its disposition is called:
    a chain of custody
    b chain of infection
    c contact precautions
    d therapeutic drug monitoring

76. Requisitions for drug screen analysis frequently originate with the individual's:
    a employer
    b nurse
    c patient
    d physician

77. A patient's blood pH is 7.28. What is the term for this patient's condition?
    a acidosis
    b alkalosis
    c ketosis
    d within reference range

78. Which of the following are electrolytes?
    a albumin, bicarbonate, blood urea nitrogen, creatinine
    b bicarbonate, calcium, chloride, sodium, potassium
    c bilirubin blood urea nitrogen, carotene, creatinine
    d calcium, chloride, osmolality, total protein

79. Urine is a(n):
    a electrolyte
    b enzyme
    c nutrient
    d waste product

80. Which of the following urine specimens would be expected to have the highest specific gravity?
    a clean-catch
    b first morning
    c random
    d evening

Nonblood Specimens   **Questions**

81. The procedure used to collect a urine specimen for routine urinalysis and to minimize contamination of the urine specimen by bacteria, genital secretions, pubic hair is called:
    - a first morning
    - b midstream
    - c postprandial
    - d random

82. The components of a routine urinalysis are:
    - a chemical analysis, dipstick analysis, description of gross characteristics
    - b osmolality, specific gravity, dipstick analysis
    - c physical assessment, chemical analysis, microscopic analysis
    - d specific gravity, microscopic analysis, physical assessment

83. Proteinuria may indicate:
    - a diabetes
    - b kidney disease
    - c myocardial infarction
    - d pregnancy

84. A patient is instructed to cleanse their genital area using soapy water before generating a urine specimen. This specimen is called a:
    - a clean-catch specimen
    - b first morning specimen
    - c midstream specimen
    - d postprandial specimen

85. In order to quantify a particular analyte in urine, the following collection technique may be employed:
    - a 12-hour urine collection
    - b 24-hour urine collection
    - c clean-catch urine
    - d culture and sensitivity

86. In order to identify a microbe causing a urinary tract infection, the following collection technique may be employed:
    - a chain-of-custody
    - b clean-catch
    - c postprandial
    - d stat

87. Which of the following agencies defines requirements for the collection, processing, and testing of urine drug screens?
    - a ASCP
    - b ASMT
    - c NIDA
    - d NIH

Questions
Nonblood Specimens

88. A specimen for drug screening was tampered with. The term describing this circumstance is:
   a abduction
   b adduction
   c adulteration
   d adventitial

89. Illegal drugs are also referred to as:
   a gateway
   b illicit
   c OSUK
   d OTC

90. What is one common name for a drug that is a benzodiazepine?
   a angel dust
   b crack
   c speed
   d valium

91. What is one common name for a drug that is an opiate?
   a angel dust
   b codeine
   c PCP
   d valium

92. Which of the following organisms can cause enteric disease?
   a *Cryptococcus* spp.
   b *Neisseria flavescens*
   c *Neisseria meningitidis*
   d *Salmonella* spp.

93. A patient is scheduled for a fecal occult blood test. Which of the following foods should he be instructed to eliminate from his diet for 3 days prior to testing?
   a bananas
   b dairy
   c gluten
   d meat

94. A patient is scheduled to collect a fecal sample for culture and sensitivity. What should the patient be instructed to wash following collection?
   a faucet handles
   b inside surface of the collection container lid
   c outside surface of the collection container
   d specimen label

©ASCP 2022   ISBN 978-089189-6876   BOC PBT & QDP Study Guide 3e

Nonblood Specimens — **Questions**

95. A fecal specimen is collected to determine the presence of an intestinal parasite. What temperature should the specimen be maintained at?
    a   −20°C
    b   4°C
    c   22°C
    d   37°C

96. Which of the following tests detects occult blood in the stool?
    a   γ-glutamyl transpeptidase
    b   gastric analysis
    c   guaiac smear
    d   serum gastrin

97. Cerebrospinal fluid is normally:
    a   clear & colorless
    b   clear & yellow
    c   cloudy & white
    d   cloudy & yellow

98. Cerebrospinal fluid is chemically similar to:
    a   amniotic fluid
    b   bronchial washing
    c   plasma
    d   urine

99. Cerebrospinal fluid is normally collected by the:
    a   phlebotomist
    b   physician
    c   nurse
    d   respiratory therapist

100. The procedure used to collect cerebrospinal fluid is called a(n):
    a   amniocentesis
    b   bronchial wash
    c   gastric analysis
    d   lumbar puncture

101. How should CSF samples be delivered to the laboratory?
    a   on dry ice
    b   priority
    c   routine
    d   stat

102. Cerebrospinal fluid analysis is most frequently ordered to diagnose:
    a   AIDS
    b   depression
    c   meningitis
    d   schizophrenia

Questions
Nonblood Specimens

103. Seminal fluid is normally:
    a. thin & clear yellow
    b. thin & yellowish white
    c. viscous & clear
    d. viscous & yellowish white

104. A male patient is being evaluated for infertility and must submit a seminal fluid sample. What instructions should he receive?
    a. ejaculate daily for at least 3 days before the test
    b. ejaculate daily for at least 7 days prior to the test
    c. sexual abstinence for at least 3 days prior to the test
    d. sexual abstinence for at least 7 days prior to the test

105. A sample for seminal fluid analyses is BEST collected in a(n):
    a. condom
    b. emesis basin
    c. sterile container
    d. syringe

106. Specimens for seminal fluid analysis should be transported at what temperature?
    a. −20°C
    b. 4°C
    c. 22°C
    d. 37°C

107. What is the maximum time that may elapse between seminal fluid collection and delivery to the laboratory?
    a. 15 minutes
    b. 30 minutes
    c. 60 minutes
    d. 120 minutes

108. Seminal fluid analysis is more commonly performed to:
    a. conduct DNA testing, evaluate infertility, or determine the reversibility of a vasectomy
    b. conduct DNA testing, confirm the effectiveness of a vasectomy, or obtain evidence in a criminal sexual investigation
    c. evaluate infertility, confirm the effectiveness of a vasectomy, or obtain evidence in a criminal sexual investigation
    d. evaluate infertility, determine the reversibility of a vasectomy, or obtain evidence in a criminal sexual investigation

109. Which of the following types of pathogens cause tuberculosis?
    a. acid-fast bacillus
    b. fungus
    c. parasite
    d. virus

Nonblood Specimens

Questions

110. When is the best time of day to collect a sputum sample from a patient?
    - a morning
    - b afternoon
    - c 1600 (military time)
    - d evening, before bed

111. What should a patient be asked to do before collecting a sputum sample to ensure a high quality specimen?
    - a fast
    - b gargle with water
    - c gargle with mouthwash
    - d urinate

112. What minimum volume of sputum sample is usually required to ensure a good quality result?
    - a 1-3 mL
    - b 3-5 mL
    - c 5-7 mL
    - d 7-9 mL

113. The body fluid that is produced in the bronchi, lungs, and trachea is called:
    - a seminal fluid
    - b serous fluid
    - c sputum
    - d synovial fluid

114. Pleural fluid is normally collected by the:
    - a phlebotomist
    - b physician
    - c nurse
    - d respiratory therapist

115. The procedure used to collect peritoneal fluid is called a(n):
    - a aspiration
    - b bronchial wash
    - c gastric analysis
    - d lavage

116. Serous fluid is normally:
    - a thin & pale yellow
    - b thin & yellowish white
    - c viscous & pale yellow
    - d viscous & yellowish white

Questions
Nonblood Specimens

117. Excess fluid accumulating in the peritoneal cavity is called a(n)
    a   diffusion
    b   effusion
    c   infusion
    d   transudate

118. Synovial fluid is found surrounding the:
    a   brain & spinal column
    b   heart
    c   joints
    d   lungs

119. Synovial fluid is normally:
    a   thin & pale yellow
    b   thin & yellowish white
    c   viscous & pale yellow
    d   viscous & yellowish white

120. An accumulation of synovial fluid may be associated with:
    a   immunoelectrophoresis
    b   immunofiltration
    c   incontinence
    d   inflammation

121. Which of the following procedures is used in the diagnosis of cystic fibrosis?
    a   dialysis
    b   diaphoresis
    c   hemapheresis
    d   iontophoresis

122. Which of the following levels is significantly and abnormally increased in the sweat of patients with cystic fibrosis?
    a   calcium
    b   chloride
    c   potassium
    d   sodium

123. The procedure used to collect amniotic fluid is called a(n):
    a   amniocentesis
    b   amniogenesis
    c   amniorrhea
    d   amniotome

Nonblood Specimens — Questions

124. Which of the following laboratory analyses is used to assess fetal development?

- a adrenocorticotropic hormone
- b α-fetoprotein
- c β-fetoprotein
- d bilirubin

125. Amniotic fluid should be transported to the laboratory:

- a at room temperature (22°C)
- b at 37°C
- c shielded from light
- d within 3 hours of collection

126. Which of the following analyses performed on amniotic fluid is a measure of fetal lung function?

- a α-fetoprotein
- b β-fetoprotein
- c bilirubin
- d L/S ratio

Explanations

Nonblood Specimens

The following items have been identified as appropriate for those preparing for the PBT examination.

1. **d** The urinary system maintains homeostasis and pH balance through the excretion of waste products of protein metabolism, and the regulation of water and electrolytes (calcium, chloride, magnesium phosphate, potassium, and sodium.
[McCall 7e, p137, 364]

2. **a** Electrolytes are chemical constituents in the blood that serve to maintain the body's acid-base balance.
[McCall 7e, p137, 364]

3. **b** The urinary system is normally composed of 2 kidneys, 2 ureters, 1 urinary bladder, and 1 urethra.
[McCall 7e, p137]

4. **b** Each kidney is composed of approximately a million nephrons, which are microscopic in size. Each nephron contains a filtration unit, called a glomerulus, which filters water, electrolytes, and waste products from the bloodstream.
[McCall 7e, p138]

5. **a** Each kidney is composed of approximately a million nephrons, which are microscopic in size. Each nephron contains a filtration unit, called a glomerulus, which filters water, electrolytes, and waste products from the bloodstream.
[McCall 7e, p138]

6. **b** Erythropoietin is a hormone that regulates red blood cell production. It is produced by the kidneys.
[McCall 7e, p137]

7. **b** Leukocytes or white blood cells (WBCs) function in fighting infection. The presence of leukocytes in the urine indicates infection.
[McCall 7e, p412]

8. **d** Ketones result when fat in the body is broken down for energy instead of carbohydrates. One condition that will produce ketones in the urine is starvation.
[McCall 7e, p415-416]

9. **b** The suffix *-ology* means "the study of." The word root *tox* means "poison." The literal meaning of *toxicology* is "the study of poison."
[McCall 7e, p357]

10. **b** Qualitative screening tests characteristically generate positive or negative results. Quantitative tests measure and report specific amounts of drugs present in a urine specimen.
[McCall 7e, p413-414]

11. **c** Qualitative screening tests characteristically generate positive or negative results. Quantitative tests measure and report specific amounts of drugs present in a urine specimen.
[McCall 7e, p413-414]

Nonblood Specimens   Explanations

12. **a**   Ethyl alcohol, ethanol, and EtOH are 3 different terms that describe the form of alcohol measured in an analysis for blood alcohol concentration (BAC).
[McCall 7e, p358]

13. **b**   Commonly referred to as "blood doping," the NCAA prohibits the use of substances that can expand oxygen carrying capacity, including erythropoietin.
[McCall 7e, p131]

14. **d**   Urine is the preferred specimen for drug testing because it can be easily collected using noninvasive methods. Additionally, drugs or metabolites commonly tested for in a drug screen may be recovered in the urine for days or weeks after ingestion.
[McCall 7e, p413]

15. **a**   Cannabinoids can be recovered in the urine for as long as a week following a single use.
[McCall 7e, p414]

16. **c**   Routine urinalysis can be performed on a random urine specimen for good quality results.
[McCall 7e, p408-410]

17. **d**   Requisitions for clinical laboratory tests originate with the patient's physician.
[McCall 7e, p215]

18. **d**   Routine urinalysis can be performed on a random urine specimen for good quality results.
[McCall 7e, p408-410]

19. **c**   The phlebotomist should always identify themselves and their department before collecting a specimen from a patient.
[McCall 7e, p221]

20. **a**   The phlebotomist should ask the patient to state their name prior to the collection procedure if capable of doing so.
[McCall 7e, p221]

21. **b**   A clean, dry collection container may be used to collect a urine specimen. The container must be free of chemicals, such as detergent, and sealed with a tightly fitting lid.
[McCall 7e, p409-410]

22. **c**   Urine specimens may be collected from babies using a plastic bag that may be placed over the urethral opening using a horseshoe shaped, hypoallergenic adhesive.
[McCall 7e, p408]

23. **b**   A clean, dry plastic container may be used to collect a urine specimen. The container must be free of chemicals, such as detergent, and sealed with a tightly fitting lid.
[McCall 7e, p409-410]

Explanations
Nonblood Specimens

24. **a** Midstream collection procedures address how to collect a urine specimen to minimize contamination by bacteria, genital secretions, and pubic hair. Patients should be instructed to begin to void into the toilet, interrupt the urine flow, position the collection container underneath the anticipated urine stream, resume voiding, and collect the remaining specimen.
[McCall 7e, p408]

25. **d** Urinalysis specimens must be delivered to the laboratory within 60 minutes of collection.
[McCall 7e, p410]

26. **c** Urinalysis specimens must be delivered to the laboratory within 60 minutes of collection.
[McCall 7e, p410]

27. **a** Labels for urinalysis specimens must always be affixed to the specimen container, never the lid. The lids will be removed prior to specimen analysis and if the label is affixed to the lid, the specimen will be unlabeled once the lid is removed.
[McCall 7e, p404]

28. **a** Standard precautions must be adhered to when transporting body fluids, including urine. The phlebotomist is required to wear gloves when transporting urine specimens.
[McCall 7e, p404]

29. **a** Labeling information on urinalysis specimens must include patient name, patient identification number, date & time of collection, phlebotomist initials supervising the collection, and "urine specimen."
[McCall 7e, p404]

30. **b** Urine specimens must be stored in the refrigerator (4°C) if they cannot be analyzed within 2 hours of collection.
[McCall 7e, p410, 411]

31. **d** Requisitions for clinical laboratory tests originate with the patient's physician.
[McCall 7e, p215]

32. **c** Normal urine is sterile. Therefore, collection procedures for urine culture and sensitivity must prevent specimen contamination. Midstream collection procedures address how to collect a urine specimen to minimize contamination by bacteria, genital secretions, and pubic hair. The additional step of providing a clean-catch urine ensures elimination of contaminants from the genital area.
[McCall 7e, p408]

33. **c** The phlebotomist should always identify themselves and their department before collecting a specimen from a patient.
[McCall 7e, p221]

34. **a** The phlebotomist should ask the patient to state their name prior to the collection procedure if capable of doing so.
[McCall 7e, p221]

Nonblood Specimens — Explanations

35. c Normal urine is sterile. Therefore, collection procedures for urine culture and sensitivity must prevent specimen contamination. Sterile containers are used to collect urine specimens for culture and sensitivity to prevent specimen contamination.
[McCall 7e, p212]

36. d The phlebotomist should provide the following explanation: Midstream clean-catch urine collection provides optimal specimens for culture and sensitivity because specimens collected in this way are free of contaminants.
[McCall 7e, p408]

37. d Normal urine is sterile. Therefore, collection procedures for urine culture and sensitivity must prevent specimen contamination. Sterile containers are used to collect urine specimens for culture and sensitivity to prevent specimen contamination.
[McCall 7e, p412]

38. d The first instruction every patient should receive prior to collecting a midstream clean-catch urine is to wash his/her hands thoroughly.
[McCall 7e, p409]

39. d Midstream collection procedures address how to collect a urine specimen to minimize contamination by bacteria, genital secretions, and pubic hair. The clean-catch procedure adds a skin cleansing step to ensure no specimen contamination. This is critically important when a specimen is analyzed for the presence of bacteria and other pathogens. The patient should be instructed to wash his hands and then, using the prepackaged cleansing agent provided, cleanse the tip of his penis in concentric circles beginning at the middle and moving outward.
[McCall 7e, p408-409]

40. d Midstream collection procedures address how to collect a urine specimen to minimize contamination by bacteria, genital secretions, and pubic hair. The clean-catch procedure adds a skin cleansing step to ensure no specimen contamination. This is critically important when a specimen is analyzed for the presence of bacteria and other pathogens. The patient should be instructed to wash his hands, retract the foreskin of his penis and then, using the prepackaged cleansing agent provided, cleanse the tip of his penis in concentric circles beginning at the middle and moving outward.
[McCall 7e, p408-409]

41. a It is likely the container was contaminated and the specimen compromised. The appropriate course of action is to recollect the specimen to ensure a good quality result.
[McCall 7e, p408-409]

42. a Urine specimens collected for culture and sensitivity should be refrigerated (4°C) immediately following collection if immediate processing is not possible.
[McCall 7e, p412]

Explanations

Nonblood Specimens

43. a Urine specimen labels must be affixed to the container, not the lid. The lids will be removed prior to specimen analysis and if the label is affixed to the lid, the specimen will be unlabeled once the lid is removed.
[McCall 7e, p404]

44. a Standard precautions must be adhered to when transporting body fluids, including urine. The phlebotomist is required to wear gloves when transporting urine specimens.
[McCall 7e, p404]

45. a Labeling information on urinalysis specimens must include patient name, patient identification number, date and time of collection, phlebotomist initials supervising the collection, and "urine C&S."
[McCall 7e, p404]

46. d At least 30 mL of urine is required to complete the analysis.
[McCall 7e, p412]

47. b Sometimes, based on specimen requirements, 24-hour urine specimens must be collected into a container containing a chemical additive. Additives should be allocated to the collection container before the collection container is issued to the patient. Additionally, the container label should include the name of the additive and safe handling instructions for the patient.
[McCall 7e, p406-407]

48. d A 24-hour urine collection procedure typically begins early in the morning, after the patient's first void of the day.
[McCall 7e, p407]

49. a The first instruction every patient should receive prior to collecting a 24-hour urine specimen is to wash his/her hands thoroughly before and after each void.
[McCall 7e, p407]

50. d Phlebotomists should provide verbal instructions to the patient for collecting a 24-hour urine specimen. Additionally, verbal instructions should be reinforced with written directions.
[McCall 7e, p405]

51. a Creatinine clearance is ordered to assess kidney function by comparing creatinine levels in the blood with creatinine levels in the urine. The procedure for creatinine clearance includes a 24-hour urine collection and a blood creatinine level collected at the midpoint of the 24-hour urine collection procedure.
[McCall 7e, p406]

52. c The phlebotomist should add any preservative required for a 24-hour urine collection to the container before issuing it to the patient. Additionally, the container label should include the name of the additive and safe handling instructions for the patient.
[McCall 7e, p407]

Nonblood Specimens — Explanations

53. **a** 5-hydroxyindoleacetic acid (HIAA) is a breakdown product of serotonin and may be measured using a 24-hour urine specimen. Patients scheduled for a 5-HIAA analysis must adhere to dietary restrictions for 4 days prior to the test. Patients should refrain from eating foods such as avocados, bananas, tomatoes, and walnuts.
[McCall 7e, p406]

54. **c** The normal range for 24-hour urine volume is 800-2,000 mL/day (with a normal fluid intake of about 2 L/day). Therefore, a 24-hour urine container must be large enough to hold a specimen of at least 2 L. Consequently, most 24-hour urine collection containers can hold a volume of at least 3 L.
[McCall 7e, p406-408]

55. **d** The patient voids the first urine specimen of the day into the toilet and notes the time to begin the 24-hour urine specimen collection. Every subsequent urine specimen, including the specimen voided at exactly the same time the following day, must be collected into the 24-hour urine collection container.
[McCall 7e, p407]

56. **a** The patient voids the first urine specimen of the day into the toilet and notes the time to begin the 24-hour urine specimen collection. Every subsequent urine specimen, including the specimen voided at exactly the same time the following day, must be collected into the 24-hour urine collection container.
[McCall 7e, p407]

57. **a** The patient voids the first urine specimen of the day into the toilet and notes the time to begin the 24-hour urine specimen collection. Every subsequent urine specimen, including the specimen voided at exactly the same time the following day, must be collected into the 24-hour urine collection container.
[McCall 7e, p406-407]

58. **c** Patients completing a 24-hour urine collection should drink normal amounts of fluid unless otherwise directed by their physician.
[McCall 7e, p407]

59. **a** A 24-hour urine specimen container (not the lid) should contain standard required labeling information, including patient first and last name, patient identification number, and the initials of the collector accepting the specimen. Additionally, the label must include start and end date and time of collection, specifying that the specimen is a 24-hour urine, and the analysis ordered by the patient's physician.
[McCall 7e, p407]

60. **a** A 24-hour urine specimen container (not the lid) should contain standard required labeling information, including patient first and last name, patient identification number, and the initials of the collector accepting the specimen. Additionally, the label must include start and end date and time of collection, specifying that the specimen is a 24-hour urine, and the analysis ordered by the patient's physician.
[McCall 7e, p407]

Explanations

Nonblood Specimens

61. **b**   A 24-hour urine specimen is typically stored at refrigerator temperatures (4°C).
[McCall 7e, p407-408]

62. **a**   Labels for 24-hour urine specimens must always be affixed to the specimen container, never the lid. The lids will be removed prior to specimen analysis and if the label is affixed to the lid, the specimen will be unlabeled once the lid is removed.
[McCall 7e, p404, 410]

63. **b**   Chain-of-custody protocols must be enacted and strictly adhered to when a specimen is submitted for forensic analysis.
[McCall 7e, p414]

64. **d**   Individuals asked to submit to a drug screen are required to sign a consent form in front of a witness.
[McCall 7e, p413-415]

65. **a**   Individuals asked to submit to a drug screen are required to present photo identification to confirm identity.
[McCall 7e, p413]

66. **c**   Individuals asked to submit to a drug screen are required to present photo identification, such as a passport, to confirm identity.
[McCall 7e, p415]

67. **d**   There are a variety of reasons an individual may present for drug screen, including pre-employment testing.
[McCall 7e, p413]

68. **c**   Phlebotomists cannot use any alcohol-based products to prepare a venipuncture site prior to collecting a sample for blood alcohol level. "Tincture" indicates a compound is dissolved in alcohol. Therefore, the only acceptable option is aqueous povidone iodine; "aqueous" indicates water is used as the solvent.
[McCall 7e, p358, 414-415]

69. **a**   Specimens should be collected in grey top sodium fluoride glass tubes. Plastic tubes are porous and gas exchange, including alcohol, can occur so glass tubes must be used for blood alcohol specimen collection. Typically, blood alcohol levels are drawn into glass, grey top sodium fluoride evacuated tubes. The additive required is determined by the procedure and equipment used to perform the analysis.
[McCall 7e, p388]

70. **b**   A markedly turbid urine specimen submitted for drug screen analysis suggests tampering. The phlebotomist specimen should not accept the specimen and follow the collection facility policies when specimen tampering is suspected.
[McCall 7e, p388, 391-392, 411]

Nonblood Specimens — Explanations

71. a The temperature of urine specimens provided for drug screen analysis must be measured within 4 minutes of collection or 0910.
[McCall 7e, p410-411]

72. b The temperature of urine specimens provided for drug screen analysis must be measured within 4 minutes of collection. The urine temperature must fall within the 90 - 100°F range to be acceptable.
[McCall 7e, p410-411]

73. d Urine specimens for drug screen analyses are sometimes divided or split for confirmatory testing.
[McCall 7e, p358]

74. d Since water is the compound most commonly used to adulterate specimens submitted for drug screen analysis, the addition of a coloring agent or "bluing" into the toilet and tank is routinely used to prevent this occurrence.
[McCall 7e, p413-414]

75. a The process maintaining accountability of a specimen from collection to disposition, including the identity of each person handling the specimen and its disposition is called chain of custody.
[Garza 10e, p628]

76. a The Department of Health and Human Services (HHS) established guidelines for drug screening for a variety of agencies, including the Department of Transportation (DOT). While most employers are not mandated to comply with the Drug-Free Workplace Act of 1988, many employers exercise their right to require drug screen as a condition of employment.
[McCall 7e, p414]

77. a The reference range for blood pH is 7.35-7.45 pH. Acidosis is the term used when a patient's blood pH is lower than 7.30.
[McCall 7e, p140]

78. b The following substances are electrolytes: bicarbonate, calcium, chloride, potassium, and sodium.
[McCall 7e, p137]

79. d Urine is produced by the urinary system as a waste product, eliminating the body of urea and functioning in water and electrolyte balance.
[McCall 7e, p137-138]

80. b The urine specimen voided first in the early morning is the most concentrated and has the highest specific gravity.
[McCall 7e, p405-406]

81. b Midstream collection procedures address how to collect a urine specimen to minimize contamination by bacteria, genital secretions and pubic hair. Patients should be instructed to begin to void into the toilet, interrupt the urine flow, position the collection container underneath the anticipated urine stream, resume voiding, and collect the remaining specimen.
[McCall 7e, p408]

Explanations
Nonblood Specimens

82. **c** A routine urinalysis typically includes 3 components: (a) a gross examination to identify the physical characteristics of the specimen (color and clarity, for example); (b) a chemical analysis typically performed using a reagent strip or "dipstick" manufactured with a series of reagent pads that measure analytes such as glucose and ketones; (c) a microscopic analysis to determine the presence of casts, cells and crystals.
[McCall 7e, p498]

83. **b** The word root *ur* means "urine." The suffix *-ia* means "condition of." The literal meaning of *proteinuria* is the condition of protein in the urine, which is an abnormal finding and indicates the possibility of kidney disease.
[Garza 10e, p167, 200]

84. **a** The clean-catch procedure adds a skin cleansing step to the midstream urine collection technique to prevent specimen contamination. This is critically important when a specimen is analyzed for the presence of bacteria and other pathogens. The patient should be instructed to wash their hands and then, using the prepackaged cleansing agent provided, cleanse the genital area as directed by the phlebotomist. The specific cleansing procedure varies by gender.
[McCall 7e, p408-409]

85. **b** A 24-hour urine collection procedure is employed to quantitatively measure a particular analyte in a patient's urine over a 24-hour time frame.
[McCall 7e, p406-408]

86. **b** Normal urine is sterile. Therefore, collection procedures for a urine culture and sensitivity must prevent specimen contamination. Midstream collection procedures address how to collect a urine specimen to minimize contamination by bacteria, genital secretions, and pubic hair. The clean-catch procedure adds a skin cleansing step to ensure no specimen contamination. This is critically important when a specimen is analyzed for the presence of bacteria and other pathogens. The patient should be instructed to wash his hands and then, using the prepackaged cleansing agent provided, cleanse the genital area as directed by the phlebotomist. The exact cleansing procedure varies by gender.
[McCall 7e, p409-410, 412]

87. **c** The National Institute on Drug Abuse (NIDA) defines patient preparation and collection procedures for specimens collected for drug screen analyses.
[McCall 7e, p414]

88. **c** Adulteration is the term used to describe tampering with a specimen submitted for a drug screen analysis.
[McCall 7e, p414]

89. **b** Illegal drugs such as heroin and cocaine are also termed illicit drugs.
[McCall 7e, p414]

90. **d** Benzodiazepine is a drug class that includes drugs such as valium, librium, and xanax.
[McCall 7e, p414]

Nonblood Specimens — Explanations

91. **b** Opiate is a drug class that includes drugs such as heroin, codeine, and morphine.
[McCall 7e, p414]

92. **d** Several organisms may cause enteric disease, including shigella, salmonella, and *Staphylococcus aureus*.
[McCall 7e, p425-426]

93. **d** A patient preparing to submit a specimen for fecal occult blood testing should be instructed to refrain from eating meat for at least 3 days prior to specimen collection. Meat by-products in a patient's stool may cause a false-positive result.
[McCall 7e, p426-427]

94. **c** The patient should be instructed to wash the outside of the specimen collection container and their hands following collection of a fecal specimen.
[McCall 7e, p426]

95. **d** The test used to screen for intestinal parasites is ova and parasites or O&P. Specimens collected for O&P analysis should be immediately transported and stored at body temperature (37°C) until analyzed.
[McCall 7e, p425-426]

96. **c** Another name for the fecal occult blood test (FOBT) is the guaiac smear test. FOBT detects the presence of blood in a patient's stool that is not in sufficient quantity to alter the obvious appearance of the stool. A positive FOBT may indicate gastrointestinal abnormalities or colorectal cancer and additional tests would be required to determine the source of the blood.
[McCall 7e, p427]

97. **a** Cerebrospinal fluid (CSF) is normally clear and colorless.
[McCall 7e, p420-421]

98. **c** Cerebrospinal fluid (CSF) is chemically similar to plasma.
[McCall 7e, p420]

99. **b** Cerebrospinal fluid (CSF) is collected by the patient's physician via lumbar puncture.
[McCall 7e, p420]

100. **d** Cerebrospinal fluid (CSF) is collected by the patient's physician via lumbar puncture.
[McCall 7e, p420]

101. **d** Cerebrospinal fluid (CSF) samples should be delivered and analyzed stat following collection.
[Garza 10e, 516]

102. **c** Cerebrospinal fluid (CSF) is ordered most frequently when meningitis is suspected. However, CSF may also be collected to assist in the diagnosis of multiple sclerosis, cancer of the central nervous system (CNS), and brain abscesses.
[McCall 7e, p420]

Explanations
Nonblood Specimens

103. d Seminal fluid is normally viscous and yellowish white.
[McCall 7e, p422]

104. c Men should be instructed to abstain from sexual activity for at least 3 days prior to the date of seminal fluid collection.
[McCall 7e, p422]

105. c The optimal collection container for a seminal fluid specimen is a sterile container from the options listed. A chemically clean container is also suitable to collect seminal fluid specimens.
[McCall 7e, p422]

106. d Seminal fluid specimens should be transported warm, ideally at body temperature (37°C).
[McCall 7e, p422]

107. d Seminal fluid specimens should be delivered to the laboratory for analysis within 2 hours (120 minutes) of collection.
[McCall 7e, p422]

108. c Seminal fluid analysis may be requisitioned to evaluate infertility, confirm the effectiveness of a vasectomy, or obtain evidence in a criminal sexual investigation.
[McCall 7e, p422]

109. a Acid-fast bacillus is the classification of organisms causing tuberculosis (TB). *Mycobacterium tuberculosis* is the specific acid-fast bacillus that causes TB.
[McCall 7e, p422]

110. a The best time to collect a sputum sample is in the morning because sputum specimens are more concentrated in the morning. Additionally, secretions accumulate overnight so a larger volume of specimen can usually be obtained in the morning.
[McCall 7e, p422-423]

111. b Patients should be instructed to rinse their mouth and gargle with water prior to sputum sample collection to minimize specimen contamination with mouth flora and saliva.
[McCall 7e, p422]

112. b The minimum volume of sputum sample required for a good quality result is 3-5 mL.
[McCall 7e, p422-423]

113. c Sputum is the body fluid generated from the lungs, bronchi, and trachea following a productive cough.
[McCall 7e, p422]

114. b Pleural fluid surrounds the lungs in the pleural cavity, providing lubrication as the lungs expand and contract. Pleural fluid is collected by the patient's physician via aspiration.
[McCall 7e, p422]

Nonblood Specimens — Explanations

115. a Peritoneal fluid surrounds the organs in the abdominal cavity. Peritoneal fluid is collected by the patient's physician via aspiration.
[McCall 7e, p422]

116. a Serous fluid is normally thin and pale yellow.
[McCall 7e, p422]

117. b Serous fluid is normally present in small amounts, but may increase in the presence of inflammation or infection. An abnormal accumulation of serous fluid is called an effusion.
[McCall 7e, p422]

118. c Synovial fluid surrounds the joints, providing lubrication as the joints move.
[McCall 7e, p423-424]

119. c Synovial fluid is normally clear yellow and viscous.
[McCall 7e, p423]

120. d Synovial fluid normally surrounds the joints in small amounts. The amount of synovial fluid may increase in the presence of inflammation.
[McCall 7e, p423-424]

121. d Iontophoresis is the procedure by which pilocarpine (a sweat-inducing medication) is transported into the skin using electrodes. The procedure is used to diagnose cystic fibrosis, a disease of the exocrine glands. Patients with cystic fibrosis have markedly elevated sweat chloride levels.
[McCall 7e, p423]

122. b Patients with cystic fibrosis have markedly elevated sweat chloride levels, often as high as 2-5× normal levels.
[McCall 7e, p423]

123. a The word suffix *-centesis* means "to puncture." Amniocentesis is the procedure by which a physician punctures the amniotic sac to withdraw amniotic fluid.
[McCall 7e, p419-420]

124. b α-fetoprotein (AFP) is present in developing human fetuses, amniotic fluid, and maternal serum. AFP levels may be used to screen for abnormalities in fetal development. Abnormal levels of AFP may indicate neural tube defects or Down syndrome.
[McCall 7e, p419-420]

125. c Amniotic fluid should be transported to the lab shielded from the light to preserve the levels of bilirubin.
[McCall 7e, p420]

126. d Amniotic fluid is analyzed for the presence of phospholipids, including lecithin. The ratio of lecithin to sphyngomyelin (L/S) is used to gauge fetal lung maturity. If the L/S ratio is less than 2, the fetus's lungs are likely immature.
[McCall 7e, p420]

Laboratory Operations

The following items have been identified as appropriate for those preparing for both PBT & QDP examinations.

1. Which of the following is a component of the 2010 National Patient Safety Goals (NPSG) by The Joint Commission (TJC)?
   a patient approach
   b patient identification
   c patient preparation
   d post-phlebotomy patient care

2. Materials and methods established to achieve intended outcomes and used during every specimen collection procedure constitute quality:
   a assurance
   b control
   c indicators
   d improvement

3. The quality of a patient's experience may be measured by evaluating the success of a medical intervention in improving the patient's condition, termed:
   a efficiency
   b efficacy
   c effectiveness
   d evaluation

4. The quality of a patient's experience as measured by the suitability of a medical intervention to address a patient's condition is:
   a adversary
   b advocacy
   c appropriateness
   d antagonism

5. The quality of a patient's experience as measured by the efficiency of addressing a patient's needs is:
   a caring function
   b concierge medicine
   c laboratory functions
   d nursing service

Laboratory Operations — Questions

6. Which of the following tasks is a quality control procedure?
   a actively engaging a patient in the identification process
   b maintaining good oral hygiene
   c tying long hair back
   d wearing a name badge

7. Which of the following tasks is a quality control procedure?
   a appropriately prioritizing specimen collection
   b maintaining good oral hygiene
   c tying long hair back
   d wearing a name badge

8. According to Clinical & Laboratory Standards Institute (CLSI), draw volumes of evacuated tubes must be within what range of the scheduled draw?
   a ±3%
   b ±5%
   c ±7%
   d ±10%

9. A phlebotomist is scheduled to collect 7 mL of specimen in an evacuated tube. According to Clinical & Laboratory Standards Institute (CLSI), what is the acceptable range of draw volume?
   a 6.8-7.2 mL
   b 6.7-7.4 mL
   c 6.5-7.5 mL
   d 6.3-7.7 mL

10. The scheduled volume of draw for evacuated tubes should be confirmed every:
    a day
    b month
    c new lot number
    d venipuncture

11. Manufacturing defects in needles are best screened for every:
    a day
    b month
    c new lot number
    d venipuncture attempt

12. Evacuated tubes manufactured at the same time are identified by:
    a expiration date
    b lot number
    c manufacturer identification number
    d Food & Drug confirmation number

Questions
Laboratory Operations

13. A phlebotomist selects a needle for a venipuncture procedure. She notices that the seal surrounding the needle is loosened. The phlebotomist should:
    a discard the needle
    b notify security
    c notify her supervisor
    d use the needle

14. Which of the following measures is most effective in assessing the function of a centrifuge?
    a relative centrifugal force
    b rotating radius
    c rotating tip radius
    d rotations per minute

15. Which of the following is used to calculate relative centrifugal force?
    a rotator angle
    b rotating radius
    c rotating tip radius
    d volume of evacuated tubes

16. A device used to measure RPMs (rotations per minute) on centrifuges is called a(n):
    a aneroid gauge
    b refractometer
    c sphygmomanometer
    d tachometer

17. When testing blood pressure cuffs for slow leaks, the mercury should not change by more than what rate to be acceptable?
    a 1 mm Hg/sec
    b 3 mm Hg/sec
    c 5 mm Hg/sec
    d 7 mm Hg/sec

18. Quality assurance indicators must be:
    a descriptive & specific
    b general & published
    c published & specific
    d specific & measurable

19. A facility has a blood culture contamination rate of 5%. This value indicates:
    a control has been completed
    b patient care is assured
    c patient care is not assured
    d staff training

Laboratory Operations   **Questions**

20. A facility has a blood culture contamination rate of 5%. What course of action does this result require?
    a   a corrective action plan must be created & implemented
    b   an incident report must be generated with the nursing service
    c   none because it is below the threshold value
    d   none because it is above the threshold value

21. During a staff meeting, a phlebotomy supervisor announces each phlebotomist must demonstrate competency in performing venipuncture. This is an example of:
    a   delta check
    b   progressive discipline
    c   quality assurance
    d   supervisor incompetence

22. A program designed to track outcomes through scheduled audits to continually improve the quality of patient care is:
    a   quality assurance
    b   quality control
    c   continuous quality improvement
    d   total quality management

23. Which of the following may be used to create continuous quality improvement program?
    a   flow charts
    b   manufacturer recommendations
    c   spot checks by supervisors
    d   surveillance cameras

24. The term used to denote specific procedures within a program designed to ensure quality patient care is:
    a   quality assurance
    b   quality control
    c   continuous quality improvement
    d   total quality management

25. The 3 components of a clinical laboratory workflow pathway are:
    a   competency, ethics, professionalism
    b   efficacy, ethics, regulations
    c   preexamination/preanalytical, examination, postexamination/postanalytical
    d   respect, service, support

26. Which of the following measures is used to evaluate quality indicators?
    a   critical (panic) values
    b   reference ranges
    c   stakeholder values
    d   threshold values

Questions   Laboratory Operations

27. The phlebotomist enters a patient's room and realizes that the patient is not there. The phlebotomist should:
   a contact the physician who ordered the test for the patient
   b contact the patient's designated healthcare provider (often a nurse)
   c immediately notify security
   d wait in the room for the patient to return

28. If a patient refuses to have his blood drawn, the phlebotomist should first:
   a ask the patient's designated healthcare provider (often a nurse) to try to enlist the patient's cooperation
   b politely leave the room
   c remind the patient his physician ordered the test
   d write "notify security" on the requisition

29. An adult male patient refuses to have their blood drawn. The phlebotomist reminds the patient the physician ordered the test and needs the results to provide proper care. The patient continues to refuse. The phlebotomist should:
   a notify the patient's designated healthcare provider (often a nurse), who may try to enlist the patient's cooperation
   b call security so the patient can be restrained
   c call a colleague to assist with restraining the patient
   d write "noncompliant" on the requisition and return the requisition to the lab

30. If a phlebotomist forcibly collects a blood specimen from a patient after the patient has refused the procedure, the phlebotomist can be charged with:
   a battery
   b malpractice
   c negligence
   d slander

31. A method of nonverbal communication commonly referred to as body language is:
   a kinesics
   b proxemics
   c sign language
   d unprofessional

32. A method of nonverbal communication involving a person's use and concept of space is:
   a body language
   b kinesics
   c proxemics
   d unprofessional

Laboratory Operations — Questions

33. Requisitions for laboratory testing originate with the:
    a. patient's designated healthcare provider (often a nurse)
    b. patient care associate
    c. physician
    d. respiratory therapist

34. What are the components of successful communication?
    a. emotions, volume adjustment, sender, receiver
    b. feedback, filters, cultural & generational differences
    c. sender, receiver, filters
    d. sender, receiver, filters, feedback

35. Barriers to communication include:
    a. cultural & generational differences, hearing impairment, emotions
    b. feedback, filters, cultural & generational differences
    c. sender, receiver, filters
    d. sender, receiver, filters, feedback

36. Telephone etiquette includes:
    a. allowing the phone to ring at least 6× before answering
    b. leaving the telephone line open while looking for the information requested
    c. saying "Hold, please" immediately after picking up the receiver
    d. using a positive tone of voice

37. When verbal and nonverbal messages do not match, it is called:
    a. empathy
    b. filter
    c. kinesic slip
    d. proxemic slip

38. An example of positive body language is:
    a. chewing gum
    b. smiling
    c. staring
    d. tapping foot

39. An example of negative body language is:
    a. erect posture
    b. maintaining eye contact
    c. sighing loudly
    d. smiling

Questions
Laboratory Operations

40. In addition to technical duties, the phlebotomist also is responsible for being the laboratory's:
    a QA officer
    b QC officer
    c public health representative
    d public relations representative

41. When working with pediatric patients, which of the following age-dependent characteristics should be considered? The patient's:
    a combativeness, restraint options, verbal ability
    b combativeness, comfort & safety
    c fears, comfort & safety
    d restraint options, safety, verbal ability

42. When working with pediatric patients, the phlebotomist may be required to consider the patient's:
    a combativeness, restraint options, verbal ability
    b communication level, safety concerns, parent behavior
    c communication level, parent behavior, restraint options
    d restraint options, safety, verbal ability

43. Communicating with a pediatric patient prior to blood collection often also involves communicating with the patient's:
    a parents
    b physicians
    c nurses
    d siblings

44. To reduce pediatric patient anxiety prior to a blood collection procedure, the phlebotomist should:
    a ask the parents to leave the room
    b involve the child's parents
    c promise the child the procedure will not hurt
    d use a papoose to immobilize the child

45. Keeping a child warm is particularly important for the comfort of:
    a neonates
    b toddlers
    c teens
    d adults

46. Children typically begin to demonstrate a fear of strangers between the ages of:
    a 0-6 months
    b 6-12 months
    c 6-12 years
    d 12 years

Laboratory Operations   **Questions**

47. Children typically begin to demonstrate the ability to understand and respond to simple commands between the ages of:
    a   0-6 months
    b   6-9 months
    c   1-3 years
    d   3-6 years

48. To communicate information about a procedure, a child may be allowed to touch and examine supplies. How old should a child be to implement this strategy?
    a   2 months
    b   4 months
    c   6 months
    d   12 months

49. Which of the following practices must be strictly adhered to when working with pediatric patients to ensure their safety?
    a   always attempt venipuncture first
    b   ask the parents to leave the room while performing the procedure
    c   use a wristband affixed to a crib handle for patient identification
    d   remove all supplies & discarded items from a child's bed

50. Which of the following practices must be strictly adhered to when working with pediatric patients to ensure their safety?
    a   always attempt venipuncture first
    b   ask the parents to leave the room while performing the procedure
    c   use a wristband affixed to a crib handle for patient identification
    d   return the safety rails to the up position

51. A phlebotomist may use role play to explain a blood collection procedure to a child beginning at age:
    a   3 months
    b   6 months
    c   3 years
    d   6 years

52. Children typically begin to express interest in the rationale for having blood drawn at age:
    a   1-3 years
    b   3-5 years
    c   6-12 years
    d   13-17 years

53. At what age do children begin to manifest hostility to mask fear?
    a   1-3 years
    b   3-5 years
    c   6-12 years
    d   13-17 years

Questions   **Laboratory Operations**

54. What patient population is projected to become the major focus of health care over the next 25 years?
    - a   geriatric
    - b   obstetric
    - c   pediatric
    - d   psychiatric

55. Geriatric patients may often experience:
    - a   amplified hearing, eyesight, taste & smell
    - b   loss of hearing, eyesight, taste & smell
    - c   thickened skin tissue & an accumulation of muscle mass
    - d   thickened skin tissue & well anchored veins

56. Which of the following conditions frequently found in geriatric patients may impair a patient's ability to straighten his/her arm in preparation for venipuncture?
    - a   arthritis
    - b   depression
    - c   hearing loss
    - d   memory loss

57. Federal legislation ensuring equal opportunities for Americans with disabilities and protecting their rights is:
    - a   Americans with Disabilities Act (ADA)
    - b   American Hospital Association (AHA)
    - c   American Nurses Association (ANA)
    - d   Older Americans Act (OAA)

58. A phlebotomist approaches an Hispanic female patient, age 50, to collect a blood specimen for a complete blood count (CBC). The sign above the patient's bed indicates that the patient is deaf. According to the Americans with Disabilities Act (ADA), what must the phlebotomist do before collecting the blood specimen?
    - a   explain the procedure in English
    - b   explain the procedure in Spanish
    - c   provide the patient with a written explanation of the procedure in English
    - d   provide the patient with a written explanation of the procedure in Spanish

Laboratory Operations — Questions

59. A phlebotomist approaches a male patient, age 90, to collect a blood specimen for an electrolyte panel. The sign above the patient's bed indicates that the patient is deaf. The phlebotomist gains the patient's attention and demonstrates she is there to collect a blood specimen by pointing to the patient's arm and holding up evacuated tubes. The patient nods his head and holds out his arm. What should the phlebotomist do next?
    a explain the procedure in English
    b proceed with the venipuncture procedure
    c provide the patient with a written explanation of the procedure in English
    d provide a sign language interpreter

60. A phlebotomist approaches a male patient, age 70, to collect a blood specimen for a cardiac enzyme panel. The sign above the patient's bed indicates that the patient is deaf. The patient requests a sign language interpreter. According to the Americans with Disabilities Act (ADA), what must the phlebotomist do before collecting the blood specimen?
    a explain the procedure in English
    b explain the procedure using motions directed at the antecubital area of her arm
    c provide the patient with a written explanation of the procedure in English
    d provide a sign language interpreter

61. A phlebotomist approaches an African American female patient, age 75, to collect a blood specimen for a complete blood count (CBC) and an electrolyte panel. The sign above the patient's bed indicates that the patient is blind and hearing impaired. According to the Americans with Disabilities Act (ADA), what must the phlebotomist do before collecting the blood specimen?
    a explain the procedure in English
    b explain the procedure in Spanish
    c provide the patient with a written explanation of the procedure in Braille
    d provide a sign language interpreter

62. What is the first rule of ethical behavior in health care, established by Hippocrates approximately in 400 BCE?
    a consistently wash your hands
    b do no harm
    c efficiency
    d proper patient identification

63. Which of the following documents are not legally binding?
    a American Society for Clinical Laboratory Science (ASCLS) Code of Ethics
    b Clinical Laboratory Improvement Amendments (CLIA) of 1988
    c Health Insurance Portability & Accountability Act (HIPAA)
    d OSHA's Bloodborne Pathogens standard

Questions

Laboratory Operations

64. A civil lawsuit based on improper treatment or negligence by a professional person is called:
    a   assault & battery
    b   malpractice
    c   negligence
    d   respondeat superior

65. Failure to exercise reasonable skill in performing a task is called:
    a   assault & battery
    b   malpractice
    c   negligence
    d   respondeat superior

66. The concept that is commonly referred to as "Let the master answer," whereby a laboratory corporation can be held responsible for a laboratory worker's negligent action is:
    a   assault & battery
    b   malpractice
    c   negligence
    d   respondeat superior

67. A person who is legally responsible for damages assigned in a legal action is:
    a   defendant
    b   liable
    c   felon
    d   tort

68. A legal term referring to a civil wrong requiring the person committing the wrong to be responsible for damages is:
    a   liability
    b   malpractice
    c   negligence
    d   tort

69. The sequence of events performed consistent with written policies and procedures is:
    a   res ipsa loquitor
    b   respondeat superior
    c   standard of care
    d   standard of proof

70. The internal process focused on minimizing injury or harm to patients and employees is:
    a   quality assurance
    b   quality control
    c   res ipsa loquitor
    d   risk management

71. A patient presents at an outpatient draw station and expresses her anxiety at having her blood drawn explaining that she "always faints" after the procedure. The phlebotomist offers reassurance stating, "That won't happen this time" and allows the patient to remain in the phlebotomy chair. After the procedure the patient faints and slides out of the chair and sustains a head injury while unconscious. The phlebotomist may be sued for:
   a   invasion of privacy
   b   nothing
   c   malpractice
   d   negligence

72. A patient presents at an outpatient draw station and expresses her anxiety at having her blood drawn explaining that she "always faints" after the procedure. The phlebotomist offers reassurance stating, "That won't happen this time" and allows the patient to remain in the phlebotomy chair. After the procedure the patient faints and slides out of the chair and sustains a head injury while unconscious.In addition to the phlebotomist, the health care facility may be sued because of:
   a   invasion of privacy
   b   nothing
   c   res ipsa loquitor
   d   respondeat superior

73. A phlebotomist inserts a needle into a patient's arm. A hematoma begins to form and the patient complains of pain. The phlebotomist elects to continue the procedure and complete the draw. If the patient sustains injury, what can the phlebotomist be charged with?
   a   invasion of privacy
   b   nothing
   c   malpractice
   d   negligence

74. The federal bill establishing regulations for clinical laboratories in the United States is the:
   a   Clinical Laboratory Improvement Amendments (CLIA) of 1988
   b   Clinical Laboratory Improvement Amendments (CLIA) of 1998
   c   Patient Bill of Rights
   d   Health Information Portability & Accountability Act

75. Which of the following agencies regulates and supervises clinical laboratories?
   a   Centers for Disease Control
   b   Food & Drug Administration
   c   Internal Revenue Service
   d   Social Security

Questions Laboratory Operations

76. Which federal agency is charged with regulating and overseeing clinical laboratories in the United States?
    a   Centers for Disease Control & Prevention (CDC)
    b   Centers for Medicare & Medicaid Services (CMS)
    c   Clinical Laboratory Improvement Amendments (CLIA) of 1998
    d   Clinical & Laboratory Standards Institute (CLSI)

77. The voluntary nongovernmental agency charged with establishing standards for the operation of hospitals and other health related facilities and services is:
    a   Centers for Disease Control & Prevention (CDC)
    b   College of American Pathologists (CAP)
    c   Occupational Safety & Health Administration (OSHA)
    d   The Joint Commission (TJC)

78. An agency which provides standards for quality improvement specific to clinical laboratories and conducts proficiency testing and laboratory inspections is the:
    a   Centers for Disease Control & Prevention (CDC)
    b   Centers for Medicare & Medicaid Services (CMS)
    c   College of American Pathologists (CAP)
    d   Clinical & Laboratory Standards Institute (CLSI)

79. Which of the following agencies has a reciprocal agreement with The Joint Commission (TJC) for the certification of clinical laboratories?
    a   Centers for Disease Control & Prevention (CDC)
    b   Centers for Medicare & Medicaid Services (CMS)
    c   College of American Pathologists (CAP)
    d   Clinical & Laboratory Standards Institute (CLSI)

80. The United States governmental agency responsible for regulating the safety and health of workers is:
    a   American Society for Clinical Pathology (ASCP)
    b   College of American Pathologists (CAP)
    c   Occupational Safety & Health Administration (OSHA)
    d   The Joint Commission (TJC)

81. Which of the following agencies developed a label designed to communicate specific dangers associated with hazardous chemicals?
    a   American Society for Clinical Pathology (ASCP)
    b   College of American Pathologists (CAP)
    c   National Fire Protection Agency (NFPA)
    d   The Joint Commission (TJC)

82. Labeling of hazardous materials is required by:
    a   OSHA's Bloodborne Pathogens standard
    b   OSHA's Hazardous Communication Standard
    c   Patient's Bill of Rights
    d   universal precautions

Laboratory Operations — Questions

83. Which of the following agencies mandated universal precautions?
    a   Centers for Disease Control & Prevention (CDC)
    b   College of American Pathologists (CAP)
    c   National Accrediting Agency for Clinical Laboratory Sciences (NAACLS)
    d   Occupational Safety & Health Administration (OSHA)

84. A consensus organization established to define global standards of practice for the clinical laboratory is:
    a   American Society for Clinical Pathology (ASCP)
    b   Clinical Laboratory Improvement Amendments of 1988 (CLIA)
    c   Clinical & Laboratory Standards Institute (CLSI)
    d   College of American Pathologists (CAP)

85. An agency which provides global procedural standards for clinical laboratory procedures is the:
    a   Centers for Disease Control & Prevention (CDC)
    b   Centers for Medicare & Medicaid Services (CMS)
    c   College of American Pathologists (CAP)
    d   Clinical & Laboratory Standards Institute (CLSI)

86. Which of the following agencies create standards of care in phlebotomy which may be used during legal proceedings?
    a   American Society for Clinical Pathology (ASCP)
    b   Clinical Laboratory Improvement Amendments of 1988 (CLIA)
    c   Clinical & Laboratory Standards Institute (CLSI)
    d   College of American Pathologists (CAP)

87. How many fundamental components are included in laboratory workflow processes and used to establish a quality management system, as defined by the Clinical & Laboratory Standards Institute (CLSI)?
    a   3
    b   6
    c   9
    d   12

88. What elements must be included in each Quality System Essential (QSE), as defined by the Clinical & Laboratory Standards Institute (CLSI)?
    a   personnel, purchasing & inventory, process control
    b   policies, processes, procedure documents
    c   purchasing & inventory, process control, occurrence management
    d   purchasing & inventory, process control, process improvement

89. The 2001 Needlestick Safety & Prevention Act requires:
    a   a written exposure control plan & employee input on selecting engineering controls
    b   a written exposure control plan & weekly fire drills
    c   weekly fire drills & green sharps containers
    d   weekly fire drills & purple sharps containers

Questions

Laboratory Operations

90. Which federal agency administrates the Centers for Disease Control & Prevention (CDC)?
    a Department of Defense
    b Department of Education
    c Department of Health & Human Services
    d Department of Homeland Security

91. The Centers for Disease Control & Prevention (CDC) are responsible for:
    a educating the American public & ensuring equal access to education
    b ensuring the safety of the American public
    c protecting the American public, through the use of military force
    d researching & controlling diseases

92. Which of the following agencies first recommended universal precautions?
    a College of American Pathologists (CAP)
    b Centers for Disease Control & Prevention (CDC)
    c National Accrediting Agency for Clinical Laboratory Sciences (NAACLS)
    d Occupational Safety & Health Administration (OSHA)

93. Which of the following agencies established recommendations for isolation procedures for hospitals and health care agencies?
    a Centers for Disease Control & Prevention (CDC)
    b Centers for Medicare & Medicaid Services (CMS)
    c College of American Pathologists (CAP)
    d Clinical & Laboratory Standards Institute (CLSI)

94. Which of the following committees provides advice and guidance to the Centers for Disease Control & Prevention regarding practices and procedures for infection control in health care settings?
    a Health Care Common Procedure Coding System
    b Healthcare Infection Control Practices Advisory Committee
    c Health Professions Network
    d National League of Nurses

95. Which of the following documents, established by The Joint Commission (TJC), recommends using at least 2 identifiers when identifying patients?
    a Occupational Safety & Health Act
    b Centers for Disease Control & Prevention universal precautions
    c Patient Care Partnership
    d National Patient Safety Goals & Recommendations

96. Blood may be collected from a patient without a standard hospital identification bracelet if the patient is in which of the following circumstances?
    a emergency department
    b operating room
    c pediatric department
    d recovery room

Laboratory Operations — Questions

97. Which of the following is ensured to the patient by the 2003 Patient Care Partnership?
    a adequate parking for visitors
    b adherence to proper patient identification procedures
    c medical records will remain confidential
    d prompt response to call lights

98. The Joint Commission (TJC) implemented changes in 2009 to increase focus on patient safety and continuous quality improvement of patient care through the use of 4 separate scoring categories. Which scoring category focuses on urgent risks to patient safety, such as a lack of adherence to quality control procedures?
    a Direct Impact Standards Requirements
    b Indirect Impact Standards Requirements
    c Situational Decision Rules
    d Immediate Threat to Health & Safety

99. The Joint Commission (TJC) implemented changes in 2009 to increase focus on patient safety and continuous quality improvement of patient care through the use of 4 separate scoring categories. Which scoring category focuses on risks to patient safety that may accumulate over time, such as a lack of professional development activities for staff?
    a Direct Impact Standards Requirements
    b Indirect Impact Standards Requirements
    c Situational Decision Rules
    d Immediate Threat to Health & Safety

100. The Joint Commission (TJC) implemented changes in 2009 to increase focus on patient safety and continuous quality improvement of patient care through the use of 4 separate scoring categories. Which scoring category focuses on risks to patient safety that may occur as a result of noncompliance of a facility with federal and state statutes?
    a Direct Impact Standards Requirements
    b Indirect Impact Standards Requirements
    c Situational Decision Rules
    d Immediate Threat to Health & Safety

101. The Joint Commission (TJC) implemented changes in 2009 to increase focus on patient safety and continuous quality improvement of patient care through the use of 4 separate scoring categories. Which scoring category focuses on direct and urgent risks to patient safety such as noncompliance with specimen labeling procedures?
    a Direct Impact Standards Requirements
    b Indirect Impact Standards Requirements
    c Situational Decision Rules
    d Immediate Threat to Health & Safety

Questions
Laboratory Operations

102. Substances that can be harmful to a person's health are called:
    a   bacteria
    b   biohazards
    c   body substance isolation
    d   universal precautions

103. Which of the following activities should NEVER occur in the laboratory?
    a   calibration
    b   eating
    c   pipetting
    d   quality control

104. Universal precautions prevents the spread of which of the following pathogens?
    a   acid-fast bacillus
    b   bloodborne
    c   respiratory
    d   tuberculosis

105. The term, "bloodborne pathogens" most commonly refers to:
    a   hepatitis A virus (HAV), hepatitis B virus (HBV) & hepatitis C virus (HCV)
    b   hepatitis A virus (HAV), hepatitis B virus (HBV) & *Plasmodium falciparum*
    c   hepatitis B virus (HBV), hepatitis C virus (HCV) & *Clostridioides difficile*
    d   hepatitis B virus (HBV), hepatitis C virus (HCV) & human immunodeficiency virus (HIV)

106. Under universal precautions, which patients are considered potentially infectious?
    a   all of them
    b   none of them
    c   patients infected with HBV
    d   patients infected with HIV

107. What term may be used instead of "universal protections"?
    a   airborne transmission precautions
    b   category-specific isolation
    c   standard precautions
    d   transmission-based precautions

108. Which of the following personal protective equipment (PPE) is required if a phlebotomist is about to enter the room of a patient in droplet precautions to collect a blood specimen?
    a   latex-free gloves
    b   mask
    c   needle shearing device
    d   N95 NIOSH certified fit-tested respirator

Laboratory Operations — Questions

109. Under standard precautions, when should a phlebotomist change gloves?
     a after every patient
     b after every second patient
     c after every third patient
     d only when soiled

110. Which of the following strategies is a healthy way to manage stress?
     a exercise regularly
     b having a few cocktails
     c keeping feelings to yourself
     d put off difficult tasks & duties as long as possible

111. Which of the following strategies is a healthy way to manage stress?
     a complete difficult tasks & duties first
     b having a few cocktails
     c make multiple life changes at one time
     d never share issues or feelings

112. Appropriately maintaining a centrifuge is an example of what kind of safety?
     a chemical
     b electrical
     c mechanical
     d radioactive

113. Which of the following fire extinguisher contents is appropriate to use on a Class A fire?
     a carbon dioxide
     b halon
     c metal X
     d pressurized water

114. What are the contents of a multipurpose (ABC) fire extinguisher?
     a carbon dioxide
     b dry chemical
     c halon
     d metal X

115. A patient remarks to a phlebotomist that she consistently develops a rash around her arm following tourniquet application and she cannot use "certain kinds of gloves" without developing a rash. The phlebotomist should:
     a call the Infection Control Department
     b complete an incident report
     c continue with the procedure
     d use latex-free products

Questions — Laboratory Operations

116. Needle safety features are mandated by:
    a   Centers for Disease Control & Prevention (CDC)
    b   Centers for Medicare & Medicaid Services (CMS)
    c   Needlestick Safety & Prevention Act (2001)
    d   OSHA's Bloodborne Pathogens Standard (1991)

117. Needle safety features must:
    a   be an accessory to the evacuated tube system
    b   be removable
    c   create a barrier between the needle and the patient's arm
    d   create a barrier between the needle and the phlebotomist's hands

118. Needle safety features must:
    a   be an accessory to the evacuated tube system
    b   be removable
    c   create a barrier between the needle and the patient's arm
    d   permanently contain a contaminated needle once a safety feature is activated

119. Which of the following practices must be eliminated to prevent needlestick injury?
    a   disposing needles in sharps containers
    b   handwashing
    c   recapping needles
    d   using transfer devices with syringes

120. To comply with safety standards when transferring blood from a syringe to an evacuated tube, the phlebotomist should:
    a   remove the stopper from the evacuated tube and eject blood into the tube using the syringe plunger
    b   use a syringe transfer device designed with an internal needle attached to the barrel
    c   use the syringe needle to pierce the evacuated tube stopper and allow the vacuum to withdraw blood from the syringe
    d   use the syringe needle to pierce the evacuated tube stopper and eject the blood into the evacuated tube using the plunger of the syringe

121. How many types of safety mechanisms are available to prevent accidental self-puncture with a contaminated winged infusion needle?
    a   0
    b   1
    c   2
    d   3

Laboratory Operations — Questions

122. To ensure maximum safety for both the phlebotomist and patient, what must the phlebotomist be sure to use?
    - a a tube holder by the same manufacturer as the needle
    - b an evacuated tube by the same manufacturer as the needle
    - c the largest needle gauge possible
    - d the smallest needle gauge possible

123. Lancet safety features must:
    - a be an accessory to the evacuated tube system
    - b be permanently retractable
    - c be reversibly retractable
    - d be used with a tube holder by the same manufacturer as the lancet

124. An evacuated tube shatters during centrifugation. What should the phlebotomist do first?
    - a call a code
    - b PASS
    - c RACE
    - d unplug the centrifuge

125. A phlebotomist is collecting blood from a patient. While the needle is in the patient's arm, the patient asks the phlebotomist to change the television channel. The phlebotomist should:
    - a immediately comply with the patient's request because it is good customer service
    - b immediately comply with the patient's request only if severe weather is threatening
    - c refuse to comply with the patient's request because it poses an electrical hazard
    - d refuse to comply with the patient's request because that is the nurse's job

126. A phlebotomist enters the laboratory to deliver patient specimens. She enters the processing area and finds a coworker on the ground with an electrical cord draped across her torso. The source of electricity cannot be accessed. The phlebotomist should immediately:
    - a activate the PASS sequence
    - b activate the RACE sequence
    - c use a forceps to remove the cord from touching her coworker
    - d use her hand inside a plastic beaker to remove the cord from touching her coworker

127. According to the National Fire Protection Agency (NFPA), which of the following fire classifications occur with ordinary combustibles?
    - a A
    - b B
    - c C
    - d D

Questions
Laboratory Operations

128. According to the National Fire Protection Agency (NFPA), which of the following fire classifications occur with flammable liquids?
    a A
    b B
    c C
    d D

129. According to the National Fire Protection Agency (NFPA), which of the following fire classifications occur with electrical equipment?
    a A
    b B
    c C
    d D

130. According to the National Fire Protection Agency (NFPA), which of the following fire classifications occur with combustible or reactive metals?
    a A
    b B
    c C
    d D

131. What is the National Fire Protection Agency (NFPA) code word for action a health care worker should take in the event of a fire?
    a EDTA
    b OSHA
    c PASS
    d RACE

132. What does the acronym RACE stand for in the event of a fire?
    a reenter, alarm, confine, extinguish
    b reenter, alert, confine, exhume
    c rescue, alarm, confine, extinguish
    d rescue, alert, confront, exhume

133. Which of the following acronyms communicates the appropriate procedure to follow when using a fire extinguisher?
    a EDTA
    b OSHA
    c PASS
    d RACE

134. What does the acronym PASS stand for in the event of a fire?
    a pull nozzle, aim pin, squeeze handle, sweep side-to-side
    b pull nozzle, aim pin, sweep side-to-side, squeeze handle
    c pull pin, aim nozzle, squeeze handle, sweep side-to-side
    d pull pin, aim nozzle, sweep side-to-side, squeeze handle

135. The symbol in the figure below communicates:

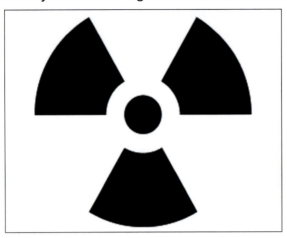

- a biohazard
- b flammability
- c mechanical hazard
- d radiation hazard

136. What are the 3 components of radiation safety?
- a alarm, confine, extinguish
- b PPE, engineering controls, education
- c stop, drop, roll
- d time, shielding, distance

137. The effects of radiation exposure:
- a are minimal
- b are immediately obvious
- c decrease over time
- d accumulate with every exposure

138. What equipment must a health care worker exposed to radiation on a regular basis wear to monitor radiation exposure?
- a dosimeter badge
- b National Institute for Occupational Safety & Health approved N75 fit-tested mask
- c National Institute for Occupational Safety & Health approved N95 fit-tested mask
- d self-contained breathing apparatus (SBCA)

139. Which of the following phlebotomists must exercise additional caution when entering areas displaying the radiation symbol? The phlebotomist who is:
- a anorexic
- b obese
- c pregnant
- d receiving chemotherapy

Questions — Laboratory Operations

140. What agency uses the label pictured in the figure below?

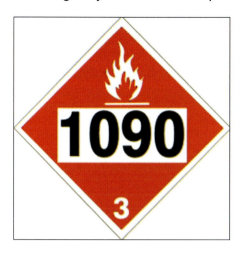

- a Centers for Disease Control & Prevention
- b Department of Transportation
- c National Fire Protection Agency
- d Occupational Safety & Health Administration

141. The symbol indicated by the arrow in the figure below is:

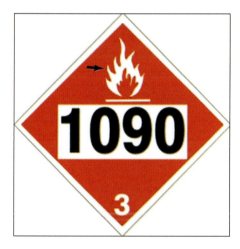

- a hazard class symbol
- b hazard identification
- c instability hazard
- d United Nations hazard number

142. The symbol indicated by the arrow in the figure below is:

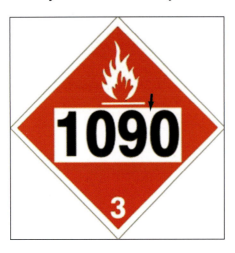

 a hazard class symbol
 b hazard identification
 c instability hazard
 d United Nations hazard number

143. The symbol indicated by the arrow in the below above is:

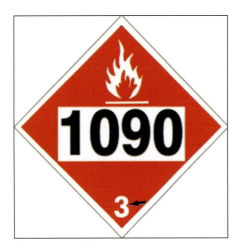

 a hazard class symbol
 b hazard identification
 c instability hazard
 d United Nations hazard number

Questions

Laboratory Operations

144. What agency uses the label pictured in the figure below?

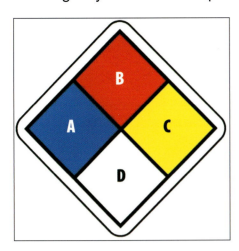

- a Centers for Disease Control & Prevention
- b Department of Transportation
- c National Fire Protection Agency
- d Occupational Safety & Health Administration

145. The diamond labeled "A" in the figure below is blue in color and communicates:

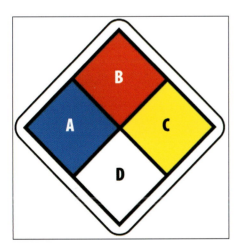

- a fire hazard
- b health hazard
- c instability hazard
- d specific hazard

146. The diamond labeled "B" in the figure below is red in color and communicates:

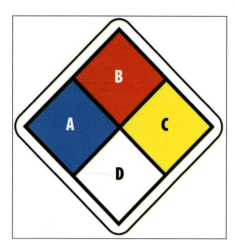

   a   fire hazard
   b   health hazard
   c   instability hazard
   d   specific hazard

147. The diamond labeled "C" in the figure below is yellow in color and communicates:

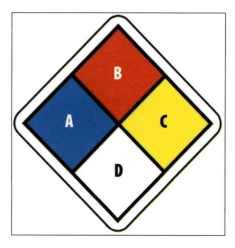

   a   fire hazard
   b   health hazard
   c   instability hazard
   d   specific hazard

Questions — **Laboratory Operations**

148. The diamond labeled "D" in the figure below is white in color and communicates:

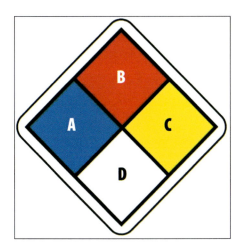

- a fire hazard
- b health hazard
- c instability hazard
- d special hazard

149. The zeros in the symbol in the figure below indicate that the chemical is:

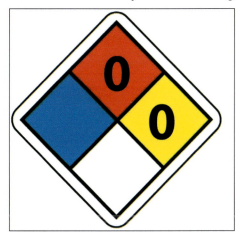

- a a serious health & stability hazard
- b a serious fire & instability hazard
- c inflammable & very stable
- d very flammable & highly unstable

150. Standards for chemical safety in the workplace are mandated by:
- a Centers for Disease Control & Prevention universal precautions
- b National Safety Goals & Recommendations
- c Occupational Safety & Health Administration Bloodborne Pathogens standard
- d Occupational Safety & Health Administration Hazard Communication Standard

151. The bill often referred to as the "Right to Know Law" regarding chemical safety in the workplace is:
    a   Centers for Disease Control & Prevention universal precautions
    b   National Safety Goals & Recommendations
    c   Occupational Safety & Health Administration Bloodborne Pathogens standard
    d   Occupational Safety & Health Administration Hazard Communication Standard

152. A form provided by chemical manufacturers containing general information, safe handling, and emergency information regarding a particular chemical is called a(n):
    a   incident report
    b   safety data sheet
    c   procedure manual
    d   warning label

153. What information must be included on a chemical label?
    a   expiration date, nature of the hazard, precautions for safe handling, first aid recommendations
    b   lot number, nature of the hazard, precautions for safe handling, first aid recommendations
    c   warning, nature of the hazard, precautions for safe handling, first aid recommendations
    d   warning, nature of the hazard, critical (panic) values, first aid recommendations

154. When diluting acids, what sequence should be employed?
    a   always add acid to water (or other diluent)
    b   always add water (or other diluent) to acid
    c   never add acid to water (or other diluent)
    d   never dilute acids

155. Chemical spill clean-up kits contain materials that:
    a   absorb & activate
    b   absorb & neutralize
    c   exude & activate
    d   exude & neutralize

156. Chemical disposal is regulated by:
    a   Centers for Disease Control & Protection
    b   Department of Transportation
    c   Environmental Protection Agency
    d   National Fire Protection Agency

Questions — Laboratory Operations

157. The instrument used to separate blood specimens into component parts is the:
    a   centrifuge
    b   pneumatic tube
    c   sedimentation rate tube rack
    d   sphygmomanometer

158. To ensure safe operation of a centrifuge, the phlebotomist must position evacuated tubes:
    a   according to stopper color
    b   of different size & volume across from each other
    c   of similar size & volume across from each other
    d   of similar size & volume next to each other

159. To ensure safe operation of a centrifuge, the phlebotomist should place specimens in the centrifuge:
    a   in order of stopper color, with sodium citrate tubes in car 1
    b   in order of stopper color, with the sodium fluoride tube in the last car
    c   with the stoppers intact
    d   with the stoppers removed

160. When using the pneumatic tube system, what should specimens be packed in prior to transport?
    a   aluminum foil
    b   dry ice
    c   ice slurry
    d   plastic liner

161. The symbol in the figure below communicates:

    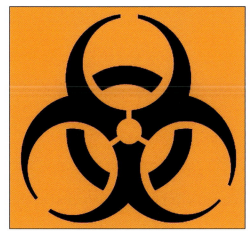

    a   biohazard
    b   flammability
    c   mechanical hazard
    d   radiation hazard

Laboratory Operations — Questions

162. An infection control program that includes monitoring specific patient population groups and classifications of infection is called:
    a surveillance
    b susceptibility
    c viability
    d virulence

163. Three components in the chain of infection are:
    a reservoir, mode of transmission, susceptible host
    b reservoir, mode of transmission, virulence
    c reservoir, viability, virulence
    d reservoir, viability, mode of transmission

164. To prevent the spread of infection, the chain of infection must be interrupted in at least how many points?
    a 1
    b 2
    c 3
    d 4

165. Microbes capable of causing infection or disease are called:
    a anaerobic
    b pasteurized
    c pathogens
    d normal flora

166. A disease resulting from the transmission of a pathogenic organism by direct or indirect contact or via airborne routes is called:
    a bloodborne
    b communicable
    c terminal
    d viable

167. What percentage of patients admitted to the hospital in the United States contract a nosocomial infection?
    a 1-3%
    b 3-5%
    c 5%-8.5%
    d 10-15%

168. The general term that applies to infections acquired in hospitals and other health care delivery facilities is:
    a bloodborne
    b chain of infection
    c transmission based
    d healthcare-associated infection (HAI)

Questions
Laboratory Operations

169. Which of the following is the most common nosocomial infection in the United States?
    a   acid-fast bacillus (AFB)
    b   bacteremia
    c   septicemia
    d   urinary tract infection (UTI)

170. A pathogen's ability to survive is:
    a   viability
    b   virulence
    c   vicarious
    d   villosity

171. A pathogen's ability to overcome the defense mechanisms of the host is its:
    a   viability
    b   vicarious
    c   villosity
    d   virulence

172. How many mechanisms may transfer an infection to a susceptible host?
    a   1
    b   3
    c   5
    d   7

173. The mode of infection transmission that requires close or intimate contact with an infected person is:
    a   airborne transmission
    b   direct contact
    c   indirect contact
    d   vector transmission

174. The mode of infection transmission that occurs when a person encounters contaminated items from a patient such as bed linens or silverware is:
    a   airborne transmission
    b   direct contact
    c   indirect contact
    d   vector transmission

175. Items that harbor pathogenic bacteria and are capable of transmitting infection are called:
    a   aerobic
    b   anaerobic
    c   fomites
    d   opportunists

176. The mode of infection transmission that occurs when a person inhales infectious droplets less than 5 μm is:
    a   airborne transmission
    b   droplet transmission
    c   vector transmission
    d   vehicle transmission

177. The mode of infection transmission that occurs when a person inhales infectious droplets greater than 5 μm in size is:
    a   airborne transmission
    b   droplet transmission
    c   vector transmission
    d   vehicle transmission

178. The mode of infection transmission involving transfer of an infectious disease by animal or insect is:
    a   airborne transmission
    b   droplet transmission
    c   vector transmission
    d   vehicle transmission

179. The mode of infection transmission involving transfer of an infectious disease by contaminated food, water, or drugs is:
    a   airborne transmission
    b   droplet transmission
    c   vector transmission
    d   vehicle transmission

180. Patients admitted to a hospital for treatment of a communicable disease are examples of what component of the chain of infection?
    a   means of transmission
    b   pathogen
    c   reservoir
    d   susceptible host

181. Patients admitted to a hospital free of infection are examples of what component of the chain of infection?
    a   means of transmission
    b   pathogen
    c   reservoir
    d   susceptible host

182. *Salmonella* organisms are examples of what component of the chain of infection?
    a   means of transmission
    b   pathogen
    c   reservoir
    d   susceptible host

Questions
Laboratory Operations

183. Which of the following is an example of a mode of transmission in the chain of infection?
    a *Salmonella*
    b *Shigella*
    c patient suffering from AIDS
    d venipuncture needle

184. Which of the following is an example of a susceptible host in the chain of infection?
    a airborne droplets
    b patient afflicted with AIDS
    c *Salmonella*
    d venipuncture needle

185. Human hands are examples of which component of the chain of infection?
    a mode of transmission
    b nosocomial infection
    c reservoir
    d susceptible host

186. Which of the following actions controls infection by safeguarding a susceptible host?
    a housekeeping, immunizations, isolation procedures
    b housekeeping, immunizations, waste disposal
    c housekeeping, laundry services, proper waste disposal
    d housekeeping, insect & rodent control, proper waste disposal

187. Which of the following actions controls infection by disrupting the mode of transmission?
    a housekeeping, immunizations, waste disposal
    b housekeeping, laundry services, proper waste disposal
    c housekeeping, insect & rodent control, proper waste disposal
    d insect & rodent control, isolation procedures, use of disposable equipment

188. Which of the following actions controls infection by protecting the patient?
    a immunizations, exercise, sound nutrition
    b immunizations, laundry services, proper waste disposal
    c insect & rodent control, proper waste disposal, sound nutrition
    d sound nutrition, isolation procedures, use of disposable equipment

189. A patient undergoing immunosuppressive therapy prior to transplant is an example of which component of the chain of infection?
    a mode of transmission
    b nosocomial infection
    c reservoir
    d susceptible host

Laboratory Operations — Questions

190. The Centers for Disease Control & Prevention recommend procedures to prevent the spread of infection due to exposure to blood, body fluids, nonintact skin, and mucous membranes called:
    a   reverse isolation
    b   social isolation
    c   standard precautions
    d   transmission-based precautions

191. The Centers for Disease Control & Prevention recommend a second level of procedures to prevent the spread of infection following exposure to patients with known or suspected infections or colonized with epidemiologically significant pathogens called:
    a   reverse isolation
    b   social isolation
    c   standard precautions
    d   transmission-based precautions

192. Under standard precautions, which patients are considered potentially infectious?
    a   all of them
    b   none of them
    c   patients infected with HBV
    d   patients infected with HIV

193. Items provided by an employer to protect the health care worker from contact with infectious materials are called:
    a   alcohol-based antiseptic hand cleaners
    b   bloodborne pathogens
    c   engineering controls
    d   personal protective equipment

194. A health care worker should use personal protective equipment whenever:
    a   a radioactive sign is posted outside a patient's room
    b   contact with patient blood or body fluids is expected
    c   leaving the laboratory
    d   leaving the lavatory

195. Which of the following PPE is required if splashing of blood or body fluids is likely?
    a   handwashing
    b   mask
    c   needle recapping
    d   respirators

Questions — Laboratory Operations

196. Which of the following PPE is required if infectious materials are likely to be spread by droplets generated by coughing or sneezing?
    a   handwashing
    b   mask
    c   needle recapping
    d   respirators

197. A phlebotomist should never:
    a   adjust the volume on a patient's television
    b   use an alcohol rinse solution as a substitute for handwashing
    c   use a foam solution as a substitute for handwashing
    d   recap a needle after use

198. Under standard precautions, a phlebotomist must wear gloves:
    a   only when a National Institute for Occupational Safety & Health approved N75 fit-tested mask is required
    b   only when a National Institute for Occupational Safety & Health approved N95 fit-tested mask is required
    c   when entering or leaving the laboratory
    d   when performing any blood collection procedure

199. Under transmission-based precautions, a phlebotomist must wear a gown:
    a   only when a National Institute for Occupational Safety & Health approved N75 fit-tested mask is required
    b   only when a National Institute for Occupational Safety & Health approved N95 fit-tested mask is required
    c   when a patient is in contact isolation
    d   when performing any blood collection procedure

200. The phlebotomist must wear gowns, gloves, and mask into a patient's transmission-precaution isolation room. What sequence should the phlebotomist use to don PPE?
    a   gloves, gown, mask
    b   gown, gloves, mask
    c   gown, mask, gloves
    d   mask, gown, gloves

201. When a phlebotomist dons a gown prior to entering a patient isolation room she must ensure that she touches the gown on the:
    a   inside surface only
    b   outside surface only
    c   sleeves only
    d   tabs & ties only

Laboratory Operations — Questions

202. When a phlebotomist chooses a gown prior to entering a patient isolation room he must ensure that the gown is large enough to cover:
    a   all of the phlebotomist's clothing
    b   from the phlebotomist's chest to her knees
    c   the phlebotomist's arms
    d   the phlebotomist's back

203. When a phlebotomist dons a gown prior to entering a patient isolation room she must ensure that the sleeves are pulled down to the:
    a   elbow
    b   fingertips
    c   forearm
    d   wrist

204. When a phlebotomist dons a gown prior to entering a patient isolation room he must ensure that the gown is securely fastened at the:
    a   neck
    b   neck & waist
    c   waist
    d   waist & wrist

205. A phlebotomist must wear a mask:
    a   only when a National Institute for Occupational Safety & Health approved N75 fit-tested mask is required
    b   only when a National Institute for Occupational Safety & Health approved N95 fit-tested mask is required
    c   when a patient requires droplet precautions
    d   when performing any blood collection procedure

206. A phlebotomist must wear a National Institute for Occupational Safety & Health approved N95 fit-tested mask when:
    a   a patient is in airborne precautions
    b   when a patient requires droplet precautions
    c   a National Institute for Occupational Safety & Health approved N95 fit-tested mask is unavailable
    d   when performing any blood collection procedure

207. Bacteria that mutate so they are no longer susceptible to antimicrobial therapy are called:
    a   antibiotic resistant
    b   immunosuppressants
    c   protease inhibitors
    d   psychiatric drugs

Questions
Laboratory Operations

208. When a phlebotomist dons a mask prior to entering a patient isolation room, he must tie the mask securely around the:
    a ears & nose
    b lower portion of the head & neck
    c middle portion of the head & neck
    d upper portion of the head & neck

209. A mask specifically fitted to each health care worker and designed to filter airborne particles is the:
    a dosimeter
    b National Institute for Occupational Safety & Health approved N75 fit-tested mask
    c National Institute for Occupational Safety & Health approved N95 fit-tested mask
    d self-contained breathing apparatus (SBCA)

210. Masks designed to filter at least 95% of airborne particles must be approved by:
    a Centers for Disease Control & Prevention
    b National Institute for Occupational Safety & Health
    c Occupational Safety & Health Administration
    d The Joint Commission (TJC)

211. National Institute for Occupational Safety & Health approved fit-tested masks are used with patients in transmission-based precautions after diagnosis of:
    a intestinal parasitic infection
    b *Salmonella* infection
    c *Shigella* infection
    d tuberculosis

212. When a phlebotomist dons gloves with a gown prior to entering an isolation room, the gloves should be:
    a pulled up over the sleeve of the gown
    b pulled up over the phlebotomist's wrist
    c rolled up & cuffed over the phlebotomist's wrist
    d tucked inside the sleeve of the gown

213. Before putting on gloves before entering the room of a patient requiring transmission-based precautions, the phlebotomist should:
    a pull the gown up to the elbows
    b remove jewelry
    c roll the gloves up, creating a cuff
    d tuck the gloves inside the sleeve of the gown

Laboratory Operations — Questions

214. A phlebotomist enters a patient's room. The patient's visitor is sneezing and coughing. The phlebotomist should:
    a immediately don a mask
    b notify the Infection Control Department
    c provide the visitor with a mask
    d instruct the visitor to cover his/her mouth & nose with a tissue

215. Under standard precautions, when should a phlebotomist change gloves?
    a after every patient
    b after every second patient
    c after every third patient
    d only when soiled

216. Under standard precautions, when should a phlebotomist sanitize his/her hands?
    a after every patient, once gloves are removed
    b between patients, without removing gloves
    c only if the gloves are soiled
    d whenever the phlebotomist wants to

217. Health care workers are required to adhere to standard precautions guidelines to avoid:
    a infection with nonpathogenic organisms
    b infection with pathogenic organisms
    c medication errors
    d patient identification errors

218. The procedure separating patients with communicable infections from other patients and limiting their contact with health care workers and visitors is called:
    a ischemia
    b isolation
    c nosocomial
    d virulence

219. A patient would be admitted to a hospital under transmission-based precautions if the patient is suspected of having an infection transmitted by:
    a airborne, contact, or droplet routes
    b airborne, contact, or vehicle routes
    c airborne, droplet, or vehicle routes
    d latex sensitivity

220. A patient would be admitted to a hospital under airborne precautions if suspected of having an infection transmitted by:
    a colonized microorganisms by directly contacting the patient
    b colonized microorganisms by contacting surfaces & patient care items
    c droplet particles less than 5 μm in diameter
    d droplet particles greater than 5 μm in diameter

Questions — Laboratory Operations

221. A patient would be admitted to a hospital under droplet precautions if suspected of having an infection transmitted by:
    a colonized microorganisms by directly contacting the patient
    b colonized microorganisms by contacting surfaces & patient care items
    c droplet particles less than 5 µm in diameter
    d droplet particles greater than 5 µm in diameter

222. A patient would be admitted to a hospital under contact precautions if suspected of having an infection transmitted by:
    a bloodborne pathogens
    b colonized microorganisms
    c droplet particles less than 5 µm in diameter
    d droplet particles greater than 5 µm in diameter

223. A patient would be admitted to a hospital under contact precautions if suspected of having an infection transmitted by equipment used in patient care such as stethoscopes or tourniquets due to:
    a bloodborne pathogens
    b colonized microorganisms
    c droplet particles less than 5 µm in diameter
    d droplet particles greater than 5 µm in diameter

224. A patient is diagnosed with *Neisseria meningitidis* infection. The patient would likely be placed in transmission-based precautions because the bacteria is transmitted via:
    a airborne route
    b contact route
    c droplet route
    d none; this condition requires reverse isolation

225. A patient is diagnosed with tuberculosis. The patient would be likely be placed in transmission-based precautions because the infection is transmitted via:
    a airborne route
    b contact route
    c droplet route
    d none; this condition requires reverse isolation

226. A patient is admitted to the hospital because of a serious decubitus infection. The patient would be likely be placed in transmission-based precautions because the infection may be transmitted via:
    a airborne route
    b contact route
    c droplet route
    d none; this condition requires reverse isolation

Laboratory Operations — Questions

227. A patient is admitted to a hospital infected with streptococcal pharyngitis (strep throat). The patient would be placed in transmission-based precautions because the infection is transmitted via:
    a   airborne route
    b   contact route
    c   droplet route
    d   none; this condition requires reverse isolation

228. A patient is admitted to the hospital with diarrhea and the physician suspects infection with *Clostridioides difficile*. The patient would be placed in transmission-based precautions because the infection is transmitted via:
    a   airborne route
    b   contact route
    c   droplet route
    d   none; this condition requires reverse isolation

229. A patient is admitted to the hospital because the physician suspects infection with *Bordetella pertussis* (whopping cough). The patient would be placed in transmission-based precautions because the infection is transmitted via:
    a   airborne route
    b   contact route
    c   droplet route
    d   none; this condition requires reverse isolation

230. A patient is admitted to the hospital because the physician suspects infection with measles (rubeola). The patient would be placed in transmission-based precautions because the infection is transmitted via:
    a   airborne route
    b   contact route
    c   droplet route
    d   none; this condition requires reverse isolation

231. A phlebotomist approaches a patient's room. How would the phlebotomist know the patient is in transmission based isolation?
    a   ask the physician who ordered the test(s)
    b   ask the patient's designated healthcare provider (often a nurse)
    c   consult the sign on the patient's door
    d   consult the Laboratory Procedure Manual

232. A phlebotomist approaches a patient's room. How would the phlebotomist know what personal protective equipment is required in addition to standard precautions?
    a   ask the physician who ordered the test(s)
    b   ask the patient's designated healthcare provider (often a nurse)
    c   consult the sign on the patient's door
    d   consult the Laboratory Procedure Manual

Questions

Laboratory Operations

233. Accidental needlestick with a contaminated needle causes what kind of exposure?
    a airborne
    b ingestion
    c percutaneous
    d permucosal

234. To prevent the spread of infection by ingestion in the clinical laboratory phlebotomists should never:
    a handle a stick of gum
    b open centrifuges before they have stopped spinning
    c pop off the stoppers of evacuated tubes
    d rub their eyes

235. To prevent the spread of infection by an airborne route in the clinical laboratory, phlebotomists should never:
    a handle a stick of gum
    b handle broken glass
    c open centrifuges before they have stopped spinning
    d rub their eyes

236. To prevent the spread of infection by a permucosal route in the clinical laboratory, phlebotomists should never:
    a handle a stick of gum
    b handle broken glass
    c open centrifuges before they have stopped spinning
    d rub their eyes

237. Which of the following would be classified as an engineering control, according to OSHA's Bloodborne Pathogens standard?
    a gloves
    b gown
    c handwashing
    d self-sheathing needle

238. Which of the following would be classified as a work practice control, according to OSHA's Bloodborne Pathogens standard?
    a handwashing policies
    b mandatory use of gown
    c self-sheathing needle
    d splash shields

Laboratory Operations — Questions

239. What personal protective equipment must a phlebotomist wear during specimen processing?
    a face shield
    b National Institute for Occupational Safety & Health approved N75 fit-tested mask
    c National Institute for Occupational Safety & Health approved N95 fit-tested mask
    d self-contained breathing apparatus (SBCA)

240. Under standard precautions, once a blood collection procedure is completed, the specimen labeled and waste discarded, the phlebotomist should remove his/her:
    a gloves
    b gown
    c N95 fit-tested mask
    d safety goggles

241. Under standard precautions, following a blood collection procedure, a phlebotomist should remove his/her gloves:
    a aerobically
    b anaerobically
    c anaphylactically
    d aseptically

242. If gloves are removed properly, the end result is:
    a 1 glove inside the other, with contaminated surfaces on the inside
    b 1 glove inside the other, with contaminated surfaces on the outside
    c 2 gloves discarded separately
    d 2 gloves discarded separately inside out

243. After a blood collection procedure is completed in a transmission based isolation room, the phlebotomist should remove personal protective equipment in the:
    a hallway
    b nurse's station
    c patient's bathroom
    d doorway of the patient's room

244. Under transmission-based precautions, once a blood collection procedure is completed, the specimen labeled and waste discarded, the phlebotomist should first remove his/her:
    a gloves
    b gown
    c mask
    d N95 fit-tested mask

Questions

Laboratory Operations

245. Under transmission-based precautions, following a blood collection procedure, a phlebotomist should remove his/her gloves:
    a aerobically
    b anaerobically
    c anaphylactically
    d aseptically

246. Under transmission-based precautions, once a blood collection procedure is completed and gloves removed, the phlebotomist should next remove his/her:
    a gloves
    b gown
    c mask
    d N95 fit-tested mask

247. Under transmission-based precautions, once a blood collection procedure is completed and gown is removed, the phlebotomist should next remove his/her:
    a gloves
    b gown
    c mask
    d N95 fit-tested mask

248. Under transmission-based precautions, a phlebotomist should remove his/her mask by touching only the:
    a front
    b inside
    c metal strip
    d strings

249. After a blood collection procedure is completed in a transmission based isolation room requiring the phlebotomist to use an National Institute for Occupational Safety & Health approved N95 fit-tested mask, the phlebotomist should remove the N95 fit-tested mask in the:
    a hallway after leaving the patient's room & closing the door
    b nurse's station
    c patient's bathroom
    d doorway of the patient's room

250. After a blood collection procedure is completed in a transmission based isolation room, the phlebotomist should transport the specimens to the laboratory:
    a following routine procedures
    b in a clean, plastic biohazard bag
    c in an ice slurry
    d stat

Laboratory Operations — Questions

251. The disease state resulting from the invasion of the body by a pathogenic microorganism is called:
     a infection
     b inflammation
     c inoculation
     d intrinsic

252. What procedure should be followed to dispose of trash and linens from an isolation room?
     a disinfection
     b double bagging
     c handwashing
     d reverse isolation

253. Chemical compounds used to remove or kill microorganisms on work surfaces or instruments are called:
     a aerosols
     b antiseptics
     c disinfectants
     d phloxine B

254. Chemicals that may be used on human skin to inhibit the growth and development of microorganisms, but not necessarily kill them, are:
     a aerosols
     b antiseptics
     c disinfectants
     d phenols

255. Which of the following is an antiseptic?
     a chloramine
     b formaldehyde
     c hypochlorite solution
     d 70% isopropyl alcohol

256. Which of the following compounds is a disinfectant?
     a 70% ethyl alcohol
     b 70% isopropyl alcohol
     c hypochlorite solution
     d tincture of iodine

257. One of the most powerful strategies to prevent the spread of infection is:
     a hand hygiene consistent with Centers for Disease Control & Prevention guidelines
     b National Institute for Occupational Safety & Health approved N95 fit-tested mask
     c requiring the use of a new gown with every patient
     d reverse isolation

Questions

Laboratory Operations

258. A phlebotomist encounters a blood spill on her hands. She should wash her hands immediately using:
   a   alcohol-based antiseptic
   b   iodine scrub
   c   soap & water
   d   tincture of green soap

259. Which agent should be used for hand hygiene, assuming the hands are not soiled with blood or body fluids?
   a   alcohol-based antiseptic
   b   iodine scrub
   c   povidone iodine
   d   tincture of green soap

260. A phlebotomist routinely uses an alcohol-based antiseptic to cleanse her hands after completing a blood collection procedure. According to the Occupational Safety & Health Administration (OSHA), the phlebotomist is required to wash her hands with soap and water after every:
   a   patient
   b   2 patients
   c   3 patients
   d   4 patients

261. Hand hygiene procedures must be completed:
   a   after returning to the laboratory following lunch break
   b   before & after every patient contact
   c   every 5 minutes
   d   every 10 minutes

262. According to the Centers for Disease Control & Prevention Guidelines for Hand Hygiene in Health Care Settings, natural fingernail length should not exceed:
   a   1/8 inch
   b   1/4 inch
   c   1/2 inch
   d   3/4 inch

263. According to the Centers for Disease Control & Prevention Guidelines for Hand Hygiene in Health Care Settings, personnel with patient contact should not use:
   a   alcohol-based antiseptic
   b   artificial nails or extenders
   c   iodine scrub
   d   tattoos

Laboratory Operations — Questions

264. A phlebotomist is preparing to leave the lab for a lunch break. She begins the hand washing procedure by wetting her hands and dispensing soap. Next she should:
    a allow the soap & water to soak on her hands for at least 20 seconds
    b allow the soap & water to soak on her hands for at least 45 seconds
    c rub her hands together vigorously for at least 20 seconds
    d rub her hands together vigorously for at least 45 seconds

265. During the rinse step of a hand wash procedure, the phlebotomist should hold her hands with the fingers pointing:
    a down
    b left
    c right
    d up

266. After the rinse step of a hand wash procedure, the phlebotomist should turn off the faucet using her:
    a glove
    b hand
    c elbow
    d paper towel

267. Health care services are often paid for by insurance companies or the federal government, called a:
    a first party payer
    b second party payer
    c third party payer
    d fourth party payer

268. The system used to provide terminology and a coding system to bill for physician office services is called:
    a current procedural terminology (CPT)
    b Health Insurance Portability & Accountability Act (HIPAA)
    c International Classification of Diseases, ninth revision, Clinical Modification (ICD9-CM)
    d International Classification of Diseases, 10th revision, Clinical Modification (ICD10-CM)

269. A system to reimburse for health care services designed to manage access, cost, and quality is called:
    a first party payer
    b second party payer
    c managed care
    d Medicare

Questions

Laboratory Operations

270. The system of reimbursement to health care facilities for services rendered based on entitlement due to employment and financed through social security is:
    a managed care
    b Medicaid
    c Medicare
    d self pay

271. The system of reimbursement to health care facilities for services rendered based on entitlement due to eligibility based in part on low income is:
    a managed care
    b Medicaid
    c Medicare
    d self pay

272. According to The Patient Care Partnership established by the American Hospital Association, what can patients expect during their hospital stay?
    a cable television
    b excellent food
    c internet access
    d protection of their privacy

273. Which law protects a patient's right to privacy?
    a Occupational Needlestick Safety & Prevention Act
    b Centers for Disease Control & Prevention Universal Precautions
    c American Hospital Association Patient Care Partnership
    d Health Insurance Portability & Accountability Act

274. A phlebotomist is assigned to the psychiatric floor. She receives a requisition for a drug screen panel on a patient, who is a member of her mother's bridge group. The phlebotomist tells her mother about the neighbor's hospitalization because she knew her mother would like to send some flowers. The phlebotomist may be charged with:
    a malpractice
    b negligence
    c nothing because this was a kind thing to do
    d respondeat superior

275. A patient's health information transmitted by electronic media or communicated or maintained in any other form or medium is:
    a current procedural terminology (CPT)
    b Health Insurance Portability & Accountability Act (HIPAA)
    c International Classification of Diseases, 10th revision, Clinical Modification (ICD10-CM)
    d protected health information

276. Health care workers must sign and comply with a confidentiality and nondisclosure statement, agreeing to:
    a   converse with patients in their native language
    b   maintain the confidentiality of all patient records
    c   use the least expensive equipment available to perform tasks & procedures
    d   use the most expensive equipment available to perform tasks & procedures

277. Health care workers must sign and comply with a confidentiality and nondisclosure statement, agreeing to:
    a   converse with patients in their native language
    b   maintain the security of computer login & password information
    c   use the least expensive equipment available to perform tasks & procedures
    d   use the most expensive equipment available to perform tasks & procedures

278. Health care workers must sign and comply with a confidentiality and nondisclosure statement, agreeing to:
    a   converse with patients in their native language
    b   maintain the security of individual patient data when using comprehensive data banks
    c   use the least expensive equipment available to perform tasks & procedures
    d   use the most expensive equipment available to perform tasks & procedures

279. Penalties for failure to adhere to the Health Information Portability & Accountability Act include:
    a   decreased vacation time
    b   fines
    c   forfeiture of annual raise
    d   promotion

280. Penalties for failure to adhere to the Health Information Portability & Accountability Act include:
    a   decreased vacation time
    b   forfeiture of annual raise
    c   incarceration
    d   promotion

Questions　　　Laboratory Operations

281. A legal claim that can be filed by a patient as the result of unauthorized release of personal information is:
    a assault
    b invasion of privacy
    c malpractice
    d respondeat superior

282. A factor causing emotional or mental strain or tension is called:
    a basal state
    b diurnal rhythm
    c rest
    d stress

283. A patient suffering from disease or injury to the central nervous system would most likely be cared for by the:
    a geriatric department
    b obstetrics department
    c orthopedic department
    d neurology department

284. A patient suffering from a mental or an emotional disorder would most likely be cared for by the:
    a neurology department
    b obstetrics department
    c pediatric department
    d psychiatry department

285. A patient experiencing complications related to pregnancy would most likely be cared for by the:
    a obstetrics department
    b odontology department
    c oncology department
    d orthopedics department

286. The field of medicine that specializes in the diagnosis and treatment of the elderly population is called:
    a geriatrics
    b oncology
    c proctology
    d rheumatology

287. The field of medicine that deals with the diagnosis and treatment of joint and tissue diseases is:
    a geriatrics
    b pediatrics
    c proctology
    d rheumatology

Laboratory Operations — **Questions**

288. The medical specialty that deals with the diagnosis and treatment of disorders of the eye is:
    a   obstetrics
    b   ophthalmology
    c   otolaryngology
    d   orthopedics

289. The field of medicine that deals with the diagnosis and treatment of diseases of the ear, nose, and throat is:
    a   obstetrics
    b   ophthalmology
    c   orthopedics
    d   otolaryngology

290. The department of medicine that specializes in the diagnosis and treatment of disorders associated with male sexual and reproductive systems and renal system for both sexes is:
    a   cardiology
    b   dermatology
    c   immunology
    d   urology

291. The medical department that specializes in the diagnosis and treatment of disorders associated with the esophagus, stomach, and intestines is:
    a   gastroenterology
    b   proctology
    c   nephrology
    d   rheumatology

292. The medical department that specializes in the treatment of disorders associated with hormone production is:
    a   endocrinology
    b   gastroenterology
    c   nephrology
    d   urology

293. The department that uses radioactive materials to treat disease processes is:
    a   medical imaging
    b   occupational therapy
    c   oncology
    d   radiotherapy

294. The department that assists patients in maintaining daily living skills, given the limitations of their physical or mental problems is:
    a   occupational therapy
    b   physical therapy
    c   psychiatric therapy
    d   radiation therapy

Questions   Laboratory Operations

295. The department that works with the patient to restore mental or physical abilities lost because of illness or accident is:
    a occupational therapy
    b physical therapy
    c psychiatric therapy
    d radiation therapy

296. A physician who specializes in the diagnosis of disease from laboratory test results, tissue evaluation, and postmortem examinations is a:
    a pathologist
    b proctologist
    c rheumatologist
    d urologist

297. A laboratory professional who enters the field after obtaining a bachelor's degree, including a year or more of study in clinical laboratory science is a:
    a medical laboratory assistant
    b medical laboratory scientist
    c medical laboratory technician
    d pathologist

298. A laboratory professional who enters the field after obtaining an associate's degree is a:
    a medical laboratory assistant
    b medical laboratory scientist
    c medical laboratory technician
    d pathologist

299. A laboratory professional trained in all aspects of blood specimen collection and transport is a:
    a medical laboratory scientist
    b medical laboratory technician
    c pathologist
    d phlebotomist

300. A clinical laboratory scientist with an advanced degree and several years experience responsible for overseeing all operations involving physician and patient services is a:
    a laboratory administrator
    b clinical laboratory scientist
    c phlebotomist
    d technical supervisor

Laboratory Operations — Explanations

The following items have been identified as appropriate for those preparing for both PBT & QDP examinations.

1. **b** The most critical step in providing quality patient care through laboratory testing is accurate patient identification as addressed in the 2010 National Patient Safety Goals (NPSG) by The Joint Commission (TJC).
[McCall 7e, p37]

2. **b** Quality control includes materials and methods established to achieve intended outcomes during every specimen collection procedure.
[Garza 10e, p635]

3. **b** Efficacy is 1 of 3 concepts (efficacy, appropriateness, and caring functions) that serve as the framework for quality assurance in heath care. Efficacy refers to the success of a medical intervention in improving a patient's condition.
[Garza 10e, p25]

4. **c** Appropriateness is 1 of 3 concepts (efficacy, appropriateness, and caring functions) that serve as the framework for quality assurance in heath care. Appropriateness refers to using the correct treatment for the patient's injury or disease.
[Garza 10e, p25]

5. **a** The caring function is 1 of 3 concepts (efficacy, appropriateness, and caring functions) that serve as the framework for quality assurance in heath care. The caring function refers to the quality of services provided to the patient and includes responsiveness, effectiveness, and understanding of a patient's needs.
[Garza 10e, p25]

6. **a** Quality control outlines the steps in a procedure all phlebotomists must follow, including a procedure for patient identification that requires at least 2 identifiers and active participation by the patient.
[Garza 10e, p25-35, 87]

7. **a** Quality control outlines the steps in a procedure all phlebotomists must follow, including a procedure for prioritizing specimen collection.
[Garza 10e, p28-29, 32-33, 35]

8. **d** According to Clinical & Laboratory Standards Institute (CLSI), draw volumes of evacuated tubes must be within ±10% of the scheduled draw. [CLSI GP39-A6, p6]

9. **d** According to Clinical & Laboratory Standards Institute (CLSI), draw volumes of evacuated tubes must be within 10% of the scheduled draw. 10% of 7 mL is 0.7 mL. Calculation: 7.0-0.7 mL = 6.3 mL and 7.0 + 0.7 mL = 7.7 mL. The acceptable range therefore is 6.3 mL - 7.7 mL. [CLSI GP39-A6, p6]

10. **c** The scheduled volume of draw for evacuated tubes should be confirmed each time a new lot number of evacuated tubes is opened for use.
[McCall 7e, p43]

Explanations **Laboratory Operations**

11. **d** Needles should be visually inspected for manufacturing defects such as burrs or barbs before every venipuncture.
[McCall 7e, p43]

12. **b** Evacuated tubes manufactured at the same time are assigned the same lot number. [CLSI GP39-A6, p6]

13. **a** Needle seals should be visually inspected before every venipuncture. If the seal is not intact, the needle should be discarded in a sharps container and another selected for use.
[McCall 7e, p43]

14. **a** Relative centrifugal force is the most effective measurement to assess centrifuge function because it includes the length of the rotating radius and the speed of rotations in the computation. [CLSI GP39-A6, p3-4]

15. **b** Relative centrifugal force is the most effective measurement to assess centrifuge function because it includes the length of the rotating radius (in centimeters) and the speed of rotations into the computation. [CLSI GP39-A6, p3-4]

16. **d** A device used to measure RPMs (rotations per minute) on centrifuges is called a tachometer.
[McCall 7e, p496]

17. **c** When testing blood pressure cuffs for slow leaks, the mercury should not change by more than 5 mm Hg/sec.
[McCall 7e, p150-151]

18. **d** To be effective, quality assurance indicators must be specific and measurable. For example, a quality assurance indicator for blood culture collection typically defines a threshold contamination rate at 3% or less.
[McCall 7e, p39-42]

19. **c** A quality assurance indicator for blood culture collection typically defines an acceptable contamination rate at 3% or less. A 5% contamination rate exceeds the 3% threshold so good quality patient care cannot be assured.
[McCall 7e, p39-42]

20. **a** A quality assurance indicator for blood culture collection typically defines a threshold for blood culture contamination rates at 3% or less. A 5% contamination rate exceeds the 3% threshold so good quality patient care cannot be assured. A corrective action plan must be created and implemented.
[McCall 7e, p39-42]

21. **c** One important method for achieving quality assurance is to periodically assess the skills and techniques of each phlebotomist to document competency in performing venipuncture regardless of length of experience or tenure at a facility.
[McCall 7e, p40-41]

Laboratory Operations — Explanations

22. **a** A program of tracking outcomes through scheduled audits to continually improve the quality of patient care is quality assurance. Quality control includes materials and methods established to achieve intended outcomes during every specimen collection procedure.
[McCall 7e, p44, 46]

23. **a** There are a number of mechanisms that may be used to create a continuous quality improvement program, including flow charts, bar graphs, scattergrams, and histograms.
[Garza 10e, p29-33]

24. **b** Quality control refers to specific procedures within a quality assurance program designed to ensure good quality patient care. An example of a quality control procedure is inspecting evacuated tubes for expiration dates before use.
[Garza 10e, p74, 76]

25. **c** To achieve standardization consistent with the International Standards Organization (ISO), the Clinical & Laboratory Standards Institute describes the laboratory work flow within the context of specimen examination processes, instead of phases. The laboratory workflow takes place in 3 processes:
1) preexamination/preanalytical process; 2) examination process; 3) postexamination/postanalytical process.
[Garza 10e, p9]

26. **d** Quality indicators generate a numerical value that is compared to the threshold value. If a quality indicator does not meet a threshold value quality patient care cannot be assured.
[McCall 7e, p40]

27. **b** The phlebotomist should first contact the patient's designated healthcare provider (often a nurse) to determine the patient's location. If the patient is temporarily unavailable, the phlebotomist may adjust the sequence of work and return for the patient before leaving for the next set of patient assignments. If the patient will not be available while the phlebotomist is on the floor, she should complete the appropriate documentation per institutional policy so the patient may be drawn after returning to the floor.
[Garza 10e, p311]

28. **c** If a patient refuses to have his blood drawn, the phlebotomist should first professionally and politely remind the patient that the blood test was ordered by the physician and the results will provide important information regarding the patient's care. If the patient continues to refuse, the phlebotomist must respect the patient's constitutional right to refuse, politely leave the patient, and complete the appropriate documentation per institutional policy. The cognizant adult patient must never be restrained or physically forced to comply.
[Garza 10e, p88, 92-93]

Explanations Laboratory Operations

29. **a** If the patient continues to refuse, the phlebotomist must respect the patient's constitutional right to refuse, politely leave the patient, and complete the appropriate documentation per institutional policy. The phlebotomist should immediately notify the patient's designated healthcare provider (often a nurse), who may also attempt to explain why the blood test is necessary. The cognizant adult patient must never be restrained or physically forced to comply.
[Garza 10e, p88, 92-93]

30. **a** The intentional touching of another person without consent is the legal definition of battery. If a patient refuses to have his blood drawn, the phlebotomist should first professionally and politely remind the patient that the blood test was ordered by the physician and the results will provide important information regarding the patient's care. The phlebotomist may immediately notify the patient's ask the patient's designated healthcare provider (often a nurse) who may also attempt to explain why the blood test is necessary. If the patient continues to refuse, the phlebotomist must respect the patient's constitutional right to refuse, politely leave the patient, and complete the appropriate documentation per institutional policy. The cognizant adult patient must never be restrained or physically forced to comply.
[Garza 10e, p88, 92-93]

31. **a** The use of nonverbal communication, including body language, is kinesics.
[McCall 7e, p11]

32. **c** A method of nonverbal communication involving a person's use and concept of space is proxemics.
[Garza 10e, p11-12]

33. **c** The preexamination/preanalytical process begins with generation of a requisition following a physician's order for a laboratory analysis.
[Garza 10e, p2, 67-68]

34. **d** Components of the communication loop include sender, receiver, filters, and feedback. Filters represent the variety of barriers that may interfere with a receiver successfully obtaining the message and includes cultural differences, generation gap, hearing impairment, and emotions.
[Garza 10e, p42]

35. **a** Successful communication requires a sender, a receiver, and feedback to confirm that the message was received. Filters represent the variety of barriers that may interfere with successful receipt of the message and include cultural differences, generation gap, hearing impairment, and emotions.
[Garza 10e, p42-43]

36. **d** Always begin a telephone conversation with a positive tone of voice. The phone should be answered as soon as possible and the response should be warm and friendly, including the name of the person to whom the caller is speaking. The line should never be left open because it could compromise confidentiality.
[Garza 10e, p53]

Laboratory Operations — Explanations

37. **c** When verbal and nonverbal messages do not match, it is called a kinesic slip. Since 80-90% of communication is nonverbal, people are more likely to respond to nonverbal cues rather than verbal communication.
[McCall 7e, p11]

38. **b** An example of positive body language is smiling.
[Garza 10e, p54-55]

39. **c** An example of negative body language is loudly sighing.
[Garza 10e, p55]

40. **d** Most patients have never seen the internal workings of a clinical laboratory or the professionals who work there. The only laboratory professional patients regularly encounter is the phlebotomist. Therefore, the phlebotomist serves as the patient's window to the laboratory and public relations is a key component of a phlebotomist's responsibilities.
[McCall 7e, p7]

41. **c** When working with the pediatric population, the phlebotomist must consider the developmental stage of the patient and take into consideration the child's fears, comfort, and safety.
[Garza 10e, p425-426]

42. **b** When a phlebotomist approaches a pediatric patient, the phlebotomist must assess the child's communication level, safety, fears, and comfort. Additionally, the phlebotomist may often interact with the parents as well as the child. Parents may prefer to assist with the blood collection process and serve as a comfort to the child during the procedure. However, some parents may prefer to leave the room during the blood collection procedure, which is also acceptable.
[Garza 10e, p425-428]

43. **a** When a phlebotomist approaches a pediatric patient, the phlebotomist must assess the child's communication level, safety, fears, and comfort. Additionally, the phlebotomist may often interact with the parents as well as the child. Parents may prefer to assist with the blood collection process and serve as a comfort to the child during the procedure. However, some parents may prefer to leave the room during the blood collection procedure, which is also acceptable.
[Garza 10e, p425-428]

44. **b** When a phlebotomist approaches a pediatric patient, the phlebotomist must assess the child's communication level, safety, fears, and comfort. Additionally, the phlebotomist may often interact with the parents as well as the child. Parents may prefer to assist with the blood collection process and serve as a comfort to the child during the procedure. However, some parents may prefer to leave the room during the blood collection procedure, which is also acceptable.
[Garza 10e, p425-428]

45. **a** Maintaining the temperature of a neonate is important so the phlebotomist must keep the baby warm during the blood collection procedure.
[Garza 10e, p425]

Explanations
Laboratory Operations

46. **b** Babies typically begin to demonstrate a fear of strangers between the ages of 6 and 12 months.
[Garza 10e, p425]

47. **c** Children are typically able to demonstrate the ability to understand and respond to simple commands between the ages of 1 and 3 years.
[Garza 10e, p426]

48. **d** Children are typically able to demonstrate the ability to understand and respond to simple commands between the ages of 1 and 3 years so a child should be at least 12 months old before being allowed to touch and examine supplies prior to a blood collection procedure.
[Garza 10e, p426]

49. **d** The phlebotomist must always be sure to return crib and bed rails to their upright position and remove all supplies and discarded items from a child's bed following a blood collection procedure to ensure the child's safety.
[Garza 10e, p425-426]

50. **d** The phlebotomist must always be sure to return crib and bed rails to their upright position and remove all supplies and discarded items from a child's bed following a blood collection procedure to ensure the child's safety.
[Garza 10e, p425-426]

51. **c** A phlebotomist may use role play to explain a blood collection procedure to a child beginning at age 3.
[Garza 10e, p426]

52. **c** Children typically begin to express interest in the rationale for having blood drawn between the ages of 6 and 12 years.
[Garza 10e, p426]

53. **d** Children typically begin to use hostility to mask fear between the ages of 13 and 17 years.
[Garza 10e, p426]

54. **a** The geriatric patient population is projected to become the major focus of health care over the next 25 years as a result of increased life expectancy and the rapidly increasing demographic of Americans age 65 and older.
[Garza 10e, p450]

55. **b** As people age, physical challenges develop including diminished sense of hearing, eyesight, taste, and smell.
[Garza 10e, p450-451]

Laboratory Operations   **Explanations**

56. **a** As people age, physical challenges may occur, including arthritis. If patients are suffering from arthritis, the mobility in their arms may be limited, preventing them from straightening an arm in preparation for venipuncture. If possible, the phlebotomist should use the other arm if it is less painful. Under no circumstances should the phlebotomist attempt to force a patient's arm into a straightened position.
[McCall 7e, p254-265]

57. **a** The Americans with Disabilities Act is federal legislation that prohibits discrimination against persons with disabilities.
[Garza 10e, p626]

58. **d** According to the Americans with Disabilities Act (ADA), the phlebotomist must effectively communicate information about the procedure before collecting the blood specimen. If the patient requests it, the phlebotomist must follow institutional protocol for providing a written explanation in their native language, where available.
[Garza 10e, p48-50, 54, 626]

59. **b** According to the Americans with Disabilities Act (ADA), the phlebotomist must effectively communicate information about the procedure before collecting the blood specimen. The phlebotomist effectively communicated what she was there to do and the patient gave consent when he extended his arm so she should proceed with the venipuncture procedure.
[Garza 10e, p54, 91-93, 626]

60. **d** According to the Americans with Disabilities Act (ADA), the phlebotomist must effectively communicate information about the procedure before collecting the blood specimen. If the patient requests it, the phlebotomist must provide a sign language interpreter, always following institutional protocol.
[Garza 10e, p48-50, 54, 626]

61. **c** According to the Americans with Disabilities Act (ADA), the phlebotomist must effectively communicate information about the procedure before collecting the blood specimen. In this case, the patient is both blind and hard of hearing. To be sure the patient understands the procedure, the phlebotomist may give the patient an explanation of the procedure written in Braille, always following institutional protocol.
[Garza 10e, p48-50, 54, 626]

62. **b** Hippocrates, the father of modern medicine, established the first rule of ethical behavior approximately in 400 BCE, "first do no harm." This tenet is the cornerstone of ethical behavior for health care workers.
[Garza 10e, p18]

63. **a** A code of ethics, such as the American Society for Clinical Laboratory Science (ASCLS) Code of Ethics, outlines behavior and conduct expected of clinical laboratory professionals but is usually not legally binding. The Clinical Laboratory Improvement Amendments (CLIA) of 1988, Health Insurance Portability & Accountability Act (HIPAA), and OSHA's Bloodborne Pathogens standard are all legally binding.
[ASCLS, p4; Garza 10e, p85-86, 628, 631, 633]

Explanations
Laboratory Operations

64. **b** Malpractice is the legal term for a civil lawsuit based on professional negligence or improper treatment by a professional person.
[Garza 10e, p89-90]

65. **c** Failure to exercise due care and reasonable skill in performing a task is negligence.
[Garza 10e, p87, 89]

66. **d** Respondeat superior is commonly referred to as "Let the master answer." By respondeat superior, a laboratory corporation can be held responsible for a laboratory worker's negligent action.
[Garza 10e, p89]

67. **b** A person who is legally responsible for damages assigned in a legal action is liable.
[Garza 10e, p89]

68. **d** Tort is the legal term referring to a civil wrong against a person or property. Tort law, which is not based on contracts, requires the person committing the wrong to be responsible for damages.
[Garza 10e, p89]

69. **c** The standard of care represents the sequence of events performed consistent with written policies and procedures. Adhering to the standard of care will prevent or minimize adverse effects or injury.
[Garza 10e, p91-92]

70. **d** Risk management is an internal process focused on minimizing injury or harm to patients and employees.
[McCall 7e, p49-51]

71. **d** In this instance, the phlebotomist may be sued for negligence. Three elements must be present to claim negligence: 1) a legal duty owed by one person to the other. In this case, the phlebotomist had a legal obligation to ensure the patient's safety; 2) failure to meet that duty. In this case, the phlebotomist did not address the patient's history of fainting by placing her on a reclining chair or a cot for the blood collection procedure; 3) harm sustained as a result. In this case, the patient sustained an head injury.
[Garza 10e, p87-90]

Laboratory Operations — Explanations

72. **d** In this instance, the phlebotomist may be sued for negligence. Additionally, the health care facility may be sued according to respondeat superior or "let the master answer," a legal doctrine that holds employers responsible for the actions of their employees. Three elements must be present to claim negligence: 1) a legal duty owed by 1 person to the other. In this case, the phlebotomist had a legal obligation to ensure the patient's safety; 2) failure to meet that duty. In this case, the phlebotomist did not address the patient's history of fainting by placing her on a reclining chair or a cot for the blood collection procedure; 3) harm sustained as a result. In this case, the patient sustained an head injury.
[Garza 10e, p87-90]

73. **d** In this instance, the phlebotomist may be sued for negligence. Three elements must be present to claim negligence: 1) a legal duty owed by one person to the other. In this case, the phlebotomist had a legal obligation to the patient; 2) failure to meet that duty. In this case, the phlebotomist did not stop the procedure when hematoma began to develop which is inconsistent with standard procedure; 3) harm sustained as a result. In this case, the patient would need to sustain an injury directly as a result of the venipuncture for a claim of negligence.
[Garza 10e, p87-90, 299]

74. **a** The Clinical Laboratory Improvement Amendments (CLIA) of 1988 is a federal bill establishing regulations for clinical laboratories in the United States.
[Garza 10e, p100, 628]

75. **b** The Food & Drug Administration is a federal agency responsible for overseeing clinical laboratories.
[Garza 10e, p99]

76. **b** The Centers for Medicare & Medicaid Services (CMS) is the federal agency charged with regulating and overseeing clinical laboratories in the United States.
[Garza 10e, p99]

77. **d** The Joint Commission (TJC) is a voluntary, nongovernmental agency charged with establishing standards of operation for hospitals and other health-related facilities and services.
[McCall 7e, p36-37]

78. **c** The College of American Pathologists (CAP) is an agency which provides standards for quality improvement specific to clinical laboratories and conducts proficiency testing and laboratory inspections.
[McCall 7e, p38-39]

79. **c** The College of American Pathologists (CAP) has a reciprocal agreement with The Joint Commission (TJC) and provides standards for quality improvement specific to clinical laboratories and conducts proficiency testing and laboratory inspections.
[McCall 7e, p38-39]

Explanations Laboratory Operations

80. **c** The Occupational Safety & Health Administration (OSHA) is the United States governmental agency responsible for regulating the safety and health of workers.
[Garza 10e, p99, 633]

81. **c** The National Fire Protection Agency (NFPA) developed a diamond shaped, color-coded label designed to communicate specific dangers associated with hazardous chemicals.
[Garza 10e, p150, 152]

82. **b** OSHA's Hazardous Communication Standard (commonly referred to as HazMat or the Right to Know Law) protects employees by requiring documentation, including labels and Safety Data Sheets (SDS), on all hazardous materials.
[Garza 10e, p150-151]

83. **d** Universal precautions are mandated by the Occupational Safety & Health Administration (OSHA) Bloodborne Pathogens standard, which was amended in 2001 to comply with OSHA's Needlestick Safety & Prevention Act. These standards are mandated by federal law to minimize the risk of occupational exposure to bloodborne pathogens.
[Garza 10e, p109-110]

84. **c** The Clinical & Laboratory Standards Institute (CLSI) is a consensus organization established to define global standards of practice for the clinical laboratory.
[CLSI GP41 7e, p2; Garza 10e, p25, 628]

85. **d** The Clinical & Laboratory Standards Institute (CLSI) is a consensus organization established to define global standards of practice for the clinical laboratory.
[CLSI GP41 7e, p2; Garza 10e, p25, 628]

86. **c** The Clinical & Laboratory Standards Institute (CLSI) is a consensus organization established to define global standards of practice for the clinical laboratory. The standards published by CLSI may be used as the standard of care in legal proceedings.
[McCall 7e, p39]

87. **a** There are 3 fundamental components included in laboratory workflow processes used to establish a quality management system, as defined by the Clinical & Laboratory Standards Institute (CLSI): preexamination/preanalytical process, examination process, and postexamination/postanalytical process.
[Garza 10e, p9]

88. **b** Policies, processes, and procedure documents must be included in each Quality System Essential (QSE), as defined by the Clinical & Laboratory Standards Institute (CLSI).
[Garza 10e, p28-30]

Laboratory Operations — Explanations

89. **a** The 2001 Needlestick Safety & Prevention Act requires revision to OSHA Bloodborne Pathogens standard in 4 areas, including a written exposure control plan, employee input on selecting engineering controls, revision of definitions related to engineering and work practice controls, and new recordkeeping standards.
[McCall 7e, p84]

90. **c** The Department of Health & Human Services administrates the Centers for Disease Control & Prevention.
[Garza 10e, p8, 99, 107, 628, 629]

91. **d** The Centers for Disease Control & Prevention (CDC) are responsible for researching and controlling diseases.
[Garza 10e, p107]

92. **b** Universal precautions were first recommended by the Centers for Disease Control & Prevention (CDC) in 1985 and later mandated by the Occupational Safety & Health Administration (OSHA) Bloodborne Pathogens standard, which was amended in 2001 to comply with OSHA's Needlestick Safety & Prevention Act. These standards are mandated by federal law to minimize the risk of occupational exposure to bloodborne pathogens.
[Garza 10e, p109-112]

93. **a** The Centers for Disease Control & Prevention (CDC) recommends isolation procedures for hospitals and health care agencies.
[Garza 10e, p119]

94. **b** Healthcare Infection Control Practices Advisory Committee provides advice and guidance to the Centers for Disease Control & Prevention regarding practices and procedures for infection control in health care settings.
[Garza 10e, p117-122]

95. **d** The Joint Commission (TJC) recommends using at least 2 identifiers when identifying patients, and incorporated accurate patient identification into the 2021 National Patient Safety Goals.
[Garza 10e, p324]

96. **a** The emergency department of the hospital is the area of patient care at highest risk for patient identification errors. Within the context of the commotion often associated with treating trauma patients, sometimes blood specimens must be collected before a patient can be absolutely identified making this area of the hospital at highest risk for patient identification errors. Some facilities may use the type and crossmatch system temporarily until a permanent wristband can be issued.
[McCall 7e, p223-224]

97. **c** The American Hospital Patient Care Partnership 2003 ensures that medical records will remain confidential.
[Garza 10e, p86]

Explanations — Laboratory Operations

98. **a** The Joint Commission (TJC) implemented changes in 2009 to increase focus on patient safety and continuous quality improvement of patient care through the use of 4 separate scoring categories, including Direct Impact Standards Requirement, Indirect Impact Standards Requirement, Situational Decision Rules, and Immediate Threat to Health & Safety. Lack of adherence to quality control procedures would be scored in the Direct Impact Standards Requirement category.
[McCall 7e, p36-37]

99. **b** The Joint Commission (TJC) implemented changes in 2009 to increase focus on patient safety and continuous quality improvement of patient care through the use of 4 separate scoring categories, including Direct Impact Standards Requirement, Indirect Impact Standards Requirement, Situational Decision Rules, and Immediate Threat to Health & Safety. Lack of professional development activities for staff would be scored in the Indirect Impact Standards Requirement category.
[McCall 7e, p36-37]

100. **c** The Joint Commission (TJC) implemented changes in 2009 to increase focus on patient safety and continuous quality improvement of patient care through the use of 4 separate scoring categories, including Direct Impact Standards Requirement, Indirect Impact Standards Requirement, Situational Decision Rules, and Immediate Threat to Health & Safety. Lack of adherence to federal and state statutes would be scored in the Situational Decision Rules category.
[McCall 7e, p36-37]

101. **d** The Joint Commission (TJC) implemented changes in 2009 to increase focus on patient safety and continuous quality improvement of patient care through the use of 4 separate scoring categories, including Direct Impact Standards Requirement, Indirect Impact Standards Requirement, Situational Decision Rules, and Immediate Threat to Health & Safety. Noncompliance with specimen labeling procedures would be scored in the Immediate Threat to Health & Safety category.
[McCall 7e, p36-37]

102. **b** Any substance that can be harmful to a person's health is called a biohazard. Biohazards are routinely encountered in the health care setting and health care workers must adhere to safety and infection control standards to work safely in that environment.
[McCall 7e, p80-82]

103. **b** A laboratory worker can be exposed to biohazards through ingestion. Eating, chewing gum, applying makeup, including lip balm, biting one's nails or putting pens or pencils in one's mouth can lead to ingestion of biohazards, and is prohibited in the clinical laboratory.
[Garza 10e, p136]

Laboratory Operations — Explanations

104. b Universal precautions were implemented to prevent the spread of bloodborne pathogens. Universal precautions were first recommended by the Centers for Disease Control & Prevention in 1985, mandated by OSHA's Bloodborne Pathogens standard in 1992 and revised and amended to include the Needlestick Safety & Prevention Act in 2001.
[Garza 10e, p109-112, 637; OSHA 2014b, p1]

105. d The term "bloodborne pathogens" refers to any pathogens that may be spread through contact with blood and most commonly refers to hepatitis B virus (HBV), hepatitis C virus (HCV) and human immunodeficiency virus (HIV).
[Garza 10e, p109, 367; OSHA 2011, p1]

106. a Under universal precautions, all patients must be treated as though they are potentially infectious.
[Garza 10e, p109, 117-118; OSHA 2011, p1]

107. c Universal precautions and standard precautions are often used interchangeably. Universal precautions recognize that blood from any patient is potentially infectious. Body substance isolation expanded universal precautions to include any body fluid as potentially infectious. The Centers for Disease Control & Prevention (CDC) and the Healthcare Infection Control Practices Advisory Committee (HICPAC) jointly recommended standard precautions when dealing with all patients, which recognizes all blood and body fluids (except sweat) as potentially infectious. Standard precautions combine infection control practices for universal precautions and body substance isolation.
[Garza 10e, p109, 637]

108. b Masks are required to protect the nose and mouth if a phlebotomist is about to enter the room of a patient requiring droplet precautions.
[Garza 10e, p119-120]

109. a Under standard precautions, gloves should be changed after every patient contact.
[Garza 10e, p118]

110. a Regular exercise is one effective strategy in managing stress.
[McCall 7e, p99-100]

111. a Procrastination can lead to increased levels of stress, so scheduling time to complete difficult or challenging tasks first is an effective strategy in managing stress.
[McCall 7e, p99-100]

112. c Appropriately maintaining a centrifuge is an example of mechanical safety.
[Garza 10e, p148]

Explanations Laboratory Operations

113. **d** Class A fire extinguishers may contain pressurized water to extinguish the fire. Fire extinguishers are manufactured based on fire classifications. Using an incorrect extinguisher on a fire is dangerous so many facilities routinely provide multipurpose (ABC) fire extinguishers containing dry chemical to use on Class A (ordinary combustibles such as paper and wood), Class B (flammable liquids such as gasoline and grease), and Class C fires (electrical).
[Garza 10e, p144]

114. **b** Fire extinguishers are manufactured to correspond to fire classifications. Using an incorrect extinguisher on a fire is dangerous so many facilities routinely provide multipurpose (ABC) fire extinguishers containing dry chemical to use on Class A (ordinary combustibles such as paper and wood), Class B (flammable liquids such as gasoline and grease), and Class C fires (electrical).
[Garza 10e, p144]

115. **d** One indication of latex allergy is skin sensitivity such as a rash subsequent to tourniquet application and the use of latex gloves. The phlebotomist should suspect a latex allergy and use latex-free products to complete the blood collection procedure.
[Garza 10e, p154-155, 311]

116. **c** Needle safety features are mandated by Needlestick Safety & Prevention Act (2001), a modification mandated by Congress to OSHA's Bloodborne Pathogens standard. The Needlestick Safety & Prevention Act (2001) mandates the use of needlestick protection devices and labels to communicate biohazard in storage, disposal, and transport containers. Updates to exposure control plans, selection of engineering controls, and recordkeeping procedures are also addressed.
[Garza 10e, p109; OSHA 2014a, p1]

117. **d** An example of an engineering control is a needlestick protection device that creates a barrier between the needle and the phlebotomist's hands. Needle safety features are mandated by Needlestick Safety & Prevention Act (2001), a modification mandated by Congress to OSHA's Bloodborne Pathogens standard. The Needlestick Safety & Prevention Act (2001) requires the use of engineering controls to eliminate or minimize employee exposure to bloodborne pathogens through accidental needlestick.
[McCall 7e, p84, 199; OSHA 2014a, p1]

118. **d** An example of an engineering control is permanent containment of a contaminated needle once a safety feature is activated. Needle safety features are mandated by Needlestick Safety & Prevention Act (2001), a modification mandated by Congress to OSHA's Bloodborne Pathogens standard. The Needlestick Safety & Prevention Act (2001) requires the use of engineering controls to eliminate or minimize employee exposure to bloodborne pathogens through accidental needlestick.
[McCall 7e, p84, 199; OSHA 2014a, p1]

Laboratory Operations — Explanations

119. **c** The following practices are never allowed: recapping, bending, breaking, or removing needles from disposable evacuated tube holders or syringes. Needle safety features are mandated by Needlestick Safety & Prevention Act (2001), a modification mandated by Congress to OSHA's Bloodborne Pathogens standard. The Needlestick Safety & Prevention Act (2001) requires the use of engineering controls to eliminate or minimize employee exposure to bloodborne pathogens through accidental needlestick.
[Garza 10e, p109-112, 127]

120. **b** To comply with safety standards while transferring blood from a syringe to an evacuated tube, the phlebotomist should use a syringe transfer device designed with an internal needle attached to the barrel.
[Garza 10e, p353]

121. **c** At least 2 different types of safety mechanisms are available to prevent accidental self-puncture with a contaminated winged infusion needle, including automatic resheathing and needle retraction.
[Garza 10e, p272-275]

122. **a** To ensure maximum safety for both the phlebotomist and patient, phlebotomists must be sure to use a tube holder and needle made by the same manufacturer.
[McCall 7e, p201-202]

123. **b** An example of an engineering control is permanent retraction of a contaminated lancet following activation. Needle safety features are mandated by Needlestick Safety & Prevention Act (2001), a modification mandated by Congress to OSHA's Bloodborne Pathogens standard. The Needlestick Safety & Prevention Act (2001) requires the use of engineering controls to eliminate or minimize employee exposure to bloodborne pathogens through accidental needlestick.
[Garza 10e, p109-112, 127, 278-279; OSHA 2011, p1]

124. **d** Electricity represents one of the major safety hazards in the clinical laboratory. If an evacuated tube shatters during centrifugation the phlebotomist should first unplug the centrifuge. Whenever electrical equipment, such as a centrifuge, has spilled liquid it must be unplugged during cleaning to prevent electrical current passing to the phlebotomist.
[Garza 10e, p146-147]

125. **c** Electricity represents one of the major safety hazards in the clinical setting. If the patient asks the phlebotomist to change the television channel during a venipuncture procedure, the phlebotomist should politely refuse to change the channel until after the procedure is completed. If a phlebotomist touches electrical equipment while holding an evacuated tube system during venipuncture, the electrical current could pass through the phlebotomist and the needle and shock the patient.
[Garza 10e, p146-147]

Explanations

Laboratory Operations

126. d The phlebotomist must use a nonconductor to remove the electrical cord from the victim. Plastic is a nonconductor, so placing a hand in a plastic beaker to remove the cord would safely remove the source of electricity from the victim.
[Garza 10e, p146-147]

127. a The National Fire Protection Agency recognizes 3 primary fire classifications. Class A fires occur with ordinary combustibles such as paper and wood.
[Garza 10e, p143-145]

128. b The National Fire Protection Agency recognizes 3 primary fire classifications. Class B fires occur with flammable liquids such as gasoline and grease.
[Garza 10e, p143-145]

129. c The National Fire Protection Agency recognizes 3 primary fire classifications. Class C fires occur with electrical equipment.
[Garza 10e, p143-145]

130. d Class D fires occur with combustible metals such as lithium, magnesium, potassium, and sodium.
[McCall 7e, p93-95]

131. d RACE is the National Fire Protection Agency (NFPA) code word for action a health care worker should take in the event of a fire and stands for Rescue, Alarm, Confine, Extinguish.
[Garza 10e, p145]

132. c RACE is the National Fire Protection Agency (NFPA) code word for action a health care worker should take in the event of a fire, and stands for Rescue, Alarm, Confine, Extinguish.
[Garza 10e, p145]

133. c PASS is the National Fire Protection Agency (NFPA) code word for using a fire extinguisher and stands for: Pull pin, Aim the nozzle at the bottom of the fire, Squeeze the handle, Sweep the nozzle side-to-side.
[Garza 10e, p144]

134. c PASS is the National Fire Protection Agency (NFPA) code word for using a fire extinguisher and stands for: Pull pin, Aim the nozzle at the bottom of the fire, Squeeze the handle, Sweep the nozzle side-to-side.
[Garza 10e, p144]

This figure is for question 135 only.

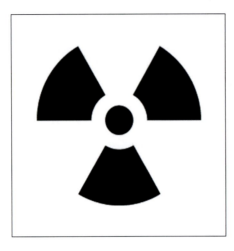

135. **d**   The symbol in the figure communicates radiation hazard.
[Garza 10e, p147]

136. **d**   The 3 components of radiation safety are time, shielding, and distance.
[Garza 10e, p147]

137. **d**   The effects of radiation accumulate with every exposure so limiting time exposed to radiation is an important element of radiation protection.
[Garza 10e, p147]

138. **a**   Dosimeter badges are used to monitor radiation exposure. Health care workers regularly exposed to radiation must wear a dosimeter badge to record radiation exposure. Badges are checked at regular intervals to monitor levels of radiation exposure in health care workers.
[Garza 10e, p147-148]

139. **c**   Radiation exposure is very hazardous to a developing fetus so pregnant phlebotomists should avoid entering areas marked with the radiation hazard symbol.
[McCall 7e, p94-96]

Explanations

Laboratory Operations

Please consult the diagram below for questions 140-143 regarding the Department of Transportation hazard label.

The Department of Transportation uses the label in the figure to communicate chemical hazard information. The symbol corresponding to the letter "A" represents the hazard class symbol. The symbol labeled "A" in the figure represents a flammable chemical. Other symbols include a bursting ball (explosive), skull and crossbones (poison), and radioactive (propeller). The number in the box labeled "B" is the four-digit chemical identification number. The number labeled "C" is the single-digit United Nations hazard class number.

[McCall 7e, p89-90]

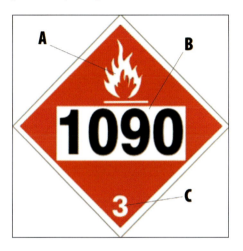

140. **b** The Department of Transportation uses the label pictured to communicate chemical hazard information
    [McCall 7e, p89-90]

141. **a** The arrow (letter A above) points to a hazard class symbol. The symbol in the figure represents a flammable chemical. Other symbols include a bursting ball (explosive), skull and crossbones (poison), and radioactive (propeller).
    [McCall 7e, p89-90]

142. **b** The arrow (letter B above) points to the four-digit chemical hazard identification number.
    [McCall 7e, p89-90]

143. **d** The arrow (letter C above) points to the single-digit United Nations hazard class number.
    [McCall 7e, p89-90]

Laboratory Operations — Explanations

Please consult the diagram below for questions 144-149 regarding the National Fire Protection Agency hazard label.

The National Fire Protection Agency (NFPA) uses the label pictured to communicate chemical hazard information. The blue diamond corresponding to the letter "A" represents health hazard. The red diamond corresponding to the letter "B" represents fire hazard. The yellow diamond corresponding to the letter "C" represents instability hazard. The white diamond corresponding to the letter "D" represents special hazards, such as radioactivity. The numbers in each diamond rank the level of hazard in each category, ranging from 0 (no hazard) to 4 (highest hazard level).

[Garza 10e, p150, 152]

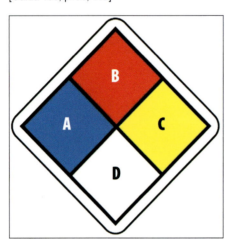

144. **c**   The National Fire Protection Agency (NFPA) uses the label in the figure to communicate chemical hazard information.
[Garza 10e, p150, 152]

145. **b**   The blue diamond corresponding to the letter "A" represents health hazard.
[Garza 10e, p150, 152]

146. **a**   The red diamond corresponding to the letter "B" represents fire hazard.
[Garza 10e, p150, 152]

147. **c**   The yellow diamond corresponding to the letter "C" represents instability hazard.
[Garza 10e, p150, 152]

148. **d**   The white diamond corresponding to the letter "D" represents special hazards, such as radioactivity.
[Garza 10e, p150, 152]

149. **c**   The zeros in the figure indicate the chemical is inflammable and very stable.
[Garza 10e, p150-152]

Explanations
Laboratory Operations

150. d Standards for chemical safety in the workplace are mandated by the Occupational Safety & Health Administration Hazard Communication Standard, also known as the OSHA HazCom standard or the "Right to Know Law."
[Garza 10e, p150-153]

151. d Standards for chemical safety in the workplace are mandated by the Occupational Safety & Health Administration Hazard Communication Standard, also known as the OSHA HazCom standard or the "Right to Know Law."
[Garza 10e, p150-153]

152. b Chemical manufacturers must use Safety Data Sheets to provide general information, safe handling, and emergency information for hazardous chemicals.
[Garza 10e, p150-153]

153. c According to the Occupational Safety & Health Administration Hazard Communication Standard, hazardous chemicals are required to be labeled. Labels must include a warning label, the nature of the hazard, safe handling instructions, and first aid recommendations.
[Garza 10e, p149]

154. a When diluting acids, always add acid to water (or other diluent) to avoid a volatile reaction.
[Garza 10e, p152]

155. b Chemical spill clean-up kits contain materials that absorb the chemical and neutralize it so it can be safely cleaned up and disposed. There are a variety of chemical spill kits available, and the laboratory worker should select the appropriate clean up kit based on the type of spill (eg, alkali, acid, mercury).
[Garza 10e, p152-153]

156. c The Environmental Protection Agency regulates chemical disposal.
[McCall 7e, p86-87]

157. a A centrifuge is the instrument used to separate blood specimens into component parts, including plasma, buffy coat (white cells and platelets), and red cell layers.
[Garza 10e, p232-233, 407-413]

158. c Specimens must be placed in a centrifuge so the centrifuge is balanced. Specimens of similar size & volume must be placed directly across from each other.
[Garza 10e, p408-409]

Laboratory Operations   Explanations

159. c Specimens should be placed in a centrifuge with the stoppers intact to prevent aerosol formation. Stopper removal carries the potential of aerosol formation. OSHA states, "All procedures involving blood or potentially infectious materials shall be performed in such a manner as to minimize splashing, spraying, splattering, and generation of droplets of these substances." To comply with this mandate, stopper removal must occur after centrifugation is completed and behind a splash shield or a full-length face shield.
[Garza 10e, p232-233, 407-413]

160. d Specimens must be placed in plastic liner labeled with the biohazard label before being placed in the pneumatic tube system for transport to the laboratory.
[Garza 10e, p400, 405]

This figure is for question 161 only.

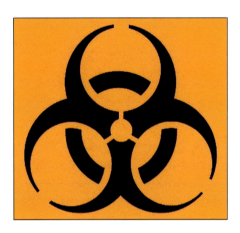

161. a The symbol in the figure communicates biohazard.
[Garza 10e, p110]

162. a An infection control program that includes monitoring specific patient population groups and classifications of infection is called surveillance.
[McCall 7e, p66-67]

163. a Three components in the chain of infection are reservoir, mode of transmission, and susceptible host.
[Garza 10e, p114-117]

164. a If the chain of infection is interrupted at 1 point, the spread of infection will be interrupted.
[Garza 10e, p117]

165. c Microbes capable of causing infection or disease are called pathogens.
[Garza 10e, p105, 633]

Explanations
Laboratory Operations

166. b A communicable disease results from the transmission of a pathogenic organism by direct or indirect contact or via airborne routes.
[Garza 10e, p105]

167. c 5%-8.5% of patients admitted to the hospital in the United States contract a health care associated (nosocomial) infection (HAI).
[McCall 7e, p61-62]

168. d Healthcare-associated infection (HAI) is a term referring to infections acquired in hospitals and other health care facilities, including home care.
[Garza 10e, p106]

169. d The most common nosocomial infection in the United States is urinary tract infection, representing 32% of all nosocomial infections.
[McCall 7e, p62]

170. a Viability refers to a pathogen's ability to survive.
[McCall 7e, p64, 498]

171. d Virulence refers to a pathogen's ability to overcome the defense mechanisms of the host.
[McCall 7e, p64, 498]

172. c Five mechanisms have been recognized to transfer an infection to a susceptible host including airborne, contact, droplet, vector, and vehicle.
[Garza 10e, p115, 118-119]

173. b The mode of infection transmission that requires close or intimate contact with an infected person is direct contact. In addition to standard precautions, health care workers may be required to wear a gown into a patient's room with contact precautions. Strict adherence to hand hygiene policies and procedures is important to prevent the spread of infections transmitted by direct contact.
[Garza 10e, p115, 119-121]

174. c The mode of infection transmission that occurs when a person encounters contaminated items from a patient, such as bed linens or silverware, is indirect contact. In addition to standard precautions, health care workers may be required to wear a gown into a patient's room with contact precautions. Strict adherence to hand hygiene policies and procedures is important to prevent the spread of infections transmitted by indirect contact.
[Garza 10e, p115, 118-119, 121-122]

175. c Fomites harbor pathogenic bacteria and are capable of transmitting infection. Examples of fomites include phlebotomy trays, tourniquets, telephones, computer keyboards, and door knobs.
[Garza 10e, p116]

Laboratory Operations — Explanations

176. a The mode of infection transmission occurring when a person inhales infectious droplets less than 5 μm in size is airborne transmission. Patients with an airborne infection are typically placed in airborne infection isolation rooms (AIIR). In addition to standard precautions, health care workers may be required to wear an N95 fit-tested mask certified by the National Institute for Occupational Safety & Health (NIOSH) when entering the room.
[McCall 7e, p64]

177. b The mode of infection transmission occurring when a person inhales infectious droplets greater than 5 μm in size is droplet transmission. In addition to standard precautions, health care workers may be required to wear a mask into a patient's room with droplet precautions.
[Garza 10e, p118-120]

178. c The mode of infection transmission involving transfer of an infectious disease by animal or insect is vector transmission. Maintaining sanitary conditions in a health care facility or a home is the best defense against spread of infection by vector transmission.
[Garza 10e, p115-116]

179. d The mode of infection transmission involving transfer of an infectious disease by contaminated food, water, or drugs is vehicle transmission.
[Garza 10e, p115-117]

180. c Patients admitted to a hospital for treatment of a communicable disease may be the reservoir component of the chain of infection.
[Garza 10e, p114]

181. d Patients admitted to a hospital free of infection may be the susceptible host component of the chain of infection.
[Garza 10e, p115-117]

182. b *Salmonella* organisms are examples of pathogenic bacteria.
[Garza 10e, p108]

183. d A venipuncture needle may be the mode of transmission component in the chain of infection.
[Garza 10e, p116]

184. b The patient afflicted with AIDS is an example of a susceptible host. AIDS patients are frequently immunocompromised and therefore susceptible to infection.
[Garza 10e, p116-117]

185. c Human hands are examples of the reservoir component in the chain of infection. Strict adherence to handwashing policies and procedures is critically important to preventing the spread of infection.
[Garza 10e, p114-115]

Explanations Laboratory Operations

186. **c** Effective housekeeping, laundry services, and proper waste disposal safeguard a susceptible host by interrupting the spread of infection.
[Garza 10e, p117]

187. **d** Insect and rodent control, isolation procedures, and use of disposable equipment disrupt the mode of transmission.
[Garza 10e, p117]

188. **a** Immunizations, exercise, and sound nutrition control infection and help patients regain their health.
[Garza 10e, p116-117]

189. **d** A patient undergoing immunosuppressive therapy prior to transplant is an example of the susceptible host component of the chain of infection.
[Garza 10e, p116-117]

190. **c** Standard precautions are the procedures recommended by the Centers for Disease Control & Prevention to prevent the spread of infection due to exposure to blood, all body fluids (except sweat), nonintact skin and mucous membranes.
[Garza 10e, p117-118, 121-122, 314]

191. **d** Transmission-based precautions are the procedures recommended by the Centers for Disease Control & Prevention to prevent the spread of infection following exposure to patients with known or suspected infections or colonized with epidemiologically significant pathogens.
[Garza 10e, p118-121]

192. **a** Under standard precautions all patient blood, body fluids (except sweat), nonintact skin, and mucous membranes must be approached as though infectious.
[Garza 10e, p117-118, 121-122, 314]

193. **d** Personal protective equipment (PPE) protects the health care worker from contact with infectious materials.
[Garza 10e, p121]

194. **b** A health care worker should use personal protective equipment (PPE) whenever contact with patient blood or body fluids is expected.
[Garza 10e, p121-122]

195. **b** A health care worker should wear a mask if splashing of blood or body fluids is likely.
[Garza 10e, p120-122]

196. **b** A health care worker should wear a mask if infectious materials are likely to be spread by droplets generated by coughing or sneezing.
[Garza 10e, p120-122]

197. **d** A phlebotomist should never recap a needle after a venipuncture procedure.
[Garza 10e, p111-112]

Laboratory Operations — Explanations

198. d Under standard precautions, a phlebotomist must wear gloves when performing any blood collection procedure.
[Garza 10e, p118, 121-127, 314]

199. c Under transmission-based precautions, a phlebotomist must wear a gown when a patient is in contact isolation.
[Garza 10e, p119, 121]

200. c The phlebotomist should put on PPE in the following order: gown, mask, gloves.
[Garza 10e, p129-130]

201. a When a phlebotomist dons a gown prior to entering a patient isolation room, she must ensure that she only touches the gown on the inside surface.
[Garza 10e, p129]

202. a When a phlebotomist chooses a gown prior to entering a patient isolation room, he must ensure that the gown is large enough to cover all of the phlebotomist's clothing. If necessary, the phlebotomist may wear 2 gowns (one to cover the front and one to cover the back) to ensure complete coverage.
[Garza 10e, p129]

203. d When a phlebotomist dons a gown prior to entering a patient isolation room, she must ensure that the sleeves are pulled down to the wrist.
[Garza 10e, p129]

204. b When a phlebotomist dons a gown prior to entering a patient isolation room, he must ensure that the gown is securely fastened at the neck and waist.
[Garza 10e, p129]

205. c A phlebotomist must wear a mask when a patient requires droplet precaution.
[Garza 10e, p119-120]

206. a A phlebotomist may be required to wear a National Institute for Occupational Safety & Health approved N95 fit-tested mask when the patient requires airborne precautions.
[McCall 7e, p64]

207. a Bacteria that mutate so they are no longer susceptible to antimicrobial therapy are called antibiotic resistant. Examples of antibiotic resistant bacteria include methicillin-resistant *Staphylococcus aureus* and vancomycin-resistant enterococcus.
[Garza 10e, p107]

208. d When a phlebotomist dons a mask prior to entering a patient isolation room, he must tie the mask securely around the upper portion of his head and neck to ensure a snug and secure fit over the nose and mouth.
[Garza 10e, p130]

Explanations Laboratory Operations

209. c The N95 respirator mask is individually fitted to each health care worker and designed to filter 95% of airborne particles less than 5 μm in diameter. N95 respirator masks must be approved by the National Institute for Occupational Safety & Health (NIOSH).
[McCall 7e, p72]

210. b The N95 respirator mask is individually fitted to each health care worker and designed to filter 95% of airborne particles less than 5 μm in diameter. N95 respirator masks must be approved by the National Institute for Occupational Safety & Health (NIOSH).
[McCall 7e, p72]

211. d The N95 respirator mask is individually fitted to each health care worker and designed to filter 95% of airborne particles less than 5 μm in diameter. Examples of diseases that may require airborne precautions and the use of an N95 respirator mask include chicken pox (varicella), *Mycobacterium tuberculosis* (TB), rubeola (measles), and SARS.
[Garza 10e, p120]

212. a When a phlebotomist dons gloves with a gown prior to entering the room of a patient requiring transmission-based precautions, the gloves should be pulled up over the sleeve of the gown.
[Garza 10e, p130]

213. b The phlebotomist should first remove any jewelry before putting on gloves prior to entering an isolation room to eliminate the risk of puncturing a glove and compromising the protective barrier required, placing the phlebotomist at risk.
[Garza 10e, p130]

214. d Respiratory hygiene and coughing etiquette were added to the practice of standard precautions. If a phlebotomist encounters anyone in the health care facility sneezing and coughing, the phlebotomist should provide the person with a tissue and politely ask them to wash their hands after discarding the tissue.
[Garza 10e, p121]

215. a Under standard precautions, a phlebotomist should change gloves after every patient encounter and immediately sanitize hands.
[Garza 10e, p314]

216. a Under standard precautions, a phlebotomist should sanitize his/her hands immediately after every patient encounter after removing gloves.
[Garza 10e, p121, 125-126, 314]

217. b Health care workers required to adhere to standard precautions to avoid infection with pathogenic organisms.
[Garza 10e, p121]

Laboratory Operations — Explanations

218. **b** Isolation is the separation of patients with communicable infections from other patients and limiting their contact with health care workers and visitors. Placing a patient in isolation carries a social stigma and can be very difficult psychologically for patients. Phlebotomists must address patients in a calm, caring, and professional manner to reduce patient feelings of isolation and apprehension.
[Garza 10e, p117, 632]

219. **a** A patient would be admitted to a hospital under transmission-based precautions if the patient is suspected of having an infection transmitted by airborne, contact, or droplet routes.
[Garza 10e, p118-119]

220. **c** A patient would be admitted to a hospital under airborne precautions if suspected of having an infection transmitted by droplet particles less than 5 μm in diameter. Examples of diseases requiring airborne precautions include chicken pox (varicella), *Mycobacterium tuberculosis* (TB), rubeola (measles), and SARS.
[Garza 10e, p118-119]

221. **d** A patient would be admitted to a hospital under droplet precautions if suspected of having an infection transmitted by particles greater than 5 μm in diameter. Examples of diseases requiring droplet precautions include *Bordetella pertussis (*whooping cough), *Neisseria meningitidis* (meningitis) and streptococcal pharyngitis (strep throat).
[Garza 10e, p118-119]]

222. **b** A patient would be admitted to a hospital under contact precautions if suspected of having an infection transmitted by direct or indirect contact with colonized microorganisms. Examples include herpes simplex, scabies, or *Staphylococcus aureus* (MRSA).
[Garza 10e, p119]

223. **b** A patient would be admitted to a hospital under contact precautions if suspected of having an infection transmitted by direct or indirect contact with colonized microorganisms. Examples include herpes simplex, scabies, or *Staphylococcus aureus* (MRSA).
[Garza 10e, p119]

224. **c** A patient would be admitted to a hospital under droplet precautions if suspected of having an infection transmitted by particles greater than 5 μm in diameter. Examples of diseases requiring droplet precautions include *Bordetella pertussis (*whooping cough), *Neisseria meningitidis* (meningitis), and streptococcal pharyngitis (strep throat).
[Garza 10e, p118-119]

Explanations *Laboratory Operations*

225. a A patient would be admitted to a hospital under airborne precautions if suspected of having an infection transmitted by droplet particles less than 5 μm in diameter. Examples of diseases requiring airborne precautions include chicken pox (varicella), *Mycobacterium tuberculosis* (TB), rubeola (measles), and SARS.
[Garza 10e, p118-119]

226. b A patient would be admitted to a hospital under contact precautions if suspected of having an infection transmitted by direct or indirect contact, such as found in wound infections. Examples include *Clostridioides difficile* or methicillin-resistant *Staphylococcus aureus* (MRSA).
[Garza 10e, p119]

227. c A patient would be admitted to a hospital under droplet precautions if suspected of having an infection transmitted by particles greater than 5 μm in diameter. Examples of diseases requiring droplet precautions include *Bordetella pertussis (*whooping cough), *Neisseria meningitidis* (meningitis), and streptococcal pharyngitis (strep throat).
[Garza 10e, p118-119]

228. b A patient would be admitted to a hospital under contact precautions if suspected of having an infection transmitted by direct or indirect contact with colonized microorganisms. Examples include herpes simplex, scabies, or *Staphylococcus aureus* (MRSA).
[Garza 10e, p119]

229. c A patient would be admitted to a hospital under droplet precautions if suspected of having an infection transmitted by particles greater than 5 μm in diameter. Examples of diseases requiring droplet precautions include *Bordetella pertussis (*whooping cough), *Neisseria meningitidis* (meningitis), and streptococcal pharyngitis (strep throat).
[Garza 10e, p118-119]

230. a A patient would be admitted to a hospital under airborne precautions if suspected of having an infection transmitted by droplet particles less than 5 μm in diameter. Examples of diseases requiring airborne precautions include chicken pox (varicella), *Mycobacterium tuberculosis* (TB), rubeola (measles), and SARS.
[Garza 10e, p118-119]

231. c Health care workers, including phlebotomists, and patient visitors are alerted to transmission-based precautions by a sign on the patient's door. Health care workers and patient visitors should adhere to the instructions on the sign on the patient's door regarding personal protective equipment (PPE) required to safely enter the patient's room. PPE required for transmission-based precautions is always in addition to standard precautions.
[Garza 10e, p119-121]

Laboratory Operations — Explanations

232. **c**   Health care workers, including phlebotomists, and patient visitors are alerted to transmission-based precautions by a sign on the patient's door. Health care workers and patient visitors should adhere to the instructions on the sign on the patient's door regarding personal protective equipment (PPE) required to safely enter the patient's room. PPE required for transmission-based precautions is always in addition to standard precautions.
[Garza 10e, p119-121]

233. **c**   Accidental needlestick with a contaminated needle causes percutaneous exposure which occurs when skin has been pierced. One strategy to avoid percutaneous exposure is the proper and consistent use of needle safety devices and biohazard disposal containers.
[Garza 10e, p109-112, 127, 136, 270-275]

234. **a**   Laboratory professionals may be exposed to biohazards through a number of routes, including airborne, ingestion, percutaneous and permucosal. To prevent the spread of infection through ingestion, eating, chewing gum, applying makeup, including lip balm, biting one's nails or putting pens or pencils in one's mouth are prohibited because these activities can lead to ingestion of biohazards.
[Garza 10e, p136-137]

235. **c**   Laboratory professionals may be exposed to biohazards through a number of routes, including airborne, ingestion, percutaneous and permucosal. To prevent the spread of infection through airborne routes, centrifuges should never be opened until after they have arrived at a complete stop.
[Garza 10e, p136, 407-409]

236. **d**   Permucosal exposure occurs when pathogens and other hazardous materials enter the body through the mucous membranes of the eyes, mouth, or nose. To prevent permucosal exposure in the clinical laboratory, phlebotomists should never rub their eyes or nose, handle contact lenses, or put contaminated fingers or hands near their eyes, mouth, or nose.
[Garza 10e, p136]

237. **d**   According to OSHA's Bloodborne Pathogens standard, engineering controls are equipment and supply mechanisms designed to separate or eliminate a bloodborne pathogen hazard. Examples of engineering controls include self-sheathing, retractable and other forms of safety needles, sharps containers, and syringe transfer devices.
[McCall 7e, p84-86]

238. **a**   According to OSHA's Bloodborne Pathogens standard, work practice controls are procedural mechanisms designed to limit the possibility of bloodborne pathogen exposure. Examples of work practice controls include handwashing and prohibiting laboratory professionals from eating, chewing gum, and applying makeup in the clinical laboratory.
[McCall 7e, p84-86]

Explanations
Laboratory Operations

239. a Airborne exposure occurs when pathogens and other hazardous materials are inhaled by the laboratory professional as aerosols or fumes are generated or when splashes occur. To prevent the spread of infection through airborne routes, face shields should be worn during specimen processing.
[Garza 10e, p136]

240. a Gloves should be removed following completion of the venipuncture procedure. Gowns, safety goggles and N95 fit-tested masks are not used for routine venipuncture procedures.
[McCall 7e, p251]

241. d Gloves should be removed aseptically (in a pathogen-free manner) following completion of a procedure.
[Garza 10e, p131]

242. a To aseptically remove gloves following a venipuncture procedure, the cuff of one glove should be grasped and pulled over the hand, inside-out and into the palm of the other hand. The other glove should be removed by slipping the fingers into the cuff of that other glove and pulling it over the first so all contaminated surfaces are contained within 1 glove once removed.
[Garza 10e, p131]

243. d After a blood collection procedure is completed in a transmission based isolation room, the phlebotomist should remove personal protective equipment in the doorway or anteroom of the patient's room.
[Garza 10e, p131]

244. a After a blood collection procedure is completed in a transmission based isolation room, the phlebotomist should remove personal protective equipment in the doorway or anteroom of the patient's room beginning with the gloves. Biohazards communicable by droplet transmission do not remain suspended in the air and carry less than 10 feet.
[Garza 10e, p131, 135]

245. d After gloves are removed, gowns should be removed aseptically (in a pathogen-free manner) following completion of a procedure.
[McCall 7e, p70-72]

246. b After gloves are removed, gowns should be removed aseptically (in a pathogen-free manner). To aseptically remove a gown following a blood collection procedure, the phlebotomist should pull the gown off from the shoulders and pulling the arms out so the gown is turned inside out, exercising care not to touch the contaminated surface with his/her hands or uniform.
[Garza 10e, p131, 135]

247. c Under transmission-based precautions, once a blood collection procedure is completed and gown is removed, the phlebotomist should next remove their mask, exercising caution to touch only the strings and never the front of the mask.
[Garza 10e, p132, 135]

Laboratory Operations — Explanations

248. d Under transmission-based precautions, once a blood collection procedure is completed and gown is removed, the phlebotomist should next remove their mask, exercising caution to touch only the strings and never the front of the mask.
[Garza 10e, p132, 135]

249. a After a blood collection procedure is completed in a transmission based isolation room requiring the phlebotomist to use an National Institute for Occupational Safety & Health approved N95 fit-tested mask, the phlebotomist should remove the N95 fit-tested mask in the hallway outside the patient's room after closing the door. Biohazards communicable by airborne transmission remain suspended in the air and may become widely dispersed.
[Garza 10e, p135]

250. b If the pneumatic tube system meets operational benchmarks and the specimen is packed properly, the pneumatic tube system serves as an efficient mechanism for transporting specimens to the laboratory for analysis. Specimens must be loaded into pneumatic tube systems using plastic bags labeled with the biohazard symbol to house the specimens and shock absorbent inserts to minimize breakage.
[Garza 10e, p405]

251. a The disease state resulting from the invasion of the body by a pathogenic microorganism is called an infection.
[Garza 10e, p631]

252. b Trash and linens from an isolation room must be safely disposed of to prevent the spread of infection. The double bag procedure involves collecting contaminated items in a red biohazard bag inside the patient's room. A second person outside the patient's room will hold a clean, red biohazard bag with the edges folded over their hands to prevent contamination. The first bag containing the contaminated items is inserted into the second bag, which is sealed and labeled with biohazard warnings before disposal.
[Garza 10e, p133]

253. c Chemical compounds used to remove or kill microorganisms on work surfaces or instruments are called disinfectants.
[Garza 10e, p137]

254. b Chemicals that may be used on human skin to inhibit the growth and development of microorganisms, but not necessarily kill them, are antiseptics. 70% isopropyl alcohol is an example of an antiseptic.
[Garza 10e, p137]

255. d Chemicals that may be used on human skin to inhibit the growth and development of microorganisms, but not necessarily kill them, are antiseptics. 70% isopropyl alcohol is an example of an antiseptic.
[Garza 10e, p137]

Explanations

Laboratory Operations

256. c Chemical compounds used to remove or kill microorganisms on work surfaces or instruments are called disinfectants. Hypochlorite solution (bleach) is a commonly used disinfectant in the clinical laboratory.
[Garza 10e, p137]

257. a Hand hygiene performed consistent with frequency and procedural recommendations is one of the most essential strategies to prevent the spread of infection.
[McCall 7e, p67-69]

258. c A phlebotomist encounters a blood spill on her hands. She should wash her hands immediately using soap and water.
[Garza 10e, p122]

259. a Alcohol-based antiseptic hand cleaners have been approved by the Centers for Disease Control & Prevention (CDC) Healthcare Infection Control Practices Advisory Committee (HICPAC) as an appropriate substitute for handwashing, assuming the hands are not soiled with blood or body fluids.
[Garza 10e, p122]

260. c A phlebotomist routinely uses an alcohol-based antiseptic to cleanse her hands after completing a blood collection procedure. According to the Occupational Safety & Health Administration (OSHA), the phlebotomist is required to wash her hands with soap and water after every third patient.
[Garza 10e, p122]

261. b Hand hygiene procedures must be completed before and after every patient contact.
[Garza 10e, p122]

262. b According to the Centers for Disease Control & Prevention Guidelines for Hand Hygiene in Health Care Settings, natural fingernail length should not exceed 1/4 inch.
[Garza 10e, p127]

263. b According to the Centers for Disease Control & Prevention Guidelines for Hand Hygiene in Health Care Settings, personnel with patient contact should not use artificial nails or extenders.
[Garza 10e, p127]

264. c A phlebotomist is preparing to leave the lab for a lunch break. She begins the hand washing procedure by wetting her hands and dispensing soap. Next she should rub her hands together vigorously for at least 20 seconds.
[Garza 10e, p123]

265. a During the rinse step of a hand wash procedure, the phlebotomist should hold her hands with the fingers pointing down.
[Garza 10e, p124]

Laboratory Operations — Explanations

266. d After the rinse step of a hand wash procedure, the phlebotomist should turn off the faucet using her paper towel.
[Garza 10e, p124]

267. c Health care services are often paid for by insurance companies or the federal government, called a third party payer.
[McCall 7e, p17]

268. a The system used to provide terminology and a coding system to bill for physician office services is called current procedural terminology (CPT).
[McCall 7e, p18]

269. c A system to reimburse for health care services designed to manage access, cost, and quality is called managed care.
[McCall 7e, p19]

270. c The system of reimbursement to health care facilities for services rendered based on entitlement due to employment and financed through social security is Medicare.
[McCall 7e, p18-19]

271. b The system of reimbursement to health care facilities for services rendered based on entitlement due to eligibility based in part on low income is Medicaid.
[McCall 7e, p18-19]

272. d According to The Patient Care Partnership established by the American Hospital Association, patients can expect their privacy to be protected during their hospital stay.
[Garza 10e, p86]

273. d The Health Insurance Portability & Accountability Act (HIPAA) is the federal law protecting a patient's right to privacy.
[Garza 10e, p90-91]

274. b The phlebotomist compromised the patient's privacy and may be charged with negligence.
[Garza 10e, p89]

275. d Protected health information includes all patient health information transmitted by electronic media or sent or stored in any other form.
[Garza 10e, p90-91]

276. b Health care workers must sign and comply with a confidentiality and nondisclosure statement, agreeing to maintain the confidentiality of all patient records.
[Garza 10e, p90]

277. b Health care workers must sign and comply with a confidentiality and nondisclosure statement, agreeing to maintain the security of computer login and password information.
[Garza 10e, p90]

Explanations
Laboratory Operations

278. **b** Health care workers must sign and comply with a confidentiality and nondisclosure statement, agreeing to maintain the security of individual patient data when using comprehensive data banks containing patient medical information.
[Garza 10e, p90]

279. **b** Penalties for failure to adhere to the Health Information Portability & Accountability Act include fines.
[McCall 7e, p9]

280. **c** Penalties for failure to adhere to the Health Information Portability & Accountability Act include incarceration.
[McCall 7e, p9]

281. **b** A legal claim that can be filed by a patient as the result of unauthorized release of personal information is invasion of privacy.
[Garza 10e, p90]

282. **d** A factor causing emotional or mental strain or tension is called stress.
[Garza 10e, p23-24]

283. **d** A patient suffering from disease or injury to the central nervous system would most likely be cared for by the neurology department.
[Garza 10e, p6]

284. **d** A patient suffering from a mental or an emotional disorder would most likely be cared for by the psychiatry department.
[Garza 10e, p6]

285. **a** A patient experiencing complications related to pregnancy would most likely be cared for by the obstetrics department.
[Garza 10e, p6]

286. **a** The field of medicine that specializes in the diagnosis and treatment of the elderly population is called geriatrics.
[Garza 10e, p6]

287. **d** The field of medicine that deals with the diagnosis and treatment of joint and tissue diseases is rheumatology.
[Garza 10e, p6]

288. **b** The medical specialty that deals with the diagnosis and treatment of disorders of the eye is ophthalmology.
[Garza 10e, p6]

289. **d** The medical specialty that deals with the diagnosis and treatment of disorders of the ear, nose, and throat is otolaryngology.
[Garza 10e, p6]

Laboratory Operations — Explanations

290. d The department of medicine that specializes in the diagnosis and treatment of disorders associated with male sexual and reproductive systems and renal system for both sexes is urology.
[Garza 10e, p6]

291. a The medical department that specializes in the diagnosis and treatment of disorders associated with the esophagus, stomach, and intestines is gastroenterology.
[Garza 10e, p5]

292. a The medical department that specializes in the treatment of disorders associated with hormone production is endocrinology.
[Garza 10e, p5]

293. d The department that uses radioactive materials to treat disease processes is radiotherapy.
[Garza 10e, p6]

294. a The department that assists patients in maintaining daily living skills, given the limitations of their physical or mental problems, is occupational therapy.
[Garza 10e, p6]

295. b The department that works with the patient to restore mental or physical abilities lost because of illness or accident is physical therapy.
[Garza 10e, p6]

296. a A physician who specializes in the diagnosis of disease from laboratory test results, tissue evaluation, and postmortem examinations is a pathologist.
[Garza 10e, p7, 10]

297. b A laboratory professional who enters the field after obtaining a bachelor's degree, including a year or more of study in clinical laboratory science, is a medical laboratory scientist (MLS).
[Garza 10e, p10]

298. c A laboratory professional who enters the field after obtaining an associate's degree is a medical laboratory technician (MLT).
[Garza 10e, p10]

299. d A laboratory professional trained in all aspects of blood specimen collection and transport is a phlebotomist.
[McCall 7e, p5]

300. a A clinical laboratory scientist with an advanced degree and several years' experience responsible for overseeing all operations involving physician and patient services is a laboratory administrator.
[McCall 7e, p30]

Chapter 7

Donor Phlebotomy

The following items have been identified as appropriate for those preparing for the QDP examination.

I. Basic Science of Blood Compatibility

1. A patient is typed as ABO group A. What ABO antigen(s) does the patient have on his red blood cells?
   - a A
   - b B
   - c A & B
   - d none

2. A patient is typed as ABO group B. What ABO antigen(s) does the patient have on his red blood cells?
   - a A
   - b B
   - c A & B
   - d none

3. A patient is typed as ABO group AB. What ABO antigen(s) does the patient have on his red blood cells?
   - a A
   - b B
   - c A & B
   - d none

4. A patient is typed as ABO group O. What ABO antigen(s) does the patient have on his red blood cells?
   - a A
   - b B
   - c A & B
   - d Neither A or B

5. A patient is typed as ABO group A. What ABO antibodies does the patient have in his serum?
   - a A
   - b B
   - c A & B
   - d none

Donor Phlebotomy   **I. Basic Science of Blood Compatibility**

6. A patient is typed as ABO group B. What ABO antibodies does the patient have in his serum?
   - a   A
   - b   B
   - c   A & B
   - d   none

7. Which of the following ABO blood types is the third most common in the United States?
   - a   A
   - b   B
   - c   AB
   - d   O

8. Which of the following ABO blood types is the least common in the United States?
   - a   A
   - b   B
   - c   AB
   - d   O

9. Which group of donors should be tested for HLA antibodies prior to donating platelets to reduce the risk of transfusion-related acute lung injury (TRALI) in recipients:
   - a   donors who have lived outside of the United States
   - b   donors who used clotting factor concentrates
   - c   donors who have a received autologous transfusions
   - d   donors who have a history of pregnancy

10. Which of the following red blood cell units is acceptable for a patient with group A positive blood?
    - a   group O positive
    - b   group B positive
    - c   group AB positive
    - d   group AB negative

11. One function of platelets is to:
    - a   treat anemia
    - b   increase blood volume
    - c   boost immune responses
    - d   form a blockage to stop bleeding

12. Transfusion of red blood cells would best be used to:
    - a   treat anemia
    - b   provide clotting factors
    - c   boost immune responses
    - d   form a blockage to stop bleeding

I. Basic Science of Blood Compatibility

Donor Phlebotomy

13. Which of the following red blood cell units is acceptable for a patient with group B positive blood?
    a   group A positive
    b   group B negative
    c   group AB positive
    d   group AB negative

14. Plasma:
    a   carries oxygen
    b   is the liquid portion of the blood
    c   provides immune response
    d   contains no clotting factors

15. White blood cells:
    a   carry oxygen
    b   are the liquid portion of the blood
    c   fight foreign bacteria
    d   contain clotting factors

16. The 4 primary ABO blood groups are:
    a   A, O, C, and AC
    b   A, B, AB, and D
    c   A, B, AB, and O
    d   A, O, B, and OB

17. In the figure below, the structure indicated by the arrow is the:

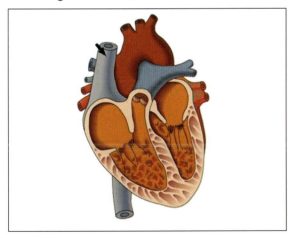

    a   pulmonary artery
    b   pulmonary vein
    c   inferior vena cava
    d   superior vena cava

18. In the figure below, the structure indicated by the arrow is the:

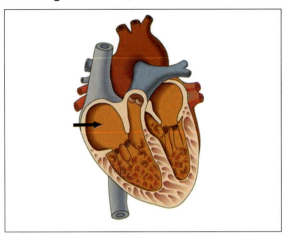

   a   right atrium
   b   left atrium
   c   right ventricle
   d   left ventricle

19. In the figure below, the structure indicated by the arrow is the:

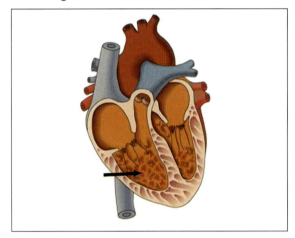

   a   right atrium
   b   left atrium
   c   right ventricle
   d   left ventricle

I. Basic Science of Blood Compatibility

20. In the figure below, the structure indicated by the arrow is the:

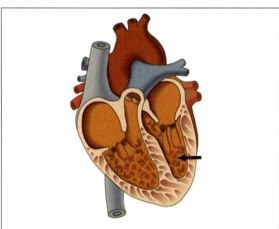

    a   right atrium
    b   left atrium
    c   right ventricle
    d   left ventricle

21. In the figure below, the structure indicated by the arrow is the:

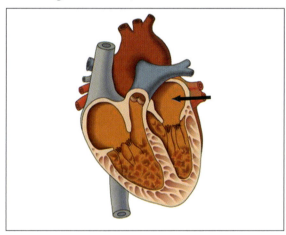

    a   right atrium
    b   left atrium
    c   right ventricle
    d   left ventricle

22. In the figure below, the structure indicated by the arrow is the:

    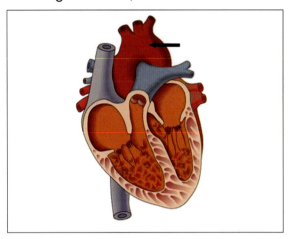

    a   aorta
    b   coronary artery
    c   pulmonary artery
    d   pulmonary vein

23. A phlebotomist performs a venipuncture as part of a whole blood collection. The blood in the tubing is bright cherry-red. What vessel did the phlebotomist likely puncture?

    a   artery
    b   capillary
    c   pulmonary artery
    d   vein

24. The blood vessel whose wall is 1 cell layer thick is the:

    a   arteriole
    b   artery
    c   capillary
    d   vein

25. Which of the following blood vessels contains a mixture of oxygenated and deoxygenated blood?

    a   arteries
    b   capillaries
    c   pulmonary arteries
    d   veins

26. Which of the following structures connect arterioles and venules?

    a   arteries
    b   pulmonary arteries
    c   capillaries
    d   veins

I. Basic Science of Blood Compatibility   **Donor Phlebotomy**

27. Which of the following blood vessels allows gas and solute exchange between blood and tissues?
    - a   capillaries
    - b   pulmonary arteries
    - c   pulmonary veins
    - d   veins

28. Which of the following specimens has the lowest concentration of oxygen?
    - a   arterial
    - b   arterialized capillary
    - c   capillary
    - d   venous

29. The blood vessels with 1-way valves in the lumen are called:
    - a   arterioles
    - b   arteries
    - c   capillaries
    - d   veins

30. Which of the following blood vessels contains deoxygenated blood?
    - a   arteries
    - b   arterioles
    - c   veins
    - d   pulmonary veins

31. After performing a routine venipuncture, the phlebotomist noticed that the blood in the evacuated tube was dark red. What vessel did the phlebotomist likely puncture?
    - a   artery
    - b   capillary
    - c   pulmonary artery
    - d   vein

32. Blood enters the right side of the heart through the:
    - a   aorta
    - b   pulmonary artery
    - c   pulmonary vein
    - d   superior vena cava

33. Blood enters the left side of the heart through the:
    - a   aorta
    - b   pulmonary arteries
    - c   pulmonary veins
    - d   inferior & superior vena cava

Donor Phlebotomy   **I. Basic Science of Blood Compatibility**

34. The 3 components of hemostasis are:
    a blood vessels, platelets, coagulation factors
    b tissue thromboplastin, platelets, antihemophiliac factor
    c fibrin split products, blood vessels, platelets
    d blood vessels, fibrin degradation products, platelets

35. Normal plasma is composed of primarily:
    a antibodies
    b fibrinogen
    c solutes
    d water

36. A blood specimen was collected into an evacuated tube containing an anticoagulant. What is the fluid portion of this blood specimen called?
    a fibrin
    b fibrinogen
    c plasma
    d serum

37. A blood specimen was collected into an evacuated tube without anticoagulant and allowed to clot. What is the fluid portion of this blood specimen called?
    a fibrin
    b fibrinogen
    c plasma
    d serum

38. The cellular element of the blood responsible for the transport of carbon dioxide from the tissues is:
    a erythrocyte
    b leukocyte
    c megakaryocyte
    d thrombocyte

39. The substance that transports oxygen in the blood is called:
    a hemoglobin
    b hematocrit
    c plasma
    d serum

40. Blood group antigens are located:
    a on the surface of erythrocytes
    b on the surface of lymphocytes
    c in plasma
    d in serum

II. Donor Identification & Selection

41. The cellular element of the blood that functions in fighting infection is:
    a   erythrocyte
    b   leukocyte
    c   megakaryocyte
    d   thrombocyte

42. The cellular element of the peripheral blood that functions in coagulation is the:
    a   erythrocyte
    b   leukocyte
    c   megakaryocyte
    d   thrombocyte

43. Which of the following proteins is found in plasma, but not serum?
    a   albumin
    b   fibrinogen
    c   fibrin
    d   globulins

44. The layer of cells that forms between red cells and plasma during centrifugation is called:
    a   agglutination
    b   buffy coat
    c   γ globulin
    d   erythropoietin

II. Donor Identification & Selection

45. The purpose of screening donors prior to blood collection is to:
    a   insure adequate blood supply and safeguard the transfusion recipient
    b   insure adequate blood supply and safeguard the donor
    c   qualify for insurance reimbursement and safeguard the transfusion recipient
    d   safeguard the donor and transfusion recipient

46. Blood components transfused from a donor that may or may not be related to the patient is:
    a   allogeneic
    b   allosteric
    c   autoimmunization
    d   autologous

47. Blood components collected from and transfused into the same person are:
    a   allogeneic
    b   allosteric
    c   autoimmunization
    d   autologous

Donor Phlebotomy — II. Donor Identification & Selection

48. A patient requests a transfusion from a specific donor during a non-emergency surgery. This is called a(n):
    a autologous donation
    b deferred donation
    c directed donation
    d exceptional medical need donation

49. Routine donor screening includes which of the following?
    a physical exam and serological testing
    b physical exam, completion of a medical questionnaire and serological testing
    c completion of a medical questionnaire and serological testing
    d completion of a medical questionnaire, serological testing and physician authorization

50. Blood centers are required to confirm donor identity and:
    a confirm physician authorization
    b connect the donor to existing donor records
    c examine the national data base for donor history of deferrals
    d examine the national data base for patient transfusion reactions after receiving blood from the donor

51. After receiving information on the donation procedure, a donor agrees to donate a unit of blood. The legal term for this exchange is:
    a Health Information Portability and Accountability Act (HIPAA)
    b informed consent
    c malpractice
    d respondeat superior

52. Which of the following topics must be included in the educational materials provided to a donor prior to donation?
    a enrollment in the hall of fame for blood donors, infectious disease tests to be performed on the donated unit
    b infectious disease tests to be performed on the donated unit, including results that must be reported to the appropriate oversight agencies
    c infectious disease tests to be performed on the donated unit, including results that must be reported to the donor's physician
    d infectious disease tests to be performed on the donated unit, including results that must be reported to the recipients' physician

53. When is the Donor History Questionnaire completed?
    a at least 1 week before the scheduled donation
    b during preregistration
    c once, before the first donation
    d on the day of donation

II. Donor Identification & Selection — Donor Phlebotomy

54. What is the minimum amount a person can weight and still donate blood?
    a   105 pounds
    b   110 pounds
    c   115 pounds
    d   120 pounds

55. A prospective donor is deferred from donating for a specified period of time. This type of deferral is termed:
    a   indefinite
    b   negligent
    c   permanent
    d   temporary

56. A prospective donor is deferred from donating for an unspecified period of time. This type of deferral is termed:
    a   indefinite
    b   negligent
    c   permanent
    d   temporary

57. A prospective donor is advised they will never be eligible to donate blood for another person. This type of deferral is termed:
    a   indefinite
    b   negligent
    c   permanent
    d   temporary

58. How long will a donor be deferred if he/she is manifesting cold symptoms?
    a   indefinitely deferred
    b   no deferral—the donor will be allowed to donate
    c   permanently deferred
    d   temporarily deferred, until symptoms subside

59. A 22-year-old female donor presents at the donor center to donate whole blood. She is on sulfamethoxazole and trimethoprim (brand name: Bactrim) to treat a UTI. What is the appropriate course of action?
    a   indefinitely deferred
    b   no deferral—the donor will be allowed to donate
    c   permanently deferred
    d   temporarily deferred

60. An 18-year-old college freshman male donor presents at the donor center to donate whole blood. He is taking tetracycline prophylactically to treat acne. What is the appropriate course of action?
    a   indefinitely deferred
    b   no deferral—the donor will be allowed to donate
    c   permanently deferred
    d   temporarily deferred

Donor Phlebotomy   **II. Donor Identification & Selection**

61. A 35-year-old mother of four presents at the donor center to donate whole blood. She is on oral contraceptives. What is the appropriate course of action?
    a   indefinitely deferred
    b   no deferral—the donor will be allowed to donate
    c   permanently deferred
    d   temporarily deferred

62. A 56-year-old prospective donor confirmed he was taking finasteridine (Proscar) to treat an enlarged prostate. What is the appropriate course of action?
    a   indefinitely deferred
    b   no deferral—the donor will be allowed to donate
    c   permanently deferred
    d   temporarily deferred

63. Which of the following medications are tetratogens and may result in donor deferral?
    a   finesteridine (Proscar), isotretoin (Accutane), dutasteroid (Avodart), etretinate (Tegison)
    b   gentamycin, vancomycin, tobramycin, erythromycin
    c   growth hormone from pituitary glands, hepatitis B immune globulin
    d   Plavix, Ticlid

64. A 35-year-old female prospective donor confirmed she was taking etretinate (Tegison) to treat psoriasis. What is the appropriate course of action?
    a   indefinitely deferred
    b   no deferral—the donor will be allowed to donate
    c   permanently deferred
    d   temporarily deferred

65. Which of the following medications interfere with platelet function and may result in donor deferral?
    a   finesteridine (Proscar), isotretoin (Accutane), dutasteroid (Avodart), etretinate (Tegison)
    b   gentamycin, vancomycin, tobramycin, erythromycin
    c   growth hormone from pituitary glands, hepatitis B immune globulin
    d   Plavix, Ticlid

66. What interval must a donor wait between whole blood donations?
    a   more than 2 days
    b   4 weeks
    c   8 weeks
    d   16 weeks

II. Donor Identification & Selection   Donor Phlebotomy

67. What interval must a donor wait between a 2-unit red cell collection?
    a   more than 2 days
    b   4 weeks
    c   8 weeks
    d   16 weeks

68. What interval must a donor wait between plateletpheresis procedures?
    a   more than 2 days
    b   4 weeks
    c   8 weeks
    d   16 weeks

69. A 25-year-old female prospective donor confirmed she had a miscarriage 12 weeks ago and is not currently pregnant. What is the appropriate course of action?
    a   indefinitely deferred
    b   no deferral—the donor will be allowed to donate
    c   permanently deferred
    d   temporarily deferred

70. A 60-year-old male prospective plateletpheresis donor indicated he had taken aspirin 4 days ago for a headache. What is the appropriate course of action?
    a   indefinitely deferred
    b   no deferral—the donor will be allowed to donate
    c   permanently deferred
    d   temporarily deferred

71. A 40-year-old construction worker indicated he had very spicy Mexican food the day before for lunch and took Pepto-Bismol for heartburn. He would like to donate platelets via plateletpheresis. What is the appropriate course of action?
    a   indefinitely deferred
    b   no deferral—the donor will be allowed to donate
    c   permanently deferred
    d   temporarily deferred

72. A laboratory worker received the third immunization in the hepatitis B series a month ago. She would like to donate whole blood. What is the appropriate course of action?
    a   indefinitely deferred
    b   no deferral—the donor will be allowed to donate
    c   permanently deferred
    d   temporarily deferred

Donor Phlebotomy   **II. Donor Identification & Selection**

73. Six weeks ago, a phlebotomist received the hepatitis B immune globulin (HBIg) following an accidental needlestick from a known hepatitis B carrier. She would like to donate whole blood. What is the appropriate course of action?
    a   indefinitely deferred
    b   no deferral—the donor will be allowed to donate
    c   permanently deferred
    d   temporarily deferred

74. A medical laboratory technician student tested non-immune for chicken pox. She received the chicken pox vaccine 3 weeks ago and presented at the donor center to donate whole blood. What is the appropriate course of action?
    a   indefinitely deferred
    b   no deferral—the donor will be allowed to donate
    c   permanently deferred
    d   temporarily deferred

75. A 34-year-old fireworks technician was involved in a serious fireworks malfunction 6 months ago and was severely burned as a result. To repair his injuries, he underwent a series of skin grafts. The fireworks technician would like to donate whole blood and presented at the donor center. What is the appropriate course of action?
    a   indefinitely deferred
    b   no deferral—the donor will be allowed to donate
    c   permanently deferred
    d   temporarily deferred

76. Extended stay in which region may require donor deferral to reduce the risk of transmitting Creutzfeld-Jakob disease (CJD) and variant Creutzfeld-Jakob disease (vCJD) through the blood supply?
    a   Africa
    b   Australia
    c   South America
    d   United Kingdom

77. Which of the following clinical conditions would indefinitely defer a donor due to increased risk of CJD?
    a   ectopic pregnancy
    b   hemochromatosis
    c   human dura mater grafts
    d   potential rabies exposure

II. Donor Identification & Selection — Donor Phlebotomy

78. Which of the following clinical conditions would indefinitely defer a donor due to increased risk of CJD?
    a ectopic pregnancy
    b hemochromatosis
    c pituitary growth hormone therapy
    d potential rabies exposure

79. Malaria is a(n):
    a nosocomial infection
    b parasitic protozoan infection
    c sexually transmitted disease
    d transmissible spongiform encephalopathy

80. Travel to which region may require donor deferral to reduce the risk of transmitting malaria through the blood supply?
    a Africa
    b Australia
    c Europe
    d Russia

81. A 45-year-old donor immigrated from India 2 years ago. He would like to donate blood in response to an American Red Cross public service announcement regarding emergency need for blood. What is the appropriate course of action?
    a indefinitely deferred
    b no deferral—the donor will be allowed to donate
    c permanently deferred
    d temporarily deferred

82. Travel to which region may require donor deferral to reduce the risk of transmitting leishmaniasis through the blood supply?
    a Australia
    b Canada
    c Costa Rica
    d Middle East

83. Which group would be most at risk for leishmaniasis?
    a diabetic patients who took insulin produced in England
    b Samoan immigrants
    c patients treated with growth hormone obtained from human pituitary glands
    d veterans of Desert Storm

Donor Phlebotomy — **II. Donor Identification & Selection**

84. A sexually transmitted disease that may be spread through blood transfusion of a contaminated unit is:
    a *Chlamydia*
    b genital herpes
    c human papillomavirus
    d syphilis

85. A 25-year-old man presented at the donor center to donate a unit of whole blood. He confirmed a diagnosis of gonorrhea 2 years ago, which was successfully treated. What is the appropriate course of action?
    a indefinitely deferred
    b no deferral—the donor will be allowed to donate
    c permanently deferred
    d temporarily deferred

86. Which of the following may be transmitted through sexual contact and intravenous drug use?
    a babesiosis
    b Chagas disease
    c human immunodeficiency virus
    d malaria

87. Which of the following may be transmitted through sexual contact and intravenous drug use?
    a babesiosis
    b hepatitis B virus
    c *Leishmania* spp
    d malaria

88. Which of the following may be transmitted through sexual contact and intravenous drug use?
    a hepatitis C virus
    b *Leishmania* spp
    c malaria
    d *Plasmodium falciparum*

89. Which of the following organisms causes Acquired Immune Deficiency Syndrome (AIDS)?
    a Epstein-Barr virus
    b human immunodeficiency virus
    c varicella zoster virus
    d Zika virus

II. Donor Identification & Selection — Donor Phlebotomy

90. A 30-year-old woman presents at the donor center to donate whole blood for her father prior to an orthopedic surgery. When asked if she had any sexual contact with anyone who used needles to inject drugs or steroids not prescribed by a doctor, she responded yes. Her ex-fiancée was a professional body builder who was disqualified from competition for the use of anabolic steroids. She had not seen him in 6 months. What is the appropriate course of action?
    a indefinitely deferred
    b no deferral—the donor will be allowed to donate
    c permanently deferred
    d temporarily deferred

91. A 24-year-old woman presents at the donor center to donate whole blood. When asked if she had any sexual contact with anyone who has hemophilia or used clotting factor concentrates, she responded yes. Her husband has hemophilia B (Christmas disease) and receives regular prophylactic infusions of Factor IX. What is the appropriate course of action?
    a indefinitely deferred
    b no deferral—the donor will be allowed to donate
    c permanently deferred
    d temporarily deferred

92. A 40-year-old sexually active homosexual male presents at the blood center to donate blood. When asked if he has ever had sex with a man, he responds yes. This is relevant to blood supply safety because it is high-risk behavior contributing to the spread of:
    a babesiosis
    b Chagas disease
    c HCV
    d malaria

93. A 35-year-old female donor affirms that she tested positive for HIV 18 months ago. What is the appropriate course of action?
    a indefinitely deferred
    b no deferral—the donor will be allowed to donate
    c permanently deferred
    d temporarily deferred

94. A prospective donor with a history of Chagas disease should be:
    a indefinitely deferred
    b no deferral—the donor will be allowed to donate
    c permanently deferred
    d temporarily deferred

Donor Phlebotomy — II. Donor Identification & Selection

95. A prospective donor with a history of babesiosis should be deferred:
    a indefinitely deferred
    b no deferral—the donor will be allowed to donate
    c permanently deferred
    d temporarily deferred

96. A 21-year-old pre-med college student presented at the blood center to donate blood. She tested positive for individual donor nucleic acid test (ID-NAT) for ZIKV (Zika virus). The donor should be:
    a eligible to donate
    b temporarily deferred for at least 60 days
    c temporarily deferred for at least 120 days
    d indefinitely deferred

97. A 28-year-old female nurse presented at the blood center to donate blood. When asked if she was ever infected with the Zika virus, she responded yes following a trip 6 weeks ago to Nicaragua. The donor should be:
    a indefinitely deferred
    b no deferral—the donor will be allowed to donate
    c permanently deferred
    d temporarily deferred

98. What is the maximum upper age limit for eligible donors?
    a 60 years old
    b 65 years old
    c 70 years old
    d There is no upper age limit

99. To be eligible to donate, a blood donor's temperature cannot exceed:
    a 37.0°C
    b 37.5°C
    c 37.8°C
    d 38°C

100. To be eligible to donate, a blood donor's temperature cannot exceed:
    a 98.6°F
    b 99.3°F
    c 99.5°F
    d 99.9°F

101. According to the FDA, what is the minimum acceptable hemoglobin concentration for female allogeneic donor eligibility?
    a 12.0 g/dL
    b 12.5 g/dL
    c 13.0 g/dL
    d 13.5 g/dL

II. Donor Identification & Selection — Donor Phlebotomy

102. According to the FDA, what is the minimum acceptable hemoglobin concentration for male allogeneic donor eligibility?
    a 12.0 g/dL
    b 12.5 g/dL
    c 13.0 g/dL
    d 13.5 g/dL

103. Which of the following donors would be deferred based on blood pressure readings?
    a 95/75 mmHg
    b 110/85 mmHg
    c 175/90 mmHg
    d 185/90 mmHg

104. Based on current AABB Standards, which of the following donors would be acceptable?
    a 17-year-old high school senior, who weighs 125 lb and took aspirin for a headache that morning
    b 35-year-old construction worker who had a tetanus shot 2 weeks prior after stepping on a rusty nail
    c 28-year-old mother of 3 who miscarried 3 weeks prior
    d 55-year-old man who is scheduled to take his last dose of Bactrim for a urinary tract infection that evening

105. A donor would be temporarily deferred for:
    a history of hepatitis C infection
    b history of being HIV positive
    c receiving human derived growth hormones
    d incarceration for 4 days following a DUI arrest

106. How long must a donor be deferred following a diptheria, tetanus, pertussis (DTAP) vaccine?
    a no deferral
    b 1 month
    c 6 months
    d 1 year

107. A donor gave a plateletpheresis donation 24 hours ago. When would he be eligible to donate again?
    a today
    b in another 24 hours
    c 8 weeks from donation
    d 16 weeks from donation

Donor Phlebotomy   **III. Donor Blood Collection & Handling**

108. A donor gave a double unit of red blood cells using an apheresis machine 24 hours ago. When can they donate again?
    - a today
    - b in another 24 hours
    - c 8 weeks from donation
    - d 16 weeks from donation

109. A donor gave whole blood unit 24 hours ago. When can they donate again?
    - a today
    - b in another 24 hours
    - c 8 weeks from donation
    - d 16 weeks from donation

110. Which vaccination would cause a 4 week deferral:
    - a rubella
    - b influenza
    - c tetanus
    - d anthrax

111. The means by which hepatitis B virus is spread is/are:
    - a contaminated food
    - b blood exposure only
    - c sexual intercourse and blood exposure
    - d airborne transmission

112. The donor's arms should be checked for signs of intravenous drug use:
    - a during blood collection
    - b when blood collection is completed
    - c before phlebotomy occurs
    - d as donor is leaving the blood drive

III. Donor Blood Collection & Handling

113. Blood collected from a voluntary donor that may be separated into component parts is termed:
    - a cryoprecipitated antihemophilic factor (AHF)
    - b platelet concentrates
    - c single-donor plasma
    - d whole blood

114. What temperature should whole blood be stored at?
    - a 1-6°C
    - b 2-8°C
    - c 3-9°C
    - d 4-10°C

III. Donor Blood Collection & Handling — Donor Phlebotomy

115. What is the shelf life of a unit of whole blood collected into citrate-phosphate-dextrose-adenine (CPDA-1)?
    a   2 weeks
    b   21 days
    c   28 days
    d   35 days

116. Platelet concentrates must be stored at what temperature?
    a   −80°C
    b   1-6°C
    c   20-24°C
    d   37°C

117. Platelet storage requires:
    a   continuous agitation
    b   deglycerolization
    c   irradiation
    d   submersion in a 37°C water bath

118. Fresh frozen plasma must be stored at what temperature?
    a   −18°C for 1 year
    b   −65°C for 10 years
    c   1-6°C
    d   20-24°C

119. Which of the following is performed to ensure donor staff retain the ability to perform their jobs well?
    a   competency assessment
    b   disaster planning
    c   equipment maintenance
    d   risk assessment

120. Which of the following may be used to identify a unit of blood?
    a   alphanumeric system
    b   color-coded system according to blood types
    c   donor initials
    d   last 4 digits of a donor's social security number

121. Which of the following must be clearly identified and linked to the donor?
    a   donor record
    b   donor's physician's contact information
    c   recipient's blood type
    d   recipient's HIV status

Donor Phlebotomy   **III. Donor Blood Collection & Handling**

122. Why is it important to maintain donor records correlating to donated blood or blood components?
    - a to insure the donor's safety
    - b to insure the recipient's safety
    - c to justify the number of blood bank employees
    - d to justify the number of laboratory supervisors

123. When applying labels to donated blood products, what should be labeled with the same identification number?
    - a blood bags, donor record, and pilot tubes
    - b daily donor log, component bags and pilot tubes
    - c daily donor log, donor record and blood bag
    - d daily donor log, pilot tubes, and donor evaluation card

124. The technique used to prepare a venipuncture site prior to donating a unit of blood is:
    - a antiseptic
    - b aseptic
    - c aerobic
    - d anaerobic

125. A phlebotomist uses a blood pressure cuff as a tourniquet during a phlebotomy to collect a unit of whole blood. The blood pressure cuff should be inflated to no more than:
    - a 40-60 mmHg
    - b 60-80 mmHg
    - c 80-90 mmHg
    - d 100-110 mmHg

126. What compound is typically used by blood centers to prepare a venipuncture site prior to donation of a unit of blood?
    - a acetone
    - b alcohol
    - c iodine
    - d tincture of green soap

127. What is the minimal length of time a phlebotomist must scrub a venipuncture site in preparation for collecting a unit of whole blood?
    - a 15 seconds
    - b 30 seconds
    - c 60 seconds
    - d 120 seconds

III. Donor Blood Collection & Handling — Donor Phlebotomy

128. After scrubbing the venipuncture site, the phlebotomist must apply an iodophor compound beginning at:
    a the periphery of the scrubbed area and moving into the puncture site using a concentric circular motion
    b the puncture site and moving outward using a concentric circular motion
    c right angles to the puncture site moving rapidly back and forth
    d once the site is scrubbed, the iodophor compound is unnecessary

129. Immediately following donation of a unit of whole blood, a donor experiences sweating and vomiting. What category of reaction is the donor likely experiencing?
    a mild
    b moderate
    c normal
    d severe

130. Immediately following donation of a unit of whole blood, a donor loses consciousness. The donor's pulse rate and systolic blood pressure are also decreased. What category of reaction is the donor likely experiencing?
    a mild
    b moderate
    c normal
    d severe

131. Immediately following a donation of a unit of whole blood, a donor loses consciousness and begins convulsing. What category of reaction is the donor likely experiencing?
    a mild
    b moderate
    c normal
    d severe

132. According to AABB Standards, what is the maximum amount of blood that may be collected per kilogram of body weight?
    a 9.0 mL
    b 9.5 mL
    c 10.0 mL
    d 10.5 mL

133. In the United States, how much blood is typically withdrawn during a routine whole blood collection procedure?
    a 350 mL
    b 375 mL
    c 400 mL
    d 450 mL

Donor Phlebotomy   **III. Donor Blood Collection & Handling**

134. What is the acceptable range of variation in whole blood collection procedures?
    - a ±5%
    - b ±10%
    - c ±15%
    - d ±20%

135. A unit of whole blood was collected into a 450 mL bag. When measured, the amount collected was 520 mL. What is the appropriate course of action?
    - a discard the unit
    - b label the unit "RBCs High Volume" and submit for processing, including physician review and approval for use
    - c label the unit "RBCs Low Volume" and submit for processing, including physician review and approval for use
    - d process the unit without special labelling

136. A unit of whole blood was collected into a 500 mL bag. When measured, the amount collected was 440 mL. What is the appropriate course of action?
    - a discard the unit
    - b label the unit "RBCs High Volume" and submit for processing, including physician review and approval for use
    - c label the unit "RBCs Low Volume" and submit for processing, including physician review and approval for use
    - d process the unit without special labelling

137. Bags used for whole blood collection from volunteer donors must be approved for use by the:
    - a Centers for Disease Control (CDC)
    - b donor
    - c pathologist
    - d Food and Drug Administration (FDA)

138. Which agency publishes requirements for labelling of blood and blood components?
    - a Centers for Disease Control (CDC)
    - b Food and Drug Administration (FDA)
    - c National Institutes of Health (NIH)
    - d Occupational Safety and Health Administration (OSHA)

139. What is the first action a phlebotomist should take upon completion of the whole blood donation process?
    - a elevate the patient's feet
    - b elevate the patient's head
    - c provide the donor with fluids
    - d withdraw the needle and activate the sheathing mechanism

III. Donor Blood Collection & Handling Donor Phlebotomy

140. Before discharging a donor, the staff should instruct the donor to avoid heavy exercise for at least:
    a 30 minutes
    b 45 minutes
    c 1 hour
    d 3 hours

141. Before discharging a donor, the staff should instruct the donor to avoid smoking for at least:
    a 30 minutes
    b 1 hour
    c 2 hours
    d 4 hours

142. Before discharging a donor, the staff should instruct the donor to increase their intake of:
    a fluids
    b glucose
    c protein
    d starches

143. Before discharging a donor, the staff should instruct the donor to avoid intake of:
    a alcohol
    b glucose
    c protein
    d starches

144. Units of red blood cells must be stored at a temperature maintained between:
    a 1-6°C
    b 1-10°C
    c 12-18°C
    d 20-24°C

145. Which testing is required for all donated blood products?
    a CMV
    b glucose
    c HIV
    d vCJD

146. What should blood donor collection kits be inspected for prior to phlebotomy?
    a unique unit numbers are applied
    b satellite bag is marked as recovered plasma
    c leaks in bags and discoloration
    d that kit fits on collection scale

Donor Phlebotomy   **III. Donor Blood Collection & Handling**

147. A donor is experiencing severe pain that is not subsiding following the venipuncture. The likely cause is:
    a needle is against the interior vein wall.
    b trauma to a nerve
    c inadequate blood flow
    d reaction to iodine scrub

148. The donor phlebotomist should periodically mix the blood with anticoagulant during the donation to prevent:
    a clotting
    b contamination
    c hemoconcentration
    d hemolysis

149. "Antecubital" means:
    a behind the elbow
    b below the skin
    c in front of the elbow
    d on the surface of the skin

150. "Fossa" means:
    a deep depression
    b deep exterior
    c shallow depression
    d thin superficial

151. The antecubital fossa is the:
    a deep depression located behind the elbow
    b deep exterior located in front of the elbow
    c superficial surface located behind the elbow
    d shallow depression located in front of the elbow

152. Approximately 70% of the population displays a venous pattern resembling which of the following letters?
    a E
    b H
    c M
    d N

III. Donor Blood Collection & Handling
Donor Phlebotomy

153. In the figure below, what is the structure indicated by the arrow?

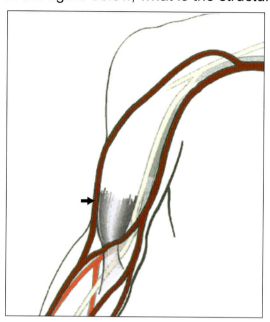

- a   basilic vein
- b   brachial artery
- c   cephalic vein
- d   median nerve

154. In the figure below, what is the structure indicated by the arrow?

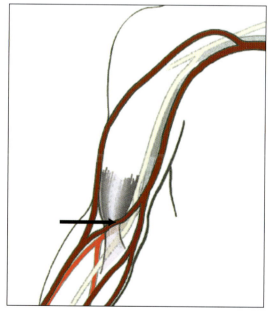

- a   basilic vein
- b   brachial artery
- c   median nerve
- d   median cubital vein

155. In the figure below, what is the structure indicated by the arrow?

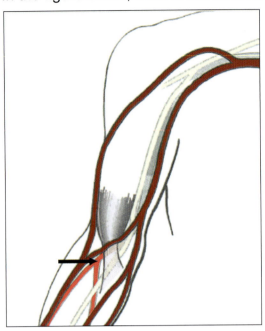

- a   basilic vein
- b   brachial artery
- c   cephalic vein
- d   median cubital vein

156. In the figure below, what is the structure indicated by the arrow?

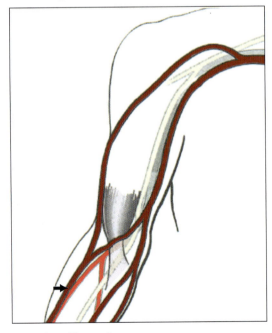

- a   basilic vein
- b   brachial artery
- c   cephalic vein
- d   median nerve

III. Donor Blood Collection & Handling — Donor Phlebotomy

157. In the figure below, what is the structure indicated by the arrow?

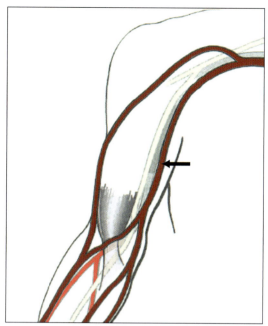

- a basilic vein
- b bicipital aponeurosis
- c brachial artery
- d median nerve

158. In the figure below, what is the structure indicated by the arrow?

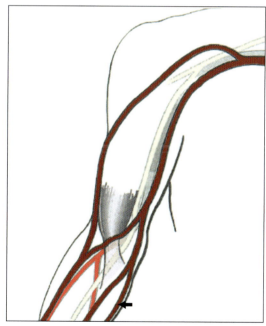

- a basilic vein
- b bicipital aponeurosis
- c brachial artery
- d median nerve

Donor Phlebotomy — III. Donor Blood Collection & Handling

159. To examine by touch or feel is to:
    a palate
    b palpate
    c palpitate
    d patency

160. A phlebotomist ties a tourniquet on a patient's arm. The phlebotomist palpates the vessels listed below. All of the vessels are the same size. Which is the most suitable for venipuncture?
    a basilic vein
    b cephalic vein
    c median vein of the forearm
    d median cubital vein

161. A phlebotomist ties a tourniquet on a patient's arm. The phlebotomist palpates the vessels listed below. All of the vessels are the same size. Which is the least suitable for venipuncture?
    a basilic vein
    b cephalic vein
    c median vein of the forearm
    d median cubital vein

162. A phlebotomist ties a tourniquet on a patient's left arm. The phlebotomist cannot palpate any veins suitable for venipuncture in the antecubital area (antecubital fossa). What site should the phlebotomist examine next for a suitable vein?
    a left antecubital area (antecubital fossa)
    b right antecubital area (antecubital fossa)
    c left wrist
    d right wrist

163. During a venipuncture procedure, a tourniquet should be tied:
    a 3-4 inches above the intended puncture site
    b for at least 2 minutes before releasing
    c like a shoelace
    d tight enough to stop all blood flow

164. Which of the following senses will the phlebotomist rely on most when selecting a site for venipuncture?
    a hearing
    b seeing
    c smell
    d touch

III. Donor Blood Collection & Handling — Donor Phlebotomy

165. When palpating for a vein, the phlebotomist should use her:
    a   index finger
    b   middle finger
    c   ring finger
    d   thumb

166. When examining a venipuncture sight, what vein characteristics does the phlebotomist palpate for?
    a   depth, direction, ease of visual recognition
    b   depth, direction, shape
    c   depth, direction, size
    d   depth, ease of visual recognition, size

167. According to CLSI Standards, which vessel must a phlebotomist attempt to locate in both arms before considering alternative venipuncture sites?
    a   brachial artery
    b   basilic vein
    c   median vein of the forearm
    d   median cubital vein

168. Which of the following veins of the antecubital area (antecubital fossa) is characteristically most stationary?
    a   basilic vein
    b   cephalic vein
    c   dorsal metacarpal vein
    d   median cubital vein

169. Which of the following structures of the antecubital area (antecubital fossa) is characteristically closer to the skin surface?
    a   bicipital aponeurosis
    b   brachial artery
    c   median cubital vein
    d   median nerve

170. The term that applies to a vein being open and turgid is:
    a   palpate
    b   palpitate
    c   patent
    d   pulse

171. What structure provides support to the median cubital vein in the antecubital area (antecubital fossa)?
    a   bicipital aponeurosis
    b   brachial artery
    c   median cutaneous nerve
    d   radial artery

Donor Phlebotomy — III. Donor Blood Collection & Handling

172. What is the correct sequence of the following steps in a venipuncture procedure?
     a apply alcohol, palpate site, apply tourniquet
     b apply tourniquet, palpate site, release tourniquet
     c palpate site, apply alcohol, apply tourniquet
     d palpate site, apply tourniquet, apply alcohol

173. What is the correct sequence of the following steps in a venipuncture procedure?
     a anchor the vein, insert the needle, uncap the needle
     b anchor the vein, uncap the needle, insert the needle
     c uncap the needle, anchor the vein, insert the needle
     d uncap the needle, insert the needle, anchor the vein

174. How should a patient's arm be positioned during venipuncture using a vein in the antecubital area (antecubital fossa)? The bicep to forearm should create a:
     a 30° angle
     b 45° angle
     c 90° angle
     d straight line from shoulder to wrist

175. Positioning the patient's arm correctly and supporting the elbow with a pillow or rolled towel will help to:
     a allow the veins to roll
     b anchor the veins
     c prevent hemolysis
     d prevent syncope

176. When anchoring a vein in the antecubital area (antecubital fossa) prior to venipuncture, the phlebotomist should place the thumb approximately 2 inches:
     a above the puncture site
     b below the puncture site
     c below the puncture site and the index finger above the puncture site
     d below the puncture site and the middle finger above the puncture site

177. When anchoring a vein in the antecubital area (antecubital fossa) prior to venipuncture, the phlebotomist should pull the skin toward the:
     a lateral side of the arm
     b medial side of the arm
     c patient's shoulder
     d patient's wrist

III. Donor Blood Collection & Handling — Donor Phlebotomy

178. During venipuncture, the needle should be inserted with the bevel turned:
     a down
     b up
     c toward the left
     d toward the right

179. During venipuncture, what angle should the needle be inserted, relative to the patient's arm?
     a 0-10°
     b 5-10°
     c 15-30°
     d 30-45°

180. During venipuncture, how should the needle be positioned immediately before the puncture, relative to the vein selected?
     a parallel, 1 inch above
     b parallel, 1 inch below
     c perpendicular
     d same direction

181. After the needle is uncapped, the phlebotomist should inspect the needle:
     a by retracting the sheath to be sure it will spring back after the needle is disengaged
     b by touching the shaft to be sure there are no burrs or gouges
     c by touching the tip to be sure there are no burrs or filaments
     d visually

182. A phlebotomist uncaps a needle and determines that a burr is present. She should:
     a determine the size of the burr; if it is small, use that needle
     b determine the size of the burr, if it is large, discard it
     c discard the needle and take another to use
     d discard the needle and notify the hospital's safety officer

183. After needle withdrawal, patients should be instructed to apply pressure to the puncture site using the gauze and:
     a a bandage
     b by bending the arm at the elbow, securing the gauze
     c keeping the arm straight
     d while holding the arm below the heart

184. Following needle withdrawal, the patient should be instructed to keep his arm:
     a bent with an alcohol prep pad positioned over the puncture site
     b bent with a dry gauze pad positioned over the puncture site
     c straight and apply pressure using an alcohol prep pad
     d straight and apply pressure using a dry gauze pad

Donor Phlebotomy   **III. Donor Blood Collection & Handling**

185. If a tourniquet is properly applied, it will:
    - a restrict all blood flow
    - b restrict arterial blood flow, but not venous blood flow
    - c restrict venous blood flow, but not arterial blood flow
    - d be tied like a shoelace

186. Which of the following may be used if a tourniquet is not available?
    - a glove
    - b rubber tubing
    - c sphygmomanometer
    - d splint

187. Which of the following needle gauges is used most often to collect units of blood from blood donors?
    - a 16-18
    - b 19-20
    - c 21-22
    - d 23-24

188. The standard for measuring the diameter of the lumen of a needle is the needle:
    - a bore
    - b brand
    - c gauge
    - d length

189. The internal space of a needle is the:
    - a bevel
    - b brand
    - c gauge
    - d lumen

190. Which of the following needle gauges represents the largest interior diameter?
    - a 18
    - b 19
    - c 20
    - d 21

191. Which of the following needle gauges represents the smallest interior diameter?
    - a 20
    - b 21
    - c 22
    - d 23

IV. Donor Considerations

192. A donor donates blood for her own use. This type of donation is:
    a   allogeneic
    b   autologous
    c   directed
    d   voluntary

193. Which of the following transfusions offers the advantage of minimizing disease transmission to the recipient?
    a   allogeneic
    b   autologous
    c   directed
    d   voluntary

194. Which of the following disadvantages is associated with autologous blood transfusion?
    a   increased cost and unit waste
    b   increased contamination and unit waste
    c   increased contamination and misidentification
    d   increased alloimmunization and contamination

195. Which of the following is required for a donor to donate an autologous unit of blood?
    a   a prescription from the patient's physician
    b   approval from the blood bank medical director
    c   consent form from the intended recipient
    d   must be age 16 or older

196. A donor presents at the donor center for preoperative autologous blood donation. What is the minimum hematocrit the donor may have to be authorized by donor room staff to donate a unit of blood?
    a   30%
    b   33%
    c   36%
    d   39%

197. At least how many hours in advance of the anticipated surgery or transfusion must a unit of blood for autologous blood donation must be collected?
    a   24
    b   48
    c   72
    d   96

198. A donor presents at the donor center with a physician's order to collect a unit of blood for autologous donation. The donor weights 95 lbs (43 kg). The appropriate volume of whole blood to collect from this donor is:
    a   0 mL because the donor does not meet the weight requirement
    b   225 mL
    c   387 mL
    d   450 mL

199. A unit of whole blood containing 400 mL was collected from a donor for autologous donation. What is the appropriate course of action for the donor room staff?
    a   discard the unit due to low volume collection
    b   follow routine procedures for allogeneic blood donation
    c   label the unit "Low Volume"
    d   label the unit "Low Volume" and "For Autologous Use Only"

200. A donor presents at the donor center with a prescription from her physician for collection of a unit of blood for autologous blood transfusion. The donor has a temperature of 38°C. What is the appropriate course of action?
    a   accept the donor and collect the unit, per the physician's order
    b   collect the unit and label the unit "Collected from Febrile Donor"
    c   defer the donor
    d   report the donor to the Centers for Disease Control

201. A unit of whole blood collected from a donor specifically for a particular patient is:
    a   autologous
    b   allogeneic
    c   directed
    d   involuntary

202. A donor presents at the donor center with a physician's order to collect a unit of blood for directed donation. The donor weights 98 lbs. (44.5 kg). The appropriate volume of whole blood to collect from this donor is:
    a   0 mL because the donor does not meet the weight requirement
    b   225 mL
    c   387 mL
    d   450 mL

203. A physician prescribes routine withdrawal of 500 mL of blood for a patient as a treatment for a pathologic condition. This is termed:
    a   autologous blood transfusion
    b   allogeneic blood transfusion
    c   malpractice
    d   therapeutic phlebotomy

IV. Donor Considerations — Donor Phlebotomy

204. Which of the following conditions is often treated by therapeutic phlebotomy?
   - a hereditary hemochromatosis and polycythemia vera
   - b hereditary hemochromatosis and idiopathic thrombocytopenic purpura
   - c Hodgkin lymphoma and polycythemia vera
   - d non-Hodgkin lymphoma and *Pneumocystis jiroveci*

205. To prevent an adverse donor reaction, donors are encouraged to:
   - a eat within 4-6 hours of donation
   - b excercise vigorously at least 12 hours prior to donation
   - c fast for 12 hours prior to donation
   - d fast for 8 hours prior to donation

206. A phlebotomist performs a venipuncture as part of a whole blood collection. The blood in the tubing is bright cherry-red and the donor bag fills in less than 4 minutes. What is the appropriate course of action for the phlebotomist?
   - a apply pressure to the venipuncture site while elevating the donor's arm
   - b loosen the donor's clothing around the neck and refer the donor to a neurologist
   - c lower the donor's head, apply a cold compress to her head
   - d provide routine post-phlebotomy care to the donor

207. Which donor reactions are most commonly reported among first-time donors and females?
   - a arterial puncture and hematoma
   - b citrate reaction and fainting
   - c presyncopal symptoms and small hematomas
   - d syncopy symptoms and local nerve injury

208. Donor room phlebotomists should remain current in:
   - a Advanced Life Support (ALS)
   - b Basic Life Support (BLS)
   - c Certified Nurse Assistant (CNA)
   - d Cardiopulmonary Resuscitation (CPR)

209. A donor collection technique involving the separation and collection of a specific blood component from whole blood and the return of the remaining blood to the donor is:
   - a apheresis
   - b aphilopony
   - c aphonogilia
   - d aphosphogenic

210. Which of the following plateletpheresis procedures differs from whole blood donation procedures?
   - a donor education
   - b informed consent
   - c testing required on donated component
   - d time between donations

Donor Phlebotomy   **V. Donor Center Operations**

211. A common adverse effect of blood donation is:
    a   HCV infection
    b   HBV infection
    c   hematoma
    d   synteny

212. After venipuncture, the patient is diaphoretic and pale. The phlebotomist should:
    a   apply ice to the venipuncture site
    b   call a code
    c   disregard these symptoms because they are normal after a venipuncture
    d   lower the patient's head and instruct her to breathe deeply

213. During a venipuncture, the patient vomits. The phlebotomist should:
    a   complete the procedure and notify housekeeping
    b   discontinue the venipuncture immediately
    c   hand the patient an emesis basin and complete the venipuncture
    d   hand the patient a tissue and complete the venipuncture

214. What response may some patients have at the sight of his/her blood being drawn?
    a   hematoma
    b   hemolysis
    c   syncope
    d   synergy

V. Donor Center Operations

215. Where are enacted federal laws published?
    a   Centers for Disease Control (CDC) web site
    b   Federal Bank Reserve (FBR)
    c   National Institutes of Health (NIH)
    d   United States Code (USC)

216. Which agency establishes regulations to ensure compliance with federal law as it relates to blood and blood products?
    a   Centers for Disease Control (CDC)
    b   Federal Bank Reserve (FBR)
    c   Food and Drug Administration (FDA)
    d   Occupational Safety and Health Administration (OSHA)

217. Where are rules governing the collection, storage and use of blood and blood products detailed?
    a   Centers for Disease Control (CDC) web site
    b   Code of Federal Regulations (CFR)
    c   Clinical Laboratory Improvement Amendments (CLIA) web site
    d   United States Code (USC)

V. Donor Center Operations — Donor Phlebotomy

218. Which of the following agencies serves as a volunteer accreditation program for blood banks?
    a   AABB
    b   Centers for Disease Control (CDC)
    c   Clinical Laboratory Improvement Amendments (CLIA)
    d   National Accrediting Agency for Clinical Laboratory Sciences (NAACLS)

219. How frequently should temperatures of refrigerators, freezers and water baths be monitored to be consistent with recommended quality control performance parameters?
    a   daily
    b   weekly
    c   monthly
    d   quarterly

220. What is a nonconforming event?
    a   a peer review of the daily quality control
    b   an incident in which the tech did not follow SOP
    c   a new FDA regulation being implemented
    d   when a donor is unable to fill out their entire questionnaire

221. Wearing gloves during donor phlebotomy procedures is mandated by:
    a   College of American Pathologists
    b   National Accrediting Agency for Clinical Laboratory Sciences
    c   Occupational Safety & Health Administration
    d   The Joint Commission (TJC)

222. Manufacturing defects in needles are best screened for every:
    a   day
    b   month
    c   new lot number
    d   venipuncture attempt

223. A phlebotomist selects a needle for a venipuncture procedure. She notices that the seal surrounding the needle is loosened. The phlebotomist should:
    a   discard the needle and blood bag
    b   notify security
    c   notify her supervisor
    d   use the needle

224. Quality assurance indicators must be:
    a   descriptive & specific
    b   general & published
    c   published & specific
    d   specific & measurable

225. A program designed to track outcomes through scheduled audits to continually improve the quality of patient care is:
    a   quality assurance
    b   quality control
    c   continuous quality improvement
    d   total quality management

226. The term used to denote specific procedures within a program designed to ensure quality patient care is:
    a   quality assurance
    b   quality control
    c   continuous quality improvement
    d   total quality management

227. A civil lawsuit based on improper treatment or negligence by a professional person is called:
    a   assault & battery
    b   malpractice
    c   negligence
    d   respondeat superior

228. Failure to exercise reasonable skill in performing a task is called:
    a   assault & battery
    b   malpractice
    c   negligence
    d   respondeat superior

229. The federal bill establishing regulations for clinical laboratories in the United States is the:
    a   Clinical Laboratory Improvement Amendments (CLIA) of 1988
    b   Clinical Laboratory Improvement Amendments (CLIA) of 1998
    c   Patient Bill of Rights
    d   Health Information Portability & Accountability Act

230. Which of the following agencies regulates and supervises clinical laboratories?
    a   Centers for Disease Control
    b   Food & Drug Administration
    c   Internal Revenue Service
    d   Social Security

231. The voluntary nongovernmental group charged with establishing standards for the operation of hospitals and other health related facilities and services is:
    a   Centers for Disease Control & Prevention (CDC)
    b   College of American Pathologists (CAP)
    c   Occupational Safety & Health Administration (OSHA)
    d   The Joint Commission (TJC)

V. Donor Center Operations

232. An organization that provides standards for quality improvement specific to clinical laboratories and conducts proficiency testing and laboratory inspections is the:
   a   Centers for Disease Control & Prevention (CDC)
   b   Centers for Medicare & Medicaid Services (CMS)
   c   College of American Pathologists (CAP)
   d   Clinical & Laboratory Standards Institute (CLSI)

233. Which of the following organizations is an outgrowth of the American Society for Clinical Pathology (ASCP)?
   a   Centers for Disease Control & Prevention (CDC)
   b   Centers for Medicare & Medicaid Services (CMS)
   c   College of American Pathologists (CAP)
   d   Clinical & Laboratory Standards Institute (CLSI)

234. The United States governmental agency responsible for regulating the safety and health of workers is:
   a   American Society for Clinical Pathology (ASCP)
   b   College of American Pathologists (CAP)
   c   Occupational Safety & Health Administration (OSHA)
   d   The Joint Commission (TJC)

235. Labeling of hazardous materials is required by:
   a   OSHA's Bloodborne Pathogens Standard
   b   OSHA's Hazardous Communication Standard
   c   Patient's Bill of Rights
   d   universal precautions

236. Which of the following organizations mandated universal precautions?
   a   Centers for Disease Control & Prevention (CDC)
   b   College of American Pathologists (CAP)
   c   National Accrediting Agency for Clinical Laboratory Sciences (NAACLS)
   d   Occupational Safety & Health Administration (OSHA)

237. The 2001 Needlestick Safety & Prevention Act requires:
   a   a written exposure control plan & employee input on selecting engineering controls
   b   a written exposure control plan & weekly fire drills
   c   weekly fire drills & green sharps containers
   d   weekly fire drills & purple sharps containers

238. Which federal agency administrates the Centers for Disease Control & Prevention (CDC)?
   a   Department of Defense
   b   Department of Education
   c   Department of Health & Human Services
   d   Department of Homeland Security

239. The Centers for Disease Control & Prevention (CDC) are responsible for:
    a   educating the American public & ensuring equal access to education
    b   ensuring the safety of the American public
    c   protecting the American public, through the use of military force
    d   researching & controlling diseases

240. Which of the following agencies first recommended universal precautions?
    a   College of American Pathologists (CAP)
    b   Centers for Disease Control & Prevention (CDC)
    c   National Accrediting Agency for Clinical Laboratory Sciences (NAACLS)
    d   Occupational Safety & Health Administration (OSHA)

241. Any substance that can be harmful to a person's health is called a:
    a   bacteria
    b   biohazard
    c   body substance isolation
    d   universal precautions

242. Universal precautions prevents the spread of which of the following pathogens?
    a   acid-fast bacillus
    b   bloodborne
    c   respiratory
    d   tuberculosis

243. The term, "bloodborne pathogens" most commonly refers to:
    a   hepatitis A virus (HAV), hepatitis B virus (HBV) & hepatitis C virus (HCV)
    b   hepatitis A virus (HAV), hepatitis B virus (HBV) & *Plasmodium falciparum*
    c   hepatitis B virus (HBV), hepatitis C virus (HCV) & *Clostridioides difficile*
    d   hepatitis B virus (HBV), hepatitis C virus (HCV) & human immunodeficiency virus (HIV)

244. Under universal precautions, which patients are considered potentially infectious?
    a   all of them
    b   none of them
    c   patients infected with HBV
    d   patients infected with HIV

245. What term may be used instead of "universal protections"?
    a   airborne transmission precautions
    b   category-specific isolation
    c   standard precautions
    d   transmission-based precautions

246. Under standard precautions, when should a phlebotomist change gloves?
    a   after every patient
    b   after every second patient
    c   after every third patient
    d   only when soiled

V. Donor Center Operations
Donor Phlebotomy

247. Which of the following fire extinguisher contents is appropriate to use on a Class A fire?
    a carbon dioxide
    b halon
    c metal X
    d pressurized water

248. What are the contents of a multipurpose (ABC) fire extinguisher?
    a carbon dioxide
    b dry chemical
    c halon
    d metal X

249. Needle safety features are mandated by:
    a Centers for Disease Control & Prevention (CDC)
    b Centers for Medicare & Medicaid Services (CMS)
    c Needlestick Safety & Prevention Act (2001)
    d OSHA's Bloodborne Pathogens Standard (1991)

250. Needle safety features must:
    a be an accessory to the evacuated tube system
    b be removable
    c create a barrier between the needle and the patient's arm
    d create a barrier between the needle and the phlebotomist's hands

251. Needle safety features must:
    a be an accessory to the evacuated tube system
    b be removable
    c create a barrier between the needle and the patient's arm
    d permanently contain a contaminated needle once a safety feature is activated

252. Which of the following practices must be eliminated to prevent needlestick injury?
    a disposing needles in sharps containers
    b handwashing
    c recapping needles
    d using transfer devices with syringes

253. According to the National Fire Protection Agency (NFPA), which of the following fire classifications occur with ordinary combustibles?
    a A
    b B
    c C
    d D

254. What does the acronym PASS stand for in the event of a fire?
- a pull nozzle, aim pin, squeeze handle, sweep side-to-side
- b pull nozzle, aim pin, sweep side-to-side, squeeze handle
- c pull pin, aim nozzle, squeeze handle, sweep side-to-side
- d pull pin, aim nozzle, sweep side-to-side, squeeze handle

255. Chemical spill clean-up kits contain materials that:
- a absorb & activate
- b absorb & neutralize
- c exude & activate
- d exude & neutralize

256. Chemical disposal is regulated by:
- a Centers for Disease Control & Protection
- b Department of Transportation
- c Environmental Protection Agency
- d National Fire Protection Agency

257. The instrument used to separate blood specimens into component parts is the:
- a centrifuge
- b pneumatic tube
- c sedimentation rate tube rack
- d sphygmomanometer

258. The symbol in the figure below communicates:

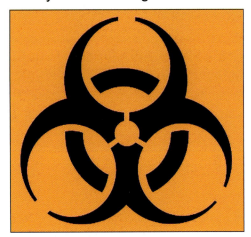

- a biohazard
- b flammability
- c mechanical hazard
- d radiation hazard

V. Donor Center Operations — Donor Phlebotomy

259. An infection control program that includes monitoring specific patient population groups and classifications of infection is called:
    a   surveillance
    b   susceptibility
    c   viability
    d   virulence

260. Three components in the chain of infection are:
    a   source, mode of transmission, susceptible host
    b   source, mode of transmission, virulence
    c   source, viability, virulence
    d   source, viability, mode of transmission

261. To prevent the spread of infection, the chain of infection must be interrupted in at least how many points?
    a   1
    b   2
    c   3
    d   4

262. Microbes capable of causing infection or disease are called:
    a   anaerobic
    b   pasteurized
    c   pathogens
    d   normal flora

263. A disease resulting from the transmission of a pathogenic organism by direct or indirect contact or via airborne routes is called:
    a   bloodborne
    b   communicable
    c   terminal
    d   viable

264. What percentage of patients admitted to the hospital in the United States contract a nosocomial infection?
    a   1-3%
    b   3-5%
    c   5-8.5%
    d   10-15%

265. The general term that applies to infections acquired in hospitals and other health care delivery facilities is:
    a   bloodborne
    b   chain of infection
    c   transmission based
    d   healthcare-associated infection (HAI)

Donor Phlebotomy — **V. Donor Center Operations**

266. A pathogen's ability to survive is:
    a viability
    b virulence
    c vicarious
    d villosity

267. Items that harbor pathogenic bacteria and are capable of transmitting infection are called:
    a aerobic
    b anaerobic
    c fomites
    d opportunists

268. Under standard precautions, which patients are considered potentially infectious?
    a all of them
    b none of them
    c patients infected with HBV
    d patients infected with HIV

269. Items provided by an employer to protect the health care worker from contact with infectious materials are called:
    a alcohol-based antiseptic hand cleaners
    b bloodborne pathogens
    c engineering controls
    d personal protective equipment

270. A phlebotomist should never:
    a adjust the volume on a patient's television
    b use an alcohol rinse solution as a substitute for handwashing
    c use a foam solution as a substitute for handwashing
    d recap a needle after use

271. Under standard precautions, when should a phlebotomist change gloves?
    a after every patient
    b after every second patient
    c after every third patient
    d only when soiled

272. Under standard precautions, when should a phlebotomist sanitize his/her hands?
    a after every patient, once gloves are removed
    b between patients, without removing gloves
    c only if the gloves are soiled
    d whenever the phlebotomist wants to

V. Donor Center Operations — Donor Phlebotomy

273. Health care workers are required to adhere to standard precautions guidelines to avoid:
     a   contact with pathogenic organisms
     b   infection with nonpathogenic organisms
     c   medication errors
     d   patient identification errors

274. To prevent the spread of infection by ingestion in the clinical laboratory phlebotomists should never:
     a   handle a stick of gum
     b   open centrifuges before they have stopped spinning
     c   pop off the stoppers of evacuated tubes
     d   rub their eyes

275. To prevent the spread of infection by an airborne route in the clinical laboratory, phlebotomists should never:
     a   handle a stick of gum
     b   handle broken glass
     c   open centrifuges before they have stopped spinning
     d   rub their eyes

276. To prevent the spread of infection by a permucosal route in the clinical laboratory, phlebotomists should never:
     a   handle a stick of gum
     b   handle broken glass
     c   open centrifuges before they have stopped spinning
     d   rub their eyes

277. Which of the following would be classified as an engineering control, according to OSHA's Bloodborne Pathogens Standard?
     a   gloves
     b   gown
     c   handwashing
     d   self-sheathing needle

278. Which of the following would be classified as a work practice control, according to OSHA's Bloodborne Pathogens Standard?
     a   handwashing policies
     b   mandatory use of gown
     c   self-sheathing needle
     d   splash shields

Donor Phlebotomy   **V. Donor Center Operations**

279. Under standard precautions, once a blood collection procedure is completed, the specimen labeled and waste discarded, the phlebotomist should remove his/her:
    - a   gloves
    - b   gown
    - c   N-95 fit-tested mask
    - d   safety goggles

280. If gloves are removed properly, the end result is:
    - a   1 glove inside the other, with contaminated surfaces on the inside
    - b   1 glove inside the other, with contaminated surfaces on the outside
    - c   2 gloves discarded separately
    - d   2 gloves discarded separately inside out

281. Chemical compounds used to remove or kill microorganisms on work surfaces or instruments are called:
    - a   aerosols
    - b   antiseptics
    - c   disinfectants
    - d   phloxine B

282. Chemicals that may be used on human skin to inhibit the growth and development of microorganisms, but not necessarily kill them, are:
    - a   aerosols
    - b   antiseptics
    - c   disinfectants
    - d   phenols

283. Which of the following is an antiseptic?
    - a   chloramine
    - b   formaldehyde
    - c   hypochlorite solution
    - d   70% isopropyl alcohol

284. Which of the following compounds is a disinfectant?
    - a   70% ethyl alcohol
    - b   70% isopropyl alcohol
    - c   hypochlorite solution
    - d   tincture of iodine

285. One of the most powerful strategies to prevent the spread of infection is:
    - a   hand hygiene consistent with Centers for Disease Control & Prevention guidelines
    - b   National Institute for Occupational Safety & Health approved N95 fit-tested mask
    - c   requiring the use of a new gown with every patient
    - d   reverse isolation

V. Donor Center Operations — Donor Phlebotomy

286. A phlebotomist encounters a blood spill on her hands. She should wash her hands immediately using:
    a alcohol-based antiseptic
    b iodine scrub
    c soap & water
    d tincture of green soap

287. Which agent should be used for hand hygiene, assuming the hands are not soiled with blood or body fluids?
    a alcohol-based antiseptic hand cleansers
    b iodine scrub
    c povidone iodine
    d tincture of green soap

288. A phlebotomist routinely uses an alcohol-based antiseptic to cleanse her hands after completing a blood collection procedure. According to the Occupational Safety & Health Administration (OSHA), the phlebotomist is required to wash her hands with soap and water after every:
    a patient
    b 2 patients
    c 3 patients
    d 4 patients

289. Hand hygiene procedures must be completed:
    a after returning to the laboratory following lunch break
    b before & after every patient contact
    c every 5 minutes
    d every 10 minutes

290. A phlebotomist is preparing to leave the lab for a lunch break. She begins the hand washing procedure by wetting her hands and dispensing soap. Next she should:
    a allow the soap & water to soak on her hands for at least 20 seconds
    b allow the soap & water to soak on her hands for at least 45 seconds
    c rub her hands together vigorously for at least 20 seconds
    d rub her hands together vigorously for at least 45 seconds

291. During the rinse step of a hand wash procedure, the phlebotomist should hold her hands with the fingers pointing:
    a down
    b left
    c right
    d up

292. After the rinse step of a hand wash procedure, the phlebotomist should turn off the faucet using the:
- **a** glove
- **b** hand
- **c** elbow
- **d** paper towel

Explanations

Donor Phlebotomy

The following items have been identified as appropriate for those preparing for the QDP examination.

I. Basic Science of Blood Compatibility

1. **a** A patient who types as group A has A antigens on the surface of their red blood cells.
 [Garza 10e, p237]

2. **b** A patient who types as group B has B antigens on the surface of their red blood cells.
 [Garza 10e, p237]

3. **c** A patient who types as group AB has A and B antigens on the surface of their red blood cells.
 [Garza 10e, p237]

4. **d** A patient who types as group O lack both A and B antigens on the surface of their red blood cells.
 [Garza 10e, p237]

5. **b** A patient who types as group A has anti-B antibodies in their plasma.
 [Garza 10e, p237]

6. **a** A patient who types as group B has anti-A antibodies in their plasma.
 [Garza 10e, p237]

7. **b** The third most common ABO blood type in the United States is Group B.
 [Garza 10e, p237]

8. **c** The least common ABO blood type in the United States is Group AB.
 [Garza 10e, p237]

9. **d** Donors who have a history of pregnancy and/or a history of receiving allogeneic transfusions are at an increased risk of developing HLA antibodies.
 [Harmening 7e, p501]

10. **a** Group A positive patients may safely receive group O positive cells.
 [Garza 10e, p238]

11. **d** Thrombocytes (platelets) are the smallest cellular element in the peripheral blood. Following an injury to a blood vessel and during the second phase of hemostasis, platelets aggregate (clump) and adhere (stick) to form a plug over the site of the injury, reducing blood flow.
 [Garza 10e, p243]

12. **a** Red blood cells treat anemia by raising the patient's hematocrit and hemoglobin levels without significantly increasing blood volume.
 [Harmening 7e, p359]

13. **b** Group B positive patients may safely receive group B negative packed cells.
 [Harmening 7e, p260]

Donor Phlebotomy   **I. Basic Science of Blood Compatibility**

14. **b**   Plasma is the liquid portion of the blood that transports nutrients, hormones, clotting factors, and blood cells through the circulatory system.
[Garza 10e, p234]

15. **c**   White blood cells (leukocytes) function by fighting infectious agents, such as foreign bacteria.
[Garza 10e, p637]

16. **c**   The general population can be divided into 4 major ABO groups: A, B, AB, and O.
[Garza 10e, p237]

Please consult the diagram below for questions 17-22 regarding identification of anatomical structures of the heart.

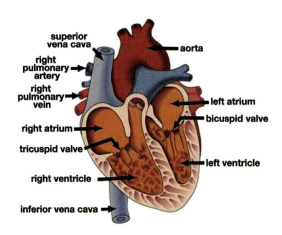

17. **d**   The superior vena cava brings deoxygenated blood from the arms, chest, head and neck to the right atrium.
[Garza 10e, p217-220]

18. **a**   The inferior and superior vena cava deliver deoxygenated blood from the tissues into the right atrium.
[Garza 10e, p217-220]

19. **c**   The right ventricle contracts, forcing blood through the pulmonary semilunar valve and closing the tricuspid valve. The pulmonary circuit begins when blood exits the right ventricle.
[Garza 10e, p217-220]

20. **d**   The left ventricle fills with oxygenated blood from the left atrium though the bicuspid valve. Contraction of the left ventricle forces blood through the aortic valve into the aorta.
[Garza 10e, p217-220]

I. Basic Science of Blood Compatibility — Donor Phlebotomy

21. **b** Pulmonary veins deposit oxygenated blood from the lungs into the left atrium.
[Garza 10e, p217-220]

22. **a** The left ventricle empties oxygenated blood into the aorta, the largest artery in the body.
[Garza 10e, p217-220]

23. **a** When arterial blood is oxygenated to normal levels, it is bright cherry red in color. If a phlebotomist inadvertently punctures an artery, the blood in the collection tube will be bright cherry red. If the phlebotomist believes an artery has been accidentally punctured, he should immediately remove the needle, and apply continuous pressure to the site for at least 5 minutes. Once the bleeding has stopped, a supervisor should be notified per the policies at the facility.
[Garza 10e, p224, 230, 493]

24. **c** Capillary vessel walls are 1 cell layer thick to allow diffusion of oxygen and nutrients from the blood to the tissues and carbon dioxide and waste products from the tissues into the bloodstream. In contrast, vessel walls of veins and arteries have 3 distinct layers (tunica adventitia, tunica media, and tunica intima).
[McCall 7e, p162-164]

25. **b** Gas and solute exchange occurs in the capillaries across the 1 cell layer thick vessel wall. As a result, blood in the capillaries is a mixture of deoxygenated and oxygenated blood.
[McCall 7e, p163]

26. **c** Capillaries are the blood vessels that connect the circuit of blood vessels by linking arterial and venous circulation.
[Garza 10e, p225]

27. **a** Capillary vessel walls are 1 cell layer thick to allow diffusion of oxygen and nutrients from the blood to the tissues and carbon dioxide and waste products from the tissues into the bloodstream. Capillaries are the only blood vessels that allow this exchange with the tissues.
[Garza 10e, p225, 229]

28. **d** Veins in the systemic circuit return deoxygenated blood to the heart. Consequently, venous specimens obtained by venipuncture contain the lowest concentration of oxygen.
[McCall 7e, p161]

29. **d** Blood moves through most of the venous network against the force of gravity. Many veins include valves composed of epithelial tissue. The valves prevent backflow of blood and ensure blood continues to move toward the heart.
[Garza 10e, p226]

7 Donor Phlebotomy — I. Basic Science of Blood Compatibility

30. **c** Veins in the systemic circuit carry deoxygenated blood to the heart. The pulmonary veins uniquely carry oxygenated blood from the lungs to the heart as part of the pulmonary circuit.
[McCall 7e, p161]

31. **d** Deoxygenated blood is dark red in color verifying that the phlebotomist punctured a vein.
[McCall 7e, p161]

32. **d** The superior vena cava brings deoxygenated blood from the arms, chest, head, and neck to the right atrium.
[Garza 10e, p217]

33. **c** Pulmonary veins deposit oxygenated blood from the lungs into the left atrium.
[Garza 10e, p219]

34. **a** There are 3 elements contributing to hemostasis *in vivo*, including blood vessels, platelets, and coagulation factors.
[Garza 10e, p243-244]

35. **d** Approximately 90% of plasma is water (H_2O).
[McCall 7e, p170, 171]

36. **c** If coagulation is prevented, the fluid portion of the blood specimen is called plasma. A variety of substances function as anticoagulants in evacuated tubes and prevent coagulation of the specimen, yielding plasma.
[Garza 10e, p233]

37. **d** If a blood specimen is collected into an evacuated tube and allowed to clot, the fluid portion of the specimen is called serum. Fibrinogen cannot be found in serum because it was converted to fibrin in the clotting process.
[Garza 10e, p233-234, 244]

38. **a** Erythrocytes (red blood cells or RBCs) contain hemoglobin, which transports oxygen to the tissues and carbon dioxide away from tissues.
[Garza 10e, p220-221, 236]

39. **a** Erythrocytes (red blood cells or RBCs) contain hemoglobin, which transports oxygen to the tissues and carbon dioxide away from tissues.
[Garza 10e, p220-221, 236]

40. **a** Blood group antigens are proteins found on the red cell membrane. The presence of blood group antigens on red cell membranes is determined genetically.
[Garza 10e, p237]

41. **b** Leukocytes or white blood cells (WBCs) function in fighting infection.
[Garza 10e, p637]

II. Donor Identification & Selection

42. **d** Thrombocytes (platelets) are the smallest cellular element in the peripheral blood and function in coagulation. Following an injury to a blood vessel and during the second phase of hemostasis, thrombocytes aggregate and adhere to form a plug over the site of injury, reducing blood flow.
[Garza 10e, p243]

43. **b** If a blood specimen is collected into an evacuated tube and allowed to clot, the fibrinogen is converted to fibrin to form the clot. Therefore, fibrinogen is not found in serum. If a blood specimen is collected into an anticoagulant and clotting is prevented, fibrinogen remains in the plasma.
[Garza 10e, p233-234, 244]

44. **b** Blood separates into 3 distinct layers following centrifugation of a blood specimen collected in anticoagulant. The heaviest cellular elements, erythrocytes, are at the bottom of the evacuated tube and the lightest element, plasma, at the top. White cells and platelets form a thin layer called a buffy coat between the erythrocytes and the plasma.
[Garza 10e, p233]

II. Donor Identification & Selection

45. **d** The purpose of donor screening is to protect the health of the donor and transfusion recipient.
[Garza 10e, p500]

46. **a** Blood components transfused from a genetically different donor of the same species are allogeneic.
[Harmening 7e, p629]

47. **d** Blood components collected from and transfused into the same person are autologous.
[Harmening 7e, p292, 501]

48. **c** A patient requests a transfusion from a specific donor during a nonemergency surgery. This is called a directed donation.
[Harmening 7e, p295]

49. **b** Routine donor screening includes a physical exam conducted consistent with AABB standards, completion of a medical questionnaire and serological testing. Results outside of acceptable parameters defined for any of these processes may disqualify a donor.
[Harmening 7e, p283-291]

50. **b** Donor centers are required to connect the donor with previous donations through existing donor records, including those given under a different name.
[AABB Technical Manual 20e, p129]

Donor Phlebotomy — II. Donor Identification & Selection

51. b Informed consent is a legal term that refers to a donor's voluntary permission to complete the donation process after receiving information about the process, including risks and consequences.
[Harmening 7e, p292]

52. b Educational materials provided to the donor prior to donation must include an explanation of the donation process, including adverse effects, infectious disease analyses to be performed on the donated unit, results that must be reported to the authorities, potential donor inclusion on the donor center's deferral registry and test limitations.
[Harmening 7e, p292]

53. d Donors must complete the medical history screening questions on the same day as donation.
[Harmening 7e, p284, 291-292]

54. b Generally, a donor must weigh at least 110 pounds to donate a unit of blood.
[Harmening 7e, p292]

55. d A temporary deferral prevents a donor from donating for a limited period of time. For example, a person who obtained a tattoo may be temporarily deferred for 12 months after obtaining the tattoo.
[Harmening 7e, p286-287]

56. a An indefinite deferral prevents a donor from donating for an unspecified time due to current regulatory guidelines, which may change in the future. For example, a person who resided in the United Kingdom for more than 3 months is deferred indefinitely due to the increased risk of Creutzfeld-Jakob disease and its variants.
[Harmening 7e, p286, 290]

57. c A permanent deferral prevents a donor from ever donating blood for another person. For example, a person who has hepatitis C is permanently deferred from blood donation.
[Harmening 7e, p286]

58. d Donors manifesting flu or cold symptoms should be temporarily deferred until the symptoms subside and the donor feels well.
[Harmening 7e, p285]

59. d Donors who are taking antibiotic to treat an existing condition are temporarily deferred until the antibiotic course is completed and the infection cleared.
[Harmening 7e, p285]

II. Donor Identification & Selection   Donor Phlebotomy

60. **b** Donors who are taking antibiotic to prophylactically treat an existing condition may be permitted to donate. For example, a donor taking tetracycline prophylactically for acne may be allowed to donate without deferral.
[Harmening 7e, p285]

61. **b** Women on oral contraceptives or using other forms of birth control are eligible to donate.
[AABB Technical Manual 20e, p135]

62. **d** Donors who are taking finasteridine (Proscar) to treat an existing condition are temporarily deferred for 1 month following the last medication dose.
[Harmening 7e, p287]

63. **a** Finesteridine (Proscar), isotretoin (Accutane), dutasteroid (Avodart) and etretinate (Tegison) are teratogens and may cause harm to a developing fetus. Donated blood could contain high enough levels to damage an unborn baby if transfused to a pregnant woman. Donors are at least temporarily deferred and possibly permanently deferred from donating blood if they had taken a teratogen.
[Harmening 7e, p286-287]

64. **c** The donor should be permanently deferred because persons who have taken Tegison are permanently deferred as blood donors.
[Harmening 7e, p287]

65. **d** Plavix and Ticlid are medications that may affect platelet function. Platelet donors taking either medication are deferred from donation for 14 days after the last dose. Deferrals apply to platelet donations only; donors taking either medication will be permitted to donate whole blood.
[Harmening 7e, p287]

66. **c** A donor must wait at least 8 weeks between whole blood donations.
[Harmening 7e, p286]

67. **d** A donor must wait at least 16 weeks between a 2-unit red cell collection.
[Harmening 7e, p286]

68. **a** A donor must wait at least 2 days between plateletpheresis procedures.
[AABB Technical Manual 20e, p149]

69. **b** A female donor must be deferred for 6 weeks following the termination of a pregnancy. Since this donor is not pregnant and miscarried 12 weeks previously, she is eligible to donate.
[Harmening 7e, p286]

70. **b** The donor is eligible to donate since he ingested aspirin more than 3 days prior to the donation.
[Harmening 7e, p286]

Donor Phlebotomy

II. Donor Identification & Selection

71. **d** The donor would be deferred for 3 days following ingestion of Pepto-Bismol because it contains salicylates (found in aspirin).
[Harmening 7e, p286]

72. **b** The hepatitis B vaccine is a synthetic viral vaccine and requires no deferral. The donor is eligible to donate.
[AABB Technical Manual 20e, p123; Harmening 7e, p286]

73. **d** Hepatitis B immune globulin (HBIg) is administered following exposure to hepatitis B to prevent hepatitis B infection. However, HBIg is not effective in every case so the donor must be temporarily deferred for at least 12 months to insure the phlebotomist is not infected because hepatitis B can be transmitted through transfusion. The donor should also be deferred for 12 months from the date of the needlestick injury to insure no exposure to other bloodborne pathogens that may be transmitted through donated blood.
[Harmening 7e, p286-287]

74. **d** The chicken pox (varicella zoster) vaccine is characteristically administered as a live attenuated viral vaccine. The donor should be temporarily deferred for 4 weeks after receiving the injection.
[Harmening 7e, p286]

75. **d** Prospective donors who received transfusions, skin grafts or an organ or tissue transplant must be temporarily deferred for 12 months from the date of receiving the blood product, tissue graft or transplant. Transfusions, skin grafts and transplant are potential sources of bloodborne pathogens and the deferral is necessary to insure the prospective donor was not infected with a bloodborne pathogen that could be transmitted via whole blood or other blood product.
[Harmening 7e, p287]

76. **d** The United Kingdom (UK) has experienced the largest number of cases of vCJD. Donors who resided in the UK for 3 months or more between 1980 and 1996 are indefinitely deferred.
[Harmening 7e, p289-290]

77. **c** CJD may be transmitted by human dura mater transplant procedures. Patients who have had a dura mater transplant must be indefinitely deferred from donating blood.
[Harmening 7e, p290-291]

78. **c** CJD may be transmitted by growth hormone obtained from the pituitary gland. Patients who have received growth hormone, even as children, must be indefinitely deferred from donating blood.
[Harmening 7e, p287]

79. **b** Malaria is an infection caused by the parasitic protozoan, *Plasmodium*, which is transmitted by mosquitos. It may also be transmitted through blood transfusions.
[Harmening 7e, p642]

II. Donor Identification & Selection — Donor Phlebotomy

80. **a** Of the regions listed, Africa is endemic for malaria. If a donor has traveled to Africa, he/she may be temporarily deferred for 1 year following the African departure date.
[Harmening 7e, p289]

81. **d** The donor should be temporarily deferred. The donor lived in an area endemic for malaria. Since he immigrated from India, it may be assumed he lived there for longer than 5 years, but donor room personnel should inquire further to confirm the dates of his residency in India. Donors who reside in an area endemic for malaria for longer than 5 years must be deferred as donors for at least 3 years from their departure date. If the donor is asymptomatic for three years after departing India, the donor may be eligible to donate if all other donor criteria are met.
[Harmening 7e, p289]

82. **c** Leishmaniasis is endemic in tropical and subtropical areas of the Middle East, Mediterranean Coast, Africa, Central and South America, and Asia.
[Harmening 7e, p290]

83. **d** Of the populations listed, veterans of Operation Desert Storm would be most at risk for leishmaniasis because the Middle East, where they were deployed, is endemic for leishmaniasis. Veterans deployed to the Middle East are deferred from donating for 12 months from their departure date.
[Harmening 7e, p290]

84. **d** Syphilis is a sexually transmitted disease caused by the spread of the *Treponema pallidum* pathogen. Donors with a history of syphilis or sexual contact with a person who takes money as payment for sex are temporarily deferred for 1 year following the last contact.
[Harmening 7e, p288]

85. **b** Diagnosis of syphilis or gonorrhea temporarily defers a donor for 12 months from the date treatment is concluded to prevent the spread of bloodborne pathogens via transfusion. In this case, the donor would be eligible to donate if documentation of successful treatment is provided to the satisfaction of the medical director.
[Harmening 7e, p288]

86. **c** The human immunodeficiency virus (HIV) may be spread via sexual contact, sharing contaminated needles for intravenous drug use and via transfusion of a contaminated unit. A donor may be deferred for 12 months from the last sexual contact with an individual who tested positive for HIV/AIDS.
[Harmening 7e, p288]

Donor Phlebotomy — II. Donor Identification & Selection

87. **b** The hepatitis B virus (HBV) may be spread via sexual contact, sharing contaminated needles for intravenous drug use and via transfusion of a contaminated unit. Identification of behaviors at high risk for transmitting HBV may result in donor deferral. A donor may be deferred for 12 months from the last sexual contact with an individual who tested positive for HBV.
[Harmening 7e, p288]

88. **a** The hepatitis C virus (HCV) may be spread via sexual contact, sharing contaminated needles for intravenous drug use and via transfusion of a contaminated unit. Consequently, the Donor History Questionnaire (DHQ) includes questions associated with behaviors at risk for contracting HCV. Identification of high-risk behaviors may result in donor deferral. A donor may be deferred for 12 months from sharing contaminated needles with an individual who tested positive for HCV.
[Harmening 7e, p288]

89. **b** The human immunodeficiency virus is the causative agent of Acquired Immune Deficiency Syndrome (AIDS).
[Garza 10e, p98, 205]

90. **d** The donor should be temporarily deferred for 12 months from her last sexual contact with her ex-fiancée. Her fiancée's use of anabolic steroids places him at high risk for HIV, which can be transmitted sexually.
[Harmening 7e, p288]

91. **d** The donor may be temporarily deferred for 12 months from the last sexual contact with her husband.
[Harmening 7e, p288]

92. **c** HCV may be spread via sexual contact. Consequently, the Donor History Questionnaire (DHQ) includes questions associated with behaviors at risk for contracting HCV. Identification of high-risk behaviors may result in donor deferral.
[Harmening 7e, p288]

93. **a** A donor who has previously tested positive for HIV must be indefinitely deferred.
[Harmening 7e, p290]

94. **a** A donor with a positive history for Chagas disease must be indefinitely deferred.
[Harmening 7e, p290-291]

95. **a** A donor with a positive history for babesiosis must be indefinitely deferred.
[Harmening 7e, p290-291]

96. **c** The donor should be temporarily deferred for 120 days. Subsequent donations must meet all eligibility criteria.
[AABB Technical Manual 20e, p188]

II. Donor Identification & Selection — Donor Phlebotomy

97. b This donor's infection was 6 weeks prior to intended donation, so she is eligible to donate. Persons infected with Zika virus are deferred for 4 weeks following infection.
[Harmening 7e, p303]

98. d There is no upper age limit for donor eligibility.
[Harmening 7e, p283]

99. b A donor's oral temperature cannot exceed 37.5°C.
[Harmening 7e, p292]

100. c A donor's oral temperature cannot exceed 99.5°F.
[Harmening 7e, p292]

101. b The minimum acceptable hemoglobin concentration for both male and female donors is 12.5 g/dL.
[Harmening 7e, p292]

102. b The minimum acceptable hemoglobin concentration for both male and female donors is 12.5 g/dL.
[Harmening 7e, p292]

103. d The donor should be deferred because his systolic blood pressure is 185, which exceeds acceptable limits. To be eligible for blood donation, blood pressure must be between 90-180 mmHg systolic, and between 50-100 mmHg diastolic.
[AABB Technical Manual 20e, p130]

104. b The construction worker is an acceptable donor. Receiving a tetanus shot does not require a deferral. The remaining donors must be temporarily deferred. The 17-year-old senior in high school took an aspirin-containing compound, which requires a 3-day deferral; the 28-year-old mother miscarried 3 weeks ago and must be deferred for at least 6 weeks; and the 55-year-old man has an active bladder infection and must be temporarily deferred until his infection is no longer active.
[Harmening 7e, p285-286]

105. d Incarceration in a correctional institution (including juvenile detention, lockup, jail, or prison) for more than 72 consecutive hours is cause for a 12-month temporary deferral.
[Harmening 7e, p288]

106. a Receipt of toxoids or killed synthetic viral, bacterial, or rickettsial vaccines (including diptheria, tetanus & pertussis [DTAP]), does not require deferral.
[Harmening 7e, p286]

107. b The donation interval following plasma-, platelet-, or leukapheresis is more than 2 days. [AABB Technical Manual 20e, p149]

108. d The donation interval following a 2-unit red cell collection is 16 weeks.
[Harmening 7e, p286]

Donor Phlebotomy   **III. Donor Blood Collection & Handling**

109. **c**   The donation interval following a whole blood donation is 8 weeks.
[Harmening 7e, p286]

110. **a**   Receipt of live attenuated viral and bacterial vaccines such as German measles (rubella) or chicken pox (varicella zoster) require a 4-week deferral. Recent receipt of flu, tetanus, and anthrax vaccines are not cause for donor deferral.
[Harmening 7e, p286]

111. **c**   Hepatitis B is a viral infection of the liver spread by contact with blood, semen, or other body fluids. HBV transmission may occur by sexual, blood transfusion, or perinatal routes.
[Harmening 7e, p309]

112. **c**   Staff must tactfully inspect both arms of the donor for evidence of illicit intravenous drug use before phlebotomy occurs. IV drug use is cause for permanent deferral.
[Harmening 7e, p292]

III. Donor Blood Collection & Handling

113. **d**   Whole blood is the term used to refer to a unit of blood collected from a voluntary blood donor for the purposes of transfusion into patients. The whole blood unit may be divided into components such as platelets and fresh frozen plasma.
[Garza 10e, p233]

114. **a**   Whole blood units should be stored at temperatures between 1-6°C.
[Harmening 7e, p335]

115. **d**   A whole blood unit collected into citrate-phosphate-dextrose-adenine (CPDA-1) has a shelf life of 35 days.
[Harmening 7e, p8, 335]

116. **c**   Platelet concentrates must be stored at 22-24°C. [Harmening 7e, 338]

117. **a**   Platelets must be continually agitated during storage.
[Harmening 7e, p338]

118. **a**   Fresh frozen plasma must be stored at –18°C or colder for 1 year. If stored at –65°C, it may be stored up to 7 years but requires FDA approval.
[Harmening 7e, p341]

119. **a**   The Human Resources (HR) Department or their designee conducts routine competency assessments to ensure staff maintain the ability to perform their jobs well.
[AABB Technical Manual 20e, p7]

III. Donor Blood Collection & Handling — Donor Phlebotomy

120. a An alphanumeric system is used to correlate the donor with the blood product donated.
[AABB Technical Manual 20e, p7; Harmening 7e, p297]

121. a An alphanumeric system is used to clearly correlate the donor with his donation history at the facility and each unit of blood or blood product he donated.
[AABB Technical Manual 20e, p129; Harmening 7e, p297]

122. b It is important to maintain donor records correlating to donated blood or blood components to insure the recipient's safety. In the event of unacceptable donor screening test results or adverse recipient reaction to transfusion, donor records will provide contact information for the donor as well as history of recipient response to transfused units from a specific donor.
[AABB Technical Manual 20e, p189-194; Harmening 7e, p299]

123. a When labelling donated blood products, labels should be affixed to blood bags, including component bags and pilot tubes and the donor record.
[Harmening 7e, p297]

124. b The technique used to prepare a venipuncture site prior to donating a unit of blood is aseptic technique.
[Harmening 7e, p298]

125. a Blood pressure cuffs may be inflated between 40 and 60 mmHg when used as a tourniquet for donor phlebotomy.
[Harmening 7e, p298]

126. c An iodine compound is typically used by blood centers to prepare a venipuncture site prior to donation of a unit of blood.
[Harmening 7e, p298]

127. b The phlebotomist must scrub the venipuncture site for at least 30 seconds using an iodine compound.
[Harmening 7e, p298]

128. b After scrubbing the venipuncture site, the phlebotomist must apply an iodophor compound beginning at the puncture site and moving outward using a concentric circular motion.
[Harmening 7e, p298]

129. a Sweating and vomiting are associated with mild donor reactions.
[Harmening 7e, p299]

130. b Loss of consciousness with decreased pulse rate and systolic blood pressure are associated with moderate donor reactions.
[Harmening 7e, p299]

Donor Phlebotomy — III. Donor Blood Collection & Handling

131. **d** Donor convulsions defines a severe donor reaction and may be caused by cerebral ischemia, marked hyperventilation, or epilepsy. Loss of consciousness with decreased pulse rate and systolic blood pressure are associated with moderate donor reactions.
[Harmening 7e, p299]

132. **d** According to AABB Standards, 10.5 mL/Kg of donor body weight may be collected.
[Harmening 7e, p292]

133. **d** In the United States, 450 mL of whole blood is typically withdrawn during a routine whole blood collection procedure.
[Harmening 7e, p293]

134. **b** Acceptable range of variation in whole blood collection procedures is ±10%.
[Harmening 7e, p293]

135. **a** Discard the unit because the anticoagulant-to-whole blood ratio will be incorrect.
[AABB Technical Manual 20e, p145]

136. **c** Label the unit "RBCs Low Volume" and submit for processing and physician review and approval for use.
[Harmening 7e, p293]

137. **d** Bags used for whole blood collection must be approved by the Food and Drug Administration (FDA).
[AABB Technical Manual 20e, p81]

138. **b** The Food and Drug Administration (FDA) requirements for labelling of blood and blood products are available in a number of publications, including but not limited to *Guideline for the Uniform Labeling of Blood and Blood Components (1985)*.
[AABB Technical Manual 20e, p164-165]

139. **d** Immediately upon completion of the donation, the phlebotomist should withdraw the needle and activate the sheathing mechanism.
[AABB Technical Manual 20e, p142]

140. **d** The staff should instruct the donor to avoid heavy exercise for at least 3 hours after the donation.
[AABB Technical Manual 20e, p143]

141. **a** The staff should instruct the donor to refrain from smoking for at least 30 minutes after the donation.
[Harmening 7e, p300]

142. **a** The staff should instruct the donor to increase their intake of fluids following blood donation.
[Harmening 7e, p300]

III. Donor Blood Collection & Handling — Donor Phlebotomy

143. a The staff should instruct the donor to avoid alcohol consumption for several hours following blood donation.
[Harmening 7e, p300]

144. a Red blood cells must be maintained between 1-6°C when in storage.
[Harmening 7e, p336]

145. c All blood products must be tested for HIV.
[Harmening 7e, p302]

146. c Blood collection kits should be checked for leaks, discoloration, needle contamination, and kinks in tubing.
[Harmening 7e, p298]

147. b Prolonged or severe pain during blood collection may indicate trauma to nerves in arm.
[McCall 7e, p290-291]

148. a The donor phlebotomist should periodically mix the blood collected with the anticoagulant to prevent clotting.
[Harmening 7e, p298]

149. c "Antecubital" means in front of, or anterior to, the elbow when the patient is in anatomic position.
[Garza 10e, p172-173, 227, 626]

150. c "Fossa" means shallow depression. The antecubital area (antecubital fossa) is the shallow depression located in front of or anterior to the elbow when the patient is in anatomic position.
[Garza 10e, p172-173, 227]

151. d The antecubital area (antecubital fossa) is the shallow depression located in front of or anterior to the elbow when the patient is in anatomic position.
[Garza 10e, p172-173, 227, 626]

152. b The venous distribution patterns of the antecubital area (antecubital fossa) resemble the letters they are named after, ie, large case H and M. The H-shaped venous pattern is found in approximately 70% of the population and includes the median cubital, cephalic, and basilic veins.
[CLSI Standard GP41, p19; Garza 10e, p330-335, 342]

Donor Phlebotomy — **III. Donor Blood Collection & Handling**

Please consult the diagram below for questions 153-158 regarding the H-shaped antecubital fossa anatomy.

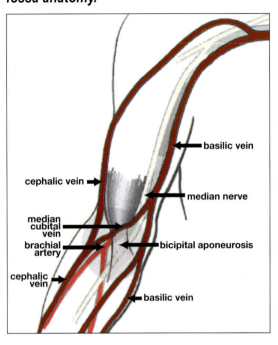

153. **c** The structure at the arrow is the cephalic vein. The cephalic vein is a large, full vein appearing on the lateral side of the antecubital fossa. The order of vein selection in the H-shaped venous pattern is: 1) median cubital vein; 2) cephalic vein; 3) basilic vein, making the cephalic vein the second choice when selecting a site for venipuncture.
[CLSI Standard GP41, p19-21; Garza 10e, p330-335]

154. **d** The structure at the arrow is the is the median cubital vein. The median cubital vein is a large, full surface vein appearing near the center of the antecubital fossa. The order of vein selection in the H-shaped venous pattern is: 1) median cubital vein; 2) cephalic vein; 3) basilic vein, making the median cubital vein the first choice when selecting a site for venipuncture. CLSI Standard GP41 requires a phlebotomist to look for a median cubital vein in both arms before selecting an alternative site for venipuncture.
[CLSI Standard GP41, p19-21; Garza 10e, p330-335]

155. **b** The structure at the arrow is the is the brachial artery. Accidental puncture of the brachial artery represents one of the risks associated with venipuncture, especially if the basilic vein is selected as a site for venipuncture.
[CLSI Standard GP41, p19-21; Garza 10e, p224-225, 230, 335, 504, 623]

III. Donor Blood Collection & Handling
Donor Phlebotomy

156. c The structure at the arrow is the is the cephalic vein. The cephalic vein is a large, full vein appearing on the lateral side of the antecubital fossa. The order of vein selection in the H-shaped venous pattern is: 1) median cubital vein; 2) cephalic vein; 3) basilic vein, making the cephalic vein the second choice when selecting a site for venipuncture.
[CLSI Standard GP41, p19-21; Garza 10e, p330-335]

157. a The structure at the arrow is the is the basilic vein. The basilic vein is a smaller vein appearing on the medial side of the antecubital fossa. The order of vein selection in the H-shaped venous pattern is: 1) median cubital vein; 2) cephalic vein; 3) basilic vein, making the basilic vein the third choice when selecting a site for venipuncture. Additionally, the basilic vein is located in proximity to the brachial artery and median nerve so other vein choices are preferred as venipuncture sites.
[CLSI Standard GP41, p19-21; Garza 10e, p330-335]

158. a The structure at the arrow is the is the basilic vein. The basilic vein is a smaller vein appearing on the medial side of the antecubital fossa. The order of vein selection in the H-shaped venous pattern is: 1) median cubital vein; 2) cephalic vein; 3) basilic vein, making the basilic vein the third choice when selecting a site for venipuncture. Additionally, the basilic vein is located in proximity to the brachial artery and median nerve so other vein choices are preferred as venipuncture sites.
[CLSI Standard GP41, p19-21; Garza 10e, p330-335]

159. b To examine by touch or feel is to palpate.
[CLSI Standard GP41, p17]

160. d The median cubital vein is a large, full surface vein appearing near the center of the antecubital fossa. The order of vein selection is: 1) median cubital vein; 2) cephalic vein, and 3) basilic vein, making the median cubital vein the first choice when selecting a site for venipuncture. CLSI Standard GP41 requires a phlebotomist to look for a median cubital vein in both arms before selecting an alternative site for venipuncture.
[CLSI Standard GP41, p19-21; Garza 10e, p330-335]

161. a The basilic vein is a smaller vein appearing on the medial side of the antecubital fossa. The order of vein selection is: 1) median cubital vein, 2) cephalic vein, and 3) basilic vein, making the basilic vein the least suitable choice when selecting a site for venipuncture. Additionally, the basilic vein is located in proximity to the brachial artery and median nerve so other choices are typically preferred. Also, venipunctures performed on the basilic vein seem more painful for the patient.
[CLSI Standard GP41, p19-21; Garza 10e, p330-335]

Donor Phlebotomy — III. Donor Blood Collection & Handling

162. b The phlebotomist should next examine the right antecubital area (antecubital fossa). CLSI Standard GP41 requires a phlebotomist to look for a median cubital vein in both arms before selecting an alternative site for venipuncture.
[CLSI Standard GP41, p19-21; Garza 10e, p330-335, 342]

163. a Tourniquets should be applied approximately 3-4 inches above the venipuncture site and away from any skin lesions.
[CLSI Standard GP41, p17]

164. d Health care workers responsible for performing venipuncture rely most heavily on their sense of touch to locate a vein.
[Garza 10e, p330]

165. a Phlebotomists should use the index fingers to palpate for a vein prior to venipuncture.
[CLSI Standard GP41, p17; Garza 10e, p319, 330, 338]

166. c When examining a site for venipuncture, a phlebotomist uses the index finger to palpate the vein and determine its depth, direction, and size.
[Garza 10e, p330, 338]

167. d CLSI Standard GP41 requires a phlebotomist to look for a median cubital vein in both arms before selecting an alternative site for venipuncture.
[CLSI Standard GP41, p20; Garza 10e, p330]

168. d The median cubital vein, a large, full, surface vein appearing near the center of the antecubital fossa, is located over the bicipital aponeurosis, which provides natural support and anchoring for the vein during venipuncture. (The phlebotomist always must also anchor the vein.) The bicipital aponeurosis is a fibrous membrane which also offers some protection to underlying arteries and nerves. CLSI Standard GP41 requires a phlebotomist to look for a median cubital vein in both arms before selecting an alternative site for venipuncture.
[CLSI Standard GP41, p19-21]

169. c The median cubital vein, a large, full, surface vein appearing near the center of the antecubital fossa, is located over the bicipital aponeurosis, which provides additional natural anchoring and support for the vein during venipuncture. (The phlebotomist always must also anchor the vein). The bicipital aponeurosis is a fibrous membrane which also offers some protection to underlying arteries and nerves. CLSI Standard GP41 requires a phlebotomist to look for a median cubital vein in both arms before selecting an alternative site for venipuncture.
[CLSI Standard GP41, p19-21]

170. c A patent vein is open, turgid and a phlebotomist will feel a bounce when palpating.
[McCall 7e, p243-244]

III. Donor Blood Collection & Handling — Donor Phlebotomy

171. a The bicipital aponeurosis, characteristically located beneath the median cubital vein, is a fibrous membrane which offers some protection to underlying arteries and nerves as well as some support to the median cubital vein during venipuncture.
[CLSI Standard GP41, p19]

172. b The correct sequence is: 1) apply tourniquet; 2) palpate site; 3) release tourniquet.
[CLSI Standard GP41, p17-18; Garza 10e, p338, 342]

173. c The correct sequence is: 1) uncap the needle; 2) anchor the vein; 3) insert the needle. The needle assembly should be held in one hand while the phlebotomist uses the other hand to anchor the vein. According to CLSI Standard GP41, the phlebotomist should anchor the vein by positioning the thumb about 1 to 2 inches below the intended puncture site and slightly to the side. Use the thumb to pull the skin toward the wrist and use the remaining fingers to hold the patient's arm away from the intended puncture site.
[CLSI Standard GP41, p23-24; Garza 10e, p342-343]

174. d The patient's arm should be positioned in a straight line from the shoulder to wrist.
[McCall 7e, p229]

175. b Positioning the patient's arm in a straight line from the shoulder to wrist during venipuncture in the antecubital area (antecubital fossa) will help to anchor the veins during venipuncture.
[McCall 7e, p229]

176. b When anchoring a vein in the antecubital area (antecubital fossa) prior to venipuncture, the phlebotomist should place the thumb 1-2 inches below the puncture site.
[CLSI Standard GP41, p23; Garza 10e, p342]

177. d When anchoring a vein in the antecubital area (antecubital fossa) prior to venipuncture, the phlebotomist should place the thumb 1-2 inches below the puncture site and pull the skin taut by stretching the skin toward the patient's wrist.
[CLSI Standard GP41, p23; Garza 10e, p342]

178. b During venipuncture, the needle should be inserted with the bevel up.
[CLSI Standard GP41, p24; Garza 10e, p343]

179. c During venipuncture, the needle should be inserted at a 30 degree angle or less. Shallow veins may require a smaller angle (15°) while deeper veins may require a larger angle (30°).
[CLSI Standard GP41, p24; Garza 10e, p343]

180. d The needle must be positioned in the same direction as the vein and at an angle of 15°-30° to the patient's arm.
[Garza 10e, p343]

Donor Phlebotomy — III. Donor Blood Collection & Handling

181. d During a venipuncture procedure after the needle is uncapped the phlebotomist should visually inspect the needle for any defects. If defects are observed, the needle should be discarded and another selected.
[McCall 7e, p237]

182. c During a venipuncture procedure, the phlebotomist should visually inspect the needle after the needle is uncapped. The needles should be discarded if imperfections, including burrs, are noted and another needle selected for use.
[McCall 7e, p237]

183. c After the needle is withdrawn, the patient should be instructed to use the gauze pad to apply pressure to the site while keeping the arm straight. Patients should not be instructed to hold the gauze in place while bending their arm up. Studies have shown this procedure actually increases the chance of bruising at the venipuncture site.
[CLSI Standard GP41, p28; Garza 10e, p335-346]

184. d After the needle is withdrawn, the patient should be instructed to use the gauze pad to apply pressure to the site while keeping the arm straight. Patients should not be instructed to hold the gauze in place while bending their arm up. Studies have shown this procedure actually increases the chance of bruising at the venipuncture site.
[CLSI Standard GP41, p28; Garza 10e, p345-346]

185. c The purpose of tourniquet administration is to diminish venous blood flow, increase venous filling, allowing for easier venipuncture site selection through palpation.
[CLSI Standard GP41, p17-18; Garza 10e, p337]

186. c A sphygmomanometer is a blood pressure cuff and may be used by those who have been trained instead of a tourniquet. When used instead of a tourniquet, the cuff should be inflated to no more than 40 mmHg.
[CLSI Standard GP41, p18]

187. a Larger gauge needles (16-18) are used for collecting units of blood (450 mL) from blood donors.
[Garza 10e, p270]

188. c The standard for measuring the diameter of the lumen of a needle is the needle gauge. The higher the gauge number, the smaller the needle; conversely, the lower the gauge, the larger the needle.
[Garza 10e, p270]

189. d The internal space of a needle is the lumen.
[McCall 7e, p490]

190. a The 18 gauge needle represents the largest needle lumen. The lower the gauge, the larger the needle and conversely, the higher the gauge, the smaller the needle.
[Garza 10e, p270]

IV. Donor Considerations

191. d The 23 gauge needle represents the smallest needle lumen. The higher the gauge number, the smaller the needle; conversely, the lower the gauge, the larger the needle.
[Garza 10e, p270]

IV. Donor Considerations

192. b A donation where a donor donates blood for her own use is termed autologous.
[Garza 10e, p501]

193. b Autologous blood transfusion offers the advantage of minimizing disease transmission to the recipient.
[Garza 10e, p501]

194. a Disadvantages associated with autologous blood transfusions include increased administrative costs and waste of unused units, which must be discarded except under circumstances approved by the medical director.
[Harmening 7e, p292-293]

195. a A patient must provide a prescription from their physician in order to donate a unit of autologous blood.
[Harmening 7e, p293]

196. b A donor must have a minimum hematocrit of 33% to be accepted as an autologous blood donor.
[Harmening 7e, p293]

197. c A unit of blood for autologous blood donation must be collected at least 72 hours in advance of the anticipated surgery or transfusion.
[Harmening 7e, p293]

198. c The amount of blood collected from the donor for autologous blood donation is 387 mL. The formula to determine the amount of blood collected is: Volume to collect = donor's weight in kg/50 × 450 mL. Units of blood containing between 300 mL and 405 mL should be labeled "Low Volume."
[Harmening 7e, p292]

199. d Units of blood containing volumes between 300 mL and 405 mL should be labelled "Low Volume." This unit was collected for autologous blood donation, so it must also be labelled "For Autologous Use Only."
[Harmening 7e, p293]

200. c The donor has a temperature of 38.3°C. The donor must be deferred for donation because of the elevated temperature, which must be equal to or less than 37.5°C (99.5°F).
[Harmening 7e, p292]

Donor Phlebotomy — IV. Donor Considerations

201. **c** A unit of whole blood collected from a donor specifically for a particular patient is directed donation.
[Harmening 7e, p295]

202. **a** The donor must be deferred from donating because they do not meet the 110 lb minimum weight requirement. Donors providing blood for directed donations must meet all of the same standards as voluntary donors.
[Harmening 7e, p292, 295]

203. **d** Routine withdrawal of whole blood for the treatment of diseases associated with the abnormal accumulation of iron stores within the body is therapeutic phlebotomy. Diseases commonly associated with therapeutic phlebotomy include hemochromatosis and polycythemia.
[Garza 10e, p502]

204. **a** Hereditary hemochromatosis and polycythemia vera are 2 conditions commonly treated using therapeutic phlebotomy.
[Garza 10e, p502]

205. **a** Donors are encouraged to eat within 4-6 hours of donation to prevent an adverse donor reaction.
[Garza 10e, p500]

206. **a** The bright cherry-red color of the blood entering the donor bag combined with the rapid filling of the donor bag with blood suggests the phlebotomist inadvertently performed an arterial puncture. The appropriate course of action is to apply pressure to the venipuncture site. The donor should be referred for ultrasound studies if hematomas appear and recur following the donation.
[AABB Technical Manual 20e, p143; Garza 10e, p230, 330, 335, 504]

207. **c** Presyncopal symptoms and small hematomas are the 2 most commonly reported adverse donor reactions.
[AABB Technical Manual 20e, p143]

208. **d** Donor room personnel should maintain current cardiopulmonary resuscitation (CPR) certification.
[Harmening 7e, p307]

209. **a** Apheresis is the donor collection technique used to separate and collect a specific blood component from whole blood and return the remaining blood to the donor.
[Harmening 7e, p630]

210. **d** The time between donations is less for plateletpheresis donors. Donors may undergo plateletpheresis 2 days after a pervious donation—not to exceed 2 donations per week or 24 donations in a 12-month period. Providing information, obtaining consent and testing procedures are the same for both whole blood and plateletpheresis products.
[Harmening 7e, p296]

V. Donor Center Operations — Donor Phlebotomy

211. c Hematomas are among the most prevalent adverse donor reactions.
[AABB Technical Manual 20e, p143]

212. d A patient who is diaphoretic is perspiring profusely. If patients are pale, they are manifesting pallor. Patient who are perspiring and pale are manifesting symptoms that may result in syncope, or fainting. The phlebotomist should lower the patient's head and instruct them to breathe deeply.
[Garza 10e, p298-299, 636; Harmening 7e, p634]

213. b If a patient vomits during venipuncture, the procedure should be discontinued immediately.
[McCall 7e, p287]

214. c Sometimes patients faint (syncope) at the thought or sight of having their blood drawn. This response may be compounded with certain other conditions such as dehydration, hypoglycemia, psychiatric issues, and certain medications.
[Garza 10e, p298-299]

V. Donor Center Operations

215. d Enacted (passed) federal laws are listed chronologically in the United States Code (USC). Rules governing the collection, storage and use of blood and blood products established by the Food and Drug Administration (FDA) and are listed in the Code of Federal Regulations (CFR).
[Harmening 7e, p256, 575]

216. c Enacted (passed) federal laws are listed chronologically in the United States Code (USC). The Food and Drug Administration (FDA) recognizes blood as both a biological and a drug and creates regulations governing the collection, storage and use of blood and blood products, which are listed in the Code of Federal Regulations (CFR).
[Harmening 7e, p282, 575]

217. b The Food and Drug Administration (FDA) recognizes blood as a pharmaceutical and creates regulations governing the collection, storage and use of blood products. Regulations for blood products are found in the Code of Federal Regulations (CFR) as decreed under the Public Health Service Act and the Federal Food, Drug, and Cosmetic Act.
[Harmening 7e, p256, 575]

Donor Phlebotomy

V. Donor Center Operations

218. a The AABB, formerly known as the American Association of Blood Banks, is an international, not-for-profit association representing individuals and institutions involved in the field of transfusion medicine. The association is committed to improving health through the development and delivery of standards designed to assist transfusion services with meeting Clinical Laboratory Improvement Amendments (CLIA) and Centers for Medicare and Medicaid Services (CMS) requirements through a variety of educational services, including publications such as the AABB Technical Manual and AABB Standards for Blood and Transfusion Services.
[Harmening 7e, p282-283]

219. a Refrigerators, freezers, plate incubators and water bath temperatures should be monitored daily to insure temperatures of these devices are within acceptable limits.
[AABB Technical Manual 20e, p29-30]

220. b A nonconforming event occurs when a technician did not follow standard operating procedures (SOPs). Donor centers should contain processes and procedures to detect, document, investigate, correct, and follow up on nonconforming events.
[AABB Technical Manual 20e, p17-20]

221. c OSHA's bloodborne pathogen standard mandates gloves must be worn during blood collection procedures.
[CLSI Standard GP41, p22; Garza 10e, p109-111, 118]

222. d Needles should be visually inspected for manufacturing defects such as burrs or barbs before every venipuncture.
[McCall 7e, p237]

223. a Needle seals should be visually inspected before every venipuncture. If the seal is not intact, the needle and blood bag should be discarded in a sharps container and another selected for use.
[McCall 7e, p237]

224. d To be effective, quality assurance indicators must be specific and measurable. For example, a quality assurance indicator for blood culture collection typically defines a threshold contamination rate at 3% or less.
[McCall 7e, p237]

225. a A program of tracking outcomes through scheduled audits to continually improve the quality of patient care is quality assurance. Quality control includes materials and methods established to achieve intended outcomes during every specimen collection procedure.
[Garza 10e, p25, 635]

V. Donor Center Operations
Donor Phlebotomy

226. **b** Quality control refers to specific procedures within a quality assurance program designed to ensure good quality patient care. An example of a quality control procedure is inspecting evacuated tubes for expiration dates before use.
[Garza 10e, p28-29, 76]

227. **b** Malpractice is the legal term for a civil lawsuit based on professional negligence or improper treatment by a professional person.
[Garza 10e, p89-90]

228. **c** Failure to exercise due care and reasonable skill in performing a task is negligence.
[Garza 10e, p89, 96-97]

229. **a** The Clinical Laboratory Improvement Amendments (CLIA) of 1988 is a federal bill establishing regulations for clinical laboratories in the United States.
[Garza 10e, p99-100]

230. **b** The Food & Drug Administration is a federal agency responsible for overseeing clinical laboratories.
[Garza 10e, p99]

231. **d** The Joint Commission (TJC) is a voluntary, nongovernmental agency charged with establishing standards of operation for hospitals and other health-related facilities and services.
[McCall 7e, p489]

232. **c** The College of American Pathologists (CAP) is an organization that provides standards for quality improvement specific to clinical laboratories and conducts proficiency testing and laboratory inspections.
[Garza 10e, p99]

233. **c** The College of American Pathologists (CAP) is an outgrowth of ASCP and provides standards for laboratory inspections.
[McCall 7e, p38-39]

234. **c** The Occupational Safety & Health Administration (OSHA) is the United States governmental agency responsible for regulating the safety and health of workers.
[Garza 10e, p633]

235. **b** OSHA's Hazardous Communication Standard (commonly referred to as HazMat or the Right to Know Law) protects employees by requiring documentation, including labels and Safety Data Sheets (SDS), on all hazardous materials.
[Garza 10e, p150-151]

Donor Phlebotomy — V. Donor Center Operations

236. **d** Universal precautions are mandated by the Occupational Safety & Health Administration (OSHA) Bloodborne Pathogens Standard, which was amended in 2001 to comply with OSHA's Needlestick Safety & Prevention Act. These standards are mandated by federal law to minimize the risk of occupational exposure to bloodborne pathogens.
[Garza 10e, p109-110]

237. **a** The 2001 Needlestick Safety & Prevention Act requires revision to OSHA Bloodborne Pathogens Standard in 4 areas, including a written exposure control plan, employee input on selecting engineering controls, revision of definitions related to engineering and work practice controls, and new recordkeeping standards.
[McCall 7e, p84]

238. **c** The Department of Health & Human Services administrates the Centers for Disease Control & Prevention.
[McCall 7e, p61]

239. **d** The Centers for Disease Control & Prevention (CDC) are responsible for researching and controlling diseases.
[Garza 10e, p106-107]

240. **b** Universal precautions were first recommended by the Centers for Disease Control & Prevention (CDC) in 1985 and later mandated by the Occupational Safety & Health Administration (OSHA) Bloodborne Pathogens Standard, which was amended in 2001 to comply with OSHA's Needlestick Safety & Prevention Act. These standards are mandated by federal law to minimize the risk of occupational exposure to bloodborne pathogens.
[Garza 10e, p109-110, 639]

241. **b** Any substance that can be harmful to a person's health is called a biohazard. Biohazards are routinely encountered in the health care setting and health care workers must adhere to safety and infection control standards to work safely in that environment.
[McCall 7e, p482]

242. **b** Universal precautions were implemented to prevent the spread of bloodborne pathogens. Universal precautions were mandated by OSHA's Bloodborne Pathogens Standard in 1992 and revised and amended to include the Needlestick Safety & Prevention Act in 2001.
[Garza 10e, p109-110, 637]

243. **d** The term "bloodborne pathogens" refers to any pathogens that may be spread through contact with blood and most commonly refers to hepatitis B virus (HBV), hepatitis C virus (HCV) and human immunodeficiency virus (HCV). Examples of other bloodborne pathogens include *Plasmodium falciparum* (malaria) and *Treponema pallidum* (syphilis).
[Garza 10e, p105-106, 627]

V. Donor Center Operations — Donor Phlebotomy

244. a Under universal precautions all patients must be treated as though they are potentially infectious.
[Garza 10e, p117-118, 636-637]

245. c Universal precautions and standard precautions are often used interchangeably. Universal precautions recognize that blood from any patient is potentially infectious. Body substance isolation expanded universal precautions to include any body fluid as potentially infectious. The Centers for Disease Control & Prevention (CDC) and the Healthcare Infection Control Practices Advisory Committee (HICPAC) jointly recommended standard precautions when dealing with all patients, which recognizes all blood and body fluids (except sweat) as potentially infectious. Standard precautions combine infection control practices for universal precautions and body substance isolation.
[Garza 10e, p636-637]

246. a Under standard precautions, gloves should be changed after every patient contact.
[Garza 10e, p118]

247. d Class A fire extinguishers may contain pressurized water to extinguish the fire. Fire extinguishers are manufactured based on fire classifications. Using an incorrect extinguisher on a fire is dangerous so many facilities routinely provide multipurpose (ABC) fire extinguishers containing dry chemical to use on Class A (ordinary combustibles such as paper and wood), Class B (flammable liquids such as gasoline and grease), and Class C fires (electrical).
[Garza 10e, p144]

248. b Fire extinguishers are manufactured to correspond to fire classifications. Using an incorrect extinguisher on a fire is dangerous so many facilities routinely provide multipurpose (ABC) fire extinguishers containing dry chemical to use on Class A (ordinary combustibles such as paper and wood), Class B (flammable liquids such as gasoline and grease), and Class C fires (electrical).
[Garza 10e, p144]

249. c Needle safety features are mandated by Needlestick Safety & Prevention Act (2001), a modification mandated by Congress to OSHA's Bloodborne Pathogens Standard. The Needlestick Safety & Prevention Act (2001) mandates the use of needlestick protection devices and labels to communicate biohazard in storage, disposal, and transport containers.
[Garza 10e, p109, 270-275]

250. **d** An example of an engineering control is a needlestick protection device that creates a barrier between the needle and the phlebotomist's hands. Needle safety features are mandated by Needlestick Safety & Prevention Act (2001), a modification mandated by Congress to OSHA's Bloodborne Pathogens Standard. The Needlestick Safety & Prevention Act (2001) requires the use of engineering controls to eliminate or minimize employee exposure to bloodborne pathogens through accidental needlestick.
[McCall 7e, p84]

251. **d** An example of an engineering control is permanent containment of a contaminated needle once a safety feature is activated. Needle safety features are mandated by Needlestick Safety & Prevention Act (2001), a modification mandated by Congress to OSHA's Bloodborne Pathogens Standard. The Needlestick Safety & Prevention Act (2001) requires the use of engineering controls to eliminate or minimize employee exposure to bloodborne pathogens through accidental needlestick.
[McCall 7e, p84]

252. **c** The following practices are never allowed: recapping, bending, breaking, or removing needles from disposable evacuated tube holders or syringes. Needle safety features are mandated by Needlestick Safety & Prevention Act (2001), a modification mandated by Congress to OSHA's Bloodborne Pathogens Standard. The Needlestick Safety & Prevention Act (2001) requires the use of engineering controls to eliminate or minimize employee exposure to bloodborne pathogens through accidental needlestick.
[Garza 10e, p109-112, 127]

253. **a** The National Fire Protection Agency recognizes 3 primary fire classifications. Class A fires occur with ordinary combustibles such as paper and wood.
[Garza 10e, p144]

254. **c** PASS is the National Fire Protection Agency (NFPA) code word for using a fire extinguisher and stands for: Pull pin, Aim the nozzle at the bottom of the fire, Squeeze the handle, Sweep the nozzle side-to-side.
[Garza 10e, p144]

255. **b** Chemical spill clean-up kits contain materials that absorb the chemical and neutralize it so it can be safely cleaned up and disposed. There are a variety of chemical spill kits available, and the laboratory worker should select the appropriate clean-up kit based on the type of spill (eg, alkali, acid, mercury).
[Garza 10e, p152-153]

256. **c** The Environmental Protection Agency regulates chemical disposal.
[McCall 7e, p86]

V. Donor Center Operations — Donor Phlebotomy

257. a A centrifuge is the instrument used to separate blood specimens into component parts, including plasma, buffy coat (white cells and platelets), and red cell layers.
[Garza 10e, p232-233, 407-413]

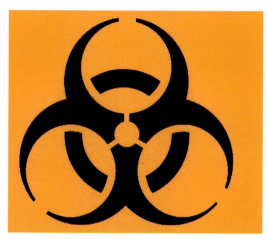

258. a The symbol in the figure communicates biohazard.
[Garza 10e, p110]

259. a An infection control program that includes monitoring specific patient population groups and classifications of infection is called surveillance.
[McCall 7e, p66-67]

260. a Three components in the chain of infection are source, mode of transmission, and susceptible host.
[Garza 10e, p114-117]

261. a If the chain of infection is interrupted at 1 point, the spread of infection will be interrupted.
[Garza 10e, p117]

262. c Microbes capable of causing infection or disease are called pathogens.
[Garza 10e, p114]

263. b A communicable disease results from the transmission of a pathogenic organism by direct or indirect contact or via airborne routes.
[Garza 10e, p105, 628]

264. c 5-8.5% of patients admitted to the hospital in the United States contract a healthcare-associated (nosocomial) infection (HAI).
[McCall 7e, p61-62]

265. d Healthcare-associated infections (HAI) is a term referring to infections acquired in hospitals and other health care facilities, including home care.
[Garza 10e, p106]

266. a Viability refers to a pathogen's ability to survive.
[McCall 7e, p64, 498]

267. c Fomites harbor pathogenic bacteria and are capable of transmitting infection. Examples of fomites include phlebotomy trays, tourniquets, telephones, computer keyboards, and door knobs.
[Garza 10e, p116]

268. a Under standard precautions all patient blood, body fluids (except sweat), nonintact skin, and mucous membranes must be approached as though infectious.
[Garza 10e, p117-118]

269. d Personal protective equipment (PPE) is provided by an employer to protect the health care worker from contact with infectious materials.
[Garza 10e, p22-23, 121-122]

270. d A phlebotomist should never recap a needle after a venipuncture procedure.
[Garza 10e, p127]

271. a Under standard precautions, a phlebotomist should change gloves after every patient encounter and immediately sanitize hands.
[Garza 10e, p121-122]

272. a Under standard precautions, a phlebotomist should sanitize his/her hands immediately after every patient encounter after removing gloves.
[Garza 10e, p121-127]

273. a Health care workers are required to adhere to standard precautions to avoid contact with pathogenic organisms.
[Garza 10e, p121]

274. a To prevent the spread of infection through ingestion, activities such as eating, chewing gum, applying makeup, including lip balm, biting one's nails or putting pens or pencils in one's mouth are prohibited because these activities can lead to ingestion of biohazards.
[Garza 10e, p112, 127, 136]

275. c To prevent the spread of infection through airborne routes, centrifuges should never be opened until after they have arrived at a complete stop.
[Garza 10e, p232-233, 407-413]

276. d Permucosal exposure occurs when pathogens and other hazardous materials enter the body through the mucous membranes of the eyes, mouth, or nose. To prevent permucosal exposure in the clinical laboratory, phlebotomists should never rub their eyes or nose, handle contact lenses, or put contaminated fingers or hands near their eyes, mouth, or nose.
[Garza 10e, p127, 136]

V. Donor Center Operations — Donor Phlebotomy

277. d According to OSHA's Bloodborne Pathogens standard, engineering controls are equipment and supply mechanisms designed to separate or eliminate a bloodborne pathogen hazard. Examples of engineering controls include self-sheathing, retractable and other forms of safety needles, sharps containers, and syringe transfer devices.
[McCall 7e, p84]

278. a According to OSHA's Bloodborne Pathogens Standard, work practice controls are procedural mechanisms designed to limit the possibility of bloodborne pathogen exposure. Examples of work practice controls include handwashing and prohibiting laboratory professionals from eating, chewing gum, and applying makeup in the clinical laboratory.
[McCall 7e, p84]

279. a Gloves should be removed following completion of the venipuncture procedure. Gowns, safety goggles and N95 fit-tested masks are not used for routine venipuncture procedures.
[McCall 7e, p70-72]

280. a To aseptically remove gloves following a venipuncture procedure, the cuff of the first glove should be grasped and pulled over the hand, inside-out and into the palm of the second hand. The second glove should be removed by slipping the fingers into the cuff of the second glove and pulling the second glove over the first so all contaminated surfaces are contained within one glove.
[Garza 10e, p120, 126; McCall 7e, p71]

281. c Chemical compounds used to remove or kill microorganisms on work surfaces or instruments are called disinfectants.
[Garza 10e, p137]

282. b Chemicals that may be used on human skin to inhibit the growth and development of microorganisms, but not necessarily kill them, are antiseptics. 70% isopropyl alcohol is an example of an antiseptic.
[Garza 10e, p137]

283. d Chemicals that may be used on human skin to inhibit the growth and development of microorganisms, but not necessarily kill them, are antiseptics. 70% isopropyl alcohol is an example of an antiseptic.
[Garza 10e, p137]

284. c Chemical compounds used to remove or kill microorganisms on work surfaces or instruments are called disinfectants. Hypochlorite solution (bleach) is a commonly used disinfectant in the clinical laboratory.
[Garza 10e, p137]

285. a Hand hygiene performed consistent with frequency and procedural recommendations is one of the most essential strategies to prevent the spread of infection.
[McCall 7e, p67-69]

Donor Phlebotomy — V. Donor Center Operations

286. c A phlebotomist encounters a blood spill on her hands. She should wash her hands immediately using soap and water.
[Garza 10e, p122]

287. a Alcohol-based antiseptic hand cleaners have been approved by the Centers for Disease Control & Prevention (CDC) Healthcare Infection Control Practices Advisory Committee (HICPAC) as an appropriate substitute for handwashing, assuming the hands are not soiled with blood or body fluids.
[Garza 10e, p122]

288. c A phlebotomist routinely uses an alcohol-based antiseptic to cleanse her hands after completing a blood collection procedure. According to the Occupational Safety & Health Administration (OSHA), the phlebotomist is required to wash her hands with soap and water after every 3 patients.
[Garza 10e, p122]

289. b Hand hygiene procedures must be completed before and after every patient contact.
[Garza 10e, p118, 122]

290. c A phlebotomist is preparing to leave the lab for a lunch break. She begins the hand washing procedure by wetting her hands and dispensing soap. Next she should rub her hands together vigorously for at least 20 seconds.
[Garza 10e, p122-123]

291. a During the rinse step of a hand wash procedure, the phlebotomist should hold their hands with the fingers pointing down.
[Garza 10e, p123-124]

292. d After the rinse step of a hand wash procedure, the phlebotomist should turn off the faucet using a paper towel.
[Garza 10e, p124]

Answer Keys

The following table shows the page numbers on which the questions, explanations, and answer keys begin for each chapter.

Chapter	Questions	Explanations	Answer Key
1 Circulatory System	1	18	490
2 Specimen Collection	29	128	491
3 Specimen Handling, Transport & Processing	203	240	492
4 Waived & Point-of-Care Testing	271	282	493
5 Nonblood Specimens	289	309	494
6 Laboratory Operations	321	372	495
7 Donor Phlebotomy	407	457	496

Circulatory System Answer Key

The following items have been identified as appropriate for those preparing for both PBT & QDP examinations.

1 d	17 a	33 d	49 b	65 b	81 d
2 a	18 d	34 c	50 c	66 d	82 a
3 b	19 a	35 b	51 c	67 d	83 c
4 a	20 a	36 a	52 d	68 b	84 b
5 d	21 b	37 a	53 a	69 a	85 d
6 c	22 a	38 b	54 c	70 c	86 c
7 c	23 a	39 d	55 b	71 a	87 d
8 d	24 a	40 c	56 a	72 c	88 d
9 b	25 c	41 d	57 c	73 d	89 d
10 b	26 b	42 b	58 c	74 a	90 c
11 a	27 c	43 a	59 d	75 a	
12 d	28 a	44 c	60 b	76 b	
13 a	29 d	45 d	61 b	77 d	
14 d	30 d	46 a	62 a	78 c	
15 a	31 c	47 a	63 d	79 b	
16 c	32 d	48 a	64 b	80 a	

Specimen Collection Answer Key

The following items have been identified as appropriate for those preparing for both PBT & QDP examinations.

1 a	53 a	105 c	157 c	209 d	261 c	313 c	365 b	417 b	469 b	521 a
2 c	54 d	106 c	158 b	210 a	262 b	314 a	366 c	418 a	470 c	522 b
3 c	55 c	107 b	159 d	211 c	263 a	315 a	367 c	419 a	471 d	523 b
4 b	56 a	108 a	160 a	212 d	264 d	316 d	368 d	420 d	472 a	524 d
5 d	57 d	109 c	161 b	213 b	265 a	317 c	369 a	421 d	473 d	525 d
6 a	58 b	110 d	162 a	214 c	266 c	318 b	370 c	422 d	474 c	526 c
7 d	59 c	111 a	163 d	215 a	267 d	319 a	371 b	423 a	475 c	527 d
8 b	60 b	112 c	164 a	216 d	268 c	320 a	372 c	424 d	476 c	528 b
9 d	61 a	113 c	165 c	217 c	269 c	321 c	373 d	425 c	477 c	529 c
10 d	62 c	114 d	166 a	218 b	270 b	322 b	374 a	426 a	478 c	530 c
11 d	63 c	115 c	167 a	219 c	271 c	323 d	375 b	427 a	479 d	531 c
12 c	64 c	116 c	168 a	220 c	272 c	324 b	376 c	428 c	480 d	532 c
13 d	65 c	117 d	169 d	221 c	273 a	325 d	377 b	429 a	481 a	533 a
14 d	66 d	118 c	170 d	222 c	274 b	326 c	378 c	430 b	482 b	534 b
15 c	67 c	119 b	171 a	223 a	275 c	327 b	379 a	431 b	483 c	535 c
16 c	68 a	120 d	172 c	224 c	276 b	328 d	380 a	432 c	484 b	536 b
17 c	69 a	121 d	173 d	225 b	277 d	329 d	381 a	433 a	485 d	537 c
18 a	70 b	122 b	174 d	226 d	278 a	330 d	382 d	434 c	486 d	538 a
19 d	71 b	123 a	175 d	227 d	279 a	331 a	383 d	435 b	487 a	539 a
20 a	72 c	124 a	176 d	228 b	280 a	332 d	384 c	436 c	488 a	540 c
21 b	73 c	125 b	177 a	229 c	281 c	333 c	385 b	437 b	489 c	541 a
22 b	74 d	126 a	178 b	230 d	282 c	334 d	386 a	438 c	490 b	542 a
23 a	75 a	127 a	179 a	231 c	283 c	335 b	387 b	439 d	491 a	543 c
24 b	76 a	128 a	180 a	232 d	284 b	336 c	388 a	440 b	492 d	544 b
25 b	77 c	129 c	181 a	233 d	285 c	337 a	389 b	441 b	493 c	545 b
26 a	78 c	130 d	182 d	234 c	286 d	338 c	390 c	442 a	494 c	546 c
27 b	79 d	131 c	183 a	235 d	287 a	339 b	391 c	443 d	495 d	547 d
28 a	80 c	132 c	184 a	236 c	288 c	340 d	392 d	444 c	496 c	548 b
29 d	81 c	133 c	185 d	237 c	289 b	341 b	393 a	445 c	497 d	549 a
30 b	82 d	134 d	186 c	238 b	290 a	342 a	394 a	446 b	498 c	550 b
31 a	83 c	135 b	187 d	239 d	291 c	343 b	395 d	447 a	499 d	551 c
32 d	84 a	136 b	188 b	240 b	292 d	344 a	396 b	448 b	500 c	552 a
33 d	85 c	137 b	189 a	241 d	293 b	345 c	397 d	449 a	501 a	553 a
34 b	86 d	138 c	190 a	242 c	294 a	346 c	398 d	450 d	502 d	554 d
35 c	87 c	139 d	191 b	243 d	295 a	347 b	399 d	451 b	503 c	555 d
36 c	88 c	140 b	192 c	244 b	296 c	348 c	400 c	452 a	504 d	556 d
37 a	89 b	141 c	193 c	245 b	297 b	349 c	401 b	453 d	505 c	557 d
38 c	90 c	142 a	194 d	246 d	298 b	350 c	402 c	454 c	506 d	558 a
39 a	91 b	143 d	195 d	247 c	299 d	351 b	403 b	455 c	507 a	559 b
40 b	92 c	144 b	196 c	248 c	300 c	352 a	404 c	456 c	508 a	560 b
41 b	93 c	145 a	197 b	249 b	301 b	353 c	405 c	457 b	509 c	561 a
42 d	94 a	146 c	198 c	250 c	302 a	354 a	406 c	458 d	510 c	
43 d	95 c	147 d	199 b	251 c	303 b	355 c	407 b	459 c	511 a	
44 a	96 d	148 b	200 d	252 d	304 b	356 d	408 c	460 c	512 d	
45 d	97 c	149 a	201 a	253 b	305 b	357 b	409 c	461 d	513 a	
46 a	98 c	150 c	202 b	254 c	306 b	358 c	410 d	462 d	514 c	
47 c	99 d	151 a	203 c	255 c	307 c	359 a	411 d	463 d	515 c	
48 b	100 d	152 a	204 c	256 c	308 b	360 c	412 c	464 b	516 a	
49 a	101 c	153 b	205 c	257 d	309 d	361 d	413 a	465 a	517 d	
50 d	102 c	154 c	206 a	258 a	310 a	362 a	414 b	466 c	518 a	
51 d	103 d	155 a	207 a	259 c	311 c	363 c	415 d	467 b	519 b	
52 d	104 b	156 b	208 c	260 d	312 c	364 d	416 c	468 b	520 d	

Specimen Handling, Transport & Processing Answer Key

The following items have been identified as appropriate for those preparing for the PBT examination.

1 a	41 c	81 c	121 c	161 d	201 b
2 a	42 d	82 c	122 c	162 a	202 b
3 d	43 c	83 a	123 a	163 b	203 a
4 c	44 b	84 a	124 d	164 b	204 b
5 b	45 c	85 a	125 b	165 d	205 d
6 c	46 c	86 a	126 c	166 d	206 a
7 c	47 c	87 d	127 a	167 d	207 d
8 c	48 d	88 c	128 b	168 d	208 b
9 a	49 d	89 c	129 d	169 b	209 d
10 d	50 c	90 a	130 d	170 d	210 d
11 d	51 d	91 a	131 d	171 c	211 b
12 a	52 c	92 a	132 a	172 d	212 b
13 b	53 b	93 c	133 c	173 c	213 c
14 c	54 d	94 c	134 a	174 d	214 b
15 b	55 d	95 a	135 d	175 a	215 d
16 b	56 c	96 a	136 a	176 d	216 b
17 c	57 b	97 c	137 c	177 a	217 d
18 c	58 b	98 c	138 d	178 a	218 b
19 c	59 a	99 c	139 b	179 a	219 b
20 d	60 a	100 a	140 c	180 a	220 d
21 d	61 d	101 b	141 d	181 d	221 a
22 a	62 a	102 d	142 d	182 b	222 b
23 a	63 c	103 c	143 b	183 b	223 c
24 a	64 b	104 d	144 c	184 d	224 c
25 d	65 a	105 b	145 c	185 d	225 d
26 c	66 b	106 d	146 d	186 b	226 c
27 c	67 a	107 d	147 d	187 a	227 a
28 d	68 d	108 a	148 b	188 c	228 d
29 b	69 d	109 a	149 c	189 a	229 c
30 c	70 a	110 c	150 b	190 a	230 a
31 c	71 d	111 c	151 b	191 c	
32 c	72 d	112 d	152 d	192 b	
33 d	73 c	113 a	153 c	193 b	
34 c	74 c	114 a	154 a	194 a	
35 a	75 a	115 d	155 a	195 c	
36 c	76 a	116 a	156 a	196 d	
37 d	77 a	117 c	157 d	197 a	
38 c	78 b	118 c	158 a	198 d	
39 c	79 c	119 d	159 b	199 a	
40 c	80 c	120 a	160 b	200 c	

Waived & Point-of-Care Testing Answer Key

The following items have been identified as appropriate for those preparing for the PBT examination.

1 d	13 a	25 b	37 b	49 a	61 a
2 c	14 c	26 a	38 b	50 b	62 d
3 a	15 d	27 b	39 a	51 c	63 d
4 d	16 b	28 b	40 b	52 a	64 c
5 a	17 a	29 a	41 c	53 b	65 b
6 c	18 d	30 a	42 c	54 d	66 b
7 d	19 b	31 d	43 c	55 d	67 d
8 b	20 c	32 d	44 c	56 d	68 c
9 b	21 c	33 c	45 a	57 d	69 d
10 b	22 d	34 a	46 c	58 c	70 b
11 c	23 c	35 b	47 a	59 a	
12 a	24 b	36 a	48 b	60 c	

Nonblood Specimens Answer Key

The following items have been identified as appropriate for those preparing for the PBT examination.

1 d	23 b	45 a	67 d	89 b	111 b
2 a	24 a	46 d	68 c	90 d	112 b
3 b	25 d	47 b	69 a	91 b	113 c
4 b	26 c	48 d	70 b	92 d	114 b
5 a	27 a	49 a	71 a	93 d	115 a
6 b	28 a	50 d	72 b	94 c	116 a
7 b	29 a	51 a	73 d	95 d	117 b
8 d	30 b	52 c	74 d	96 c	118 c
9 b	31 d	53 a	75 a	97 a	119 c
10 b	32 c	54 c	76 a	98 c	120 d
11 c	33 c	55 d	77 a	99 b	121 d
12 a	34 a	56 a	78 b	100 d	122 b
13 b	35 c	57 a	79 d	101 d	123 a
14 d	36 d	58 c	80 b	102 c	124 b
15 a	37 d	59 a	81 b	103 d	125 c
16 c	38 d	60 a	82 c	104 c	126 d
17 d	39 d	61 b	83 b	105 c	
18 d	40 d	62 a	84 a	106 d	
19 c	41 a	63 b	85 b	107 d	
20 a	42 a	64 d	86 b	108 c	
21 b	43 a	65 a	87 c	109 a	
22 c	44 a	66 c	88 c	110 a	

Laboratory Operations Answer Key

The following items have been identified as appropriate for those preparing for both PBT & QDP examinations.

1 b	51 c	101 d	151 d	201 a	251 a
2 b	52 c	102 b	152 b	202 a	252 b
3 b	53 d	103 b	153 c	203 d	253 c
4 c	54 a	104 b	154 a	204 b	254 b
5 a	55 b	105 d	155 b	205 c	255 d
6 a	56 a	106 a	156 c	206 a	256 c
7 a	57 a	107 c	157 a	207 a	257 a
8 d	58 d	108 b	158 c	208 d	258 c
9 d	59 b	109 a	159 c	209 c	259 a
10 c	60 d	110 a	160 d	210 b	260 c
11 d	61 c	111 a	161 a	211 d	261 b
12 b	62 b	112 c	162 a	212 a	262 b
13 a	63 a	113 d	163 a	213 b	263 b
14 a	64 b	114 b	164 a	214 d	264 c
15 b	65 c	115 d	165 c	215 a	265 a
16 d	66 d	116 c	166 b	216 a	266 d
17 c	67 b	117 d	167 c	217 b	267 c
18 d	68 d	118 d	168 d	218 b	268 a
19 c	69 c	119 c	169 d	219 a	269 c
20 a	70 d	120 b	170 a	220 c	270 c
21 c	71 d	121 c	171 d	221 d	271 b
22 a	72 d	122 a	172 c	222 b	272 d
23 a	73 d	123 b	173 b	223 b	273 d
24 b	74 a	124 d	174 c	224 c	274 b
25 c	75 b	125 c	175 c	225 a	275 d
26 d	76 b	126 d	176 a	226 b	276 b
27 b	77 d	127 a	177 b	227 c	277 b
28 c	78 c	128 b	178 c	228 b	278 b
29 a	79 c	129 c	179 d	229 c	279 b
30 a	80 c	130 d	180 c	230 a	280 c
31 a	81 c	131 d	181 d	231 c	281 b
32 c	82 b	132 c	182 b	232 c	282 d
33 c	83 d	133 c	183 d	233 c	283 d
34 d	84 c	134 c	184 b	234 a	284 d
35 a	85 d	135 d	185 c	235 c	285 a
36 d	86 c	136 d	186 c	236 d	286 a
37 c	87 a	137 d	187 d	237 d	287 d
38 b	88 b	138 a	188 a	238 a	288 b
39 c	89 a	139 c	189 d	239 a	289 d
40 d	90 c	140 b	190 c	240 a	290 d
41 c	91 d	141 a	191 d	241 d	291 a
42 b	92 b	142 b	192 a	242 a	292 a
43 a	93 a	143 d	193 d	243 d	293 d
44 b	94 b	144 c	194 b	244 a	294 a
45 a	95 d	145 b	195 b	245 d	295 b
46 b	96 a	146 a	196 b	246 b	296 a
47 c	97 c	147 c	197 d	247 c	297 b
48 d	98 a	148 d	198 d	248 d	298 c
49 d	99 b	149 c	199 c	249 a	299 d
50 d	100 c	150 d	200 c	250 b	300 a

Donor Phlebotomy Answer Key

The following items have been identified as appropriate for those preparing for the QDP examination.

I. Basic Science of Blood Compatibility
1. a
2. b
3. c
4. d
5. b
6. a
7. b
8. c
9. d
10. a
11. d
12. a
13. b
14. b
15. c
16. c
17. d
18. a
19. c
20. d
21. b
22. a
23. a
24. c
25. b
26. c
27. a
28. d
29. d
30. c
31. d
32. d
33. c
34. a
35. d
36. c
37. d
38. a
39. a
40. a
41. b
42. d
43. b
44. b

II. Donor Identification & Selection
45. d
46. a
47. d
48. c
49. b
50. b
51. b
52. b
53. d
54. b
55. d
56. a
57. c
58. d
59. d
60. b
61. b
62. d
63. a
64. c
65. d
66. c
67. d
68. a
69. b
70. b
71. d
72. b
73. d
74. d
75. d
76. d
77. c
78. c
79. b
80. a
81. d
82. c
83. d
84. d
85. b
86. c
87. b
88. a
89. b
90. d
91. d
92. c
93. a
94. a
95. a
96. c
97. b
98. d
99. b
100. c
101. b
102. b
103. d
104. b
105. d
106. a
107. b
108. d
109. c
110. a
111. c
112. c

III. Donor Blood Collection & Handling
113. d
114. a
115. d
116. c
117. a
118. a
119. a
120. a
121. a
122. b
123. a
124. b
125. a
126. c
127. b
128. b
129. a
130. b
131. d
132. d
133. b
134. b
135. a
136. c
137. d
138. b
139. d
140. d
141. a
142. a
143. a
144. a
145. c
146. c
147. b
148. a
149. c
150. c
151. d
152. b
153. c
154. d
155. b
156. c
157. a
158. a
159. b
160. d
161. a
162. b
163. a
164. d
165. a
166. c
167. d
168. d
169. d
170. d
171. a
172. b
173. c
174. d
175. b
176. b
177. d
178. b
179. c
180. d
181. d
182. c
183. c
184. d
185. c
186. c
187. a
188. c
189. d
190. a
191. d

IV. Donor Considerations
192. b
193. b
194. a
195. a
196. b
197. c
198. c
199. d
200. c
201. c
202. a
203. d
204. a
205. a
206. a
207. c
208. d
209. a
210. d
211. c
212. d
213. b
214. c

V. Donor Center Operations
215. d
216. c
217. b
218. a
219. a
220. b
221. c
222. d
223. a
224. d
225. a
226. b
227. b
228. c
229. a
230. b
231. d
232. c
233. c
234. c
235. b
236. d
237. a
238. c
239. d
240. b
241. b
242. b
243. d
244. a
245. c
246. a
247. d
248. b
249. c
250. d
251. d
252. c
253. a
254. c
255. b
256. c
257. a
258. a
259. a
260. a
261. a
262. c
263. b
264. c
265. d
266. a
267. c
268. a
269. d
270. d
271. a
272. a
273. a
274. a
275. c
276. d
277. d
278. a
279. a
280. a
281. c
282. b
283. d
284. c
285. a
286. c
287. a
288. c
289. b
290. c
291. a
292. d